LIVER DISEASES IN INFANCY AND CHILDHOOD

Dedicated to the memory of Professor Marcel Lelong

LIVER DISEASES IN INFANCY AND CHILDHOOD

edited by

SAMUEL R. BERENBERG, M.D.

1976

MARTINUS NIJHOFF MEDICAL DIVISION - THE HAGUE

ISBN-13:978-94-010-1419-9   e-ISBN-13:978-94-010-1417-5
DOI: 10.1007/978-94-010-1417-5

Softcover reprint of the hardcover 1st edition 1976

PREFACE

For almost four decades the Josiah Macy, Jr. Foundation has been convening conferences relating to medicine, medical education, and health care in their broadest contexts. During the 1940s and 1950s the conferences focused on biomedical research, which was at that time in its golden age in the United States. As medical care and medical education ascended in importance, since the mid-1960s the conferences have been largely concentrated on topics in these fields.

The Macy Foundation also fosters international conferences, and a major effort in recent years has been a rewarding collaboration with France's most distinguished medical statesman, Professor Robert Debré, and the International Children's Centre in Paris, which he founded and directs. Nineteen seventy-five was an especially busy year for this Franco-American alliance: in April there was a seminar on 'The Family Doctor: France and the United States'; and, in June, a conference on 'Diseases of the Liver in Infancy and Childhood'. Earlier Franco-American conferences have been on 'Brain Development' (1972) and on 'Puberty' (1974).

As with the others the participants in this conference on Liver Disease in Infancy and Childhood were drawn from the United States and Europe. We were especially pleased to have as three of the participants men who hold sabbatical awards as Macy Foundation Faculty Scholars, Ivan Diamond, M.D., Ph.D., Thomas Starzl, M.D., Ph.D. and M. Michael Thaler, M.D.

Our continuing pleasure is the rewarding liaison with Professor Robert Debré who has made so many enduring contributions to medicine and health in France and elsewhere in the world.

John Z. Bowers, M.D.

CONTENTS

PARTICIPANTS

Øystein Aagenaes, M.D., Pediatric Department, Rikshospitalet, Barneklinikken, Universitetsklinikk, Oslo, Norway

William H. Admirand, M.D., Department of Medicine, School of Medicine, San Francisco General Hospital, San Francisco, California, U.S.A.

Daniel Alagille, M.D., Hôpital d'Enfants de Bicêtre, Clinique de Pédiatrie, Bicêtre, France

Irwin M. Arias, M.D., Division of Gastroenterology and Liver Disease, Albert Einstein College of Medicine of Yeshiva University, Bronx, New York, U.S.A.

Henri Bismuth, M.D., Chirurgien des Hopitaux de Paris, Groupe Hospitalier Paul Brousse, Villejuif, France

R. Brodersen, Ph.D., Institute of Medical Biochemistry. University of Aarhus, Århus, Denmark

H. William Clatworthy jr., M.D., Department of Surgery, College of Medicine, The Ohio State University, Columbus, Ohio, U.S.A.

Y. E. Cossart, M.D., Virus Reference Laboratory, Central Public Health Laboratory, London, England

Ivan Diamond, M.D., Ph.D., Department of Neurology, School of Medicine, University of California, San Francisco, California, U.S.A.

Jean-Marie Dupuy, M.D., Unité de Recherche d'Hepatologie Infantile, INSERM, Kremlin-Bicêtre, France

Marthe Gautier, M.D., Hôpital d'Enfants de Bicêtre, Clinique de Pédiatrie, Bicêtre, France.

Sydney S. Gellis, M.D., Department of Pediatrics, School of Medicine, Tufts University, Boston, Massachusetts, U.S.A.

William P. Longmire jr., M.D., Department of Surgery, School of Medicine, University of California, Los Angeles, California, U.S.A.

Alex P. Mowat, M.D., Department of Child Health, King's College Hospital, Medical School, London, England

Malte K. Neidhardt, M.D., Kinderklinik, Augsburg, West Germany

A. Nowoslawski, Ph.D., Department of Immunopathology, National Institute of Hygiene, Warsaw, Poland

Gerard B. Odell, M.D., Department of Pediatrics, School of Medicine The Johns Hopkins University, Baltimore, Maryland, U.S.A.

Michel Odièvre, M.D., Hôpital d'Enfants de Bicêtre, Clinique de Pédiatrie, Bicêtre, France

Hans Popper, M.D., Ph.D., Mount Sinai School of Medicine of the City University of New York, New York, U.S.A.

M. Schmid, M.D., Medizinische Klinik, Stadtspital Waid Zürich, Zürich, Switzerland

William K. Schubert, M.D., Department of Pediatrics, Children's Hospital Medical Center, University of Cincinnatti, Cincinnatti, Ohio, U.S.A.

Fenton Schaffner, M.D., Division of Liver Diseases, Mount Sinai School of Medicine of the City University of New York, New York, U.S.A.

Harvey L. Sharp, M.D., Department of Pediatrics, University of Minnesota Hospitals, Minneapolis, Minnesota, U.S.A.

Thomas E. Starzl, M.D., Ph.D., Department of Surgery, School of Medicine, The University of Colorado, Denver, Colorado, U.S.A.

M. Michael Thaler, M.D., Department of Pediatrics, School of Medicine, University of California, San Francisco, California, U.S.A.

J. Valayer, M.D., Service de Chirurgie Pédiatrique, Hôpital St. Vincent de Paul, Paris, France

Arie J. Zuckerman, M.D., D.Sc., Department of Virology, London School of Tropical Medicine, London, England

ABBREVIATIONS

ALG	=	antilymphocytic globulin
ALS	=	antilymphocytic serum
α-1 AT	=	α-1 antitrypsin
ATP	=	adenosine triphosphate
Brb	=	bilirubin
Brb - Alb	=	bilirubin - albumin
BSA	=	bovine serum albumin
BSP	=	sulfobromophthalein
CD	=	circular dichroism
CMV	=	cytomegalic virus
CNS	=	central nervous system
CoA	=	coenzyme A
CPS	=	carbamyl phosphate synthetase
DBSP	=	dibromsulfophthalein
DDT	=	1,1,1 Trichloro-2,2-bis (P-chlorophenyl ethane)
DNA	=	deoxyribonucleic acid
ER	=	endoplasmic reticulum
FSH	=	follicle stimulating hormone
GI	=	gastrointestinal
GSH transferase	=	glutathione transferase
H and E	=	hemotoxylin and eosin (stain)
HBABA	=	parahydroxybenzeneazobenzoic acid
HBcAb	=	hepatitis B core antibody
HbcAg	=	hepatitis core antigen
HBSAB	=	hepatitis B surface antibody
HBsAg	=	hepatitis B surface antigen
HBV	=	hepatitis B virus
HPC	=	hepatoporto/cholecystostomy

HPE	=	hepatoporto/enterostomy
HPS	=	hepatoporto/stomy
HSA	=	human serum albumin
ICG	=	indocyanine green
Ig	=	immune globulin
IgG	=	immunoglobulin class G
I.P.	=	intraperitoneal
K1, K2	=	first order rate constants for influx and efflux
L.D.	=	lethal dose
MHV	=	mouse hepatitis virus
NRS	=	normal rabbit serum
O.T.	=	orthoptic transplant
OTC	=	ornithine transcarbamylase
PAPS	=	3′ phosphoadenosine 5′ phosphosulfate
PAS	=	periodic acid Schiff (reaction)
QAE-A	=	quarternary aminoethyl cellulose ion exchange resin
RNA	=	ribonucleic acid
RSA	=	rat serum albumin
S	=	storage capacity
S.D.	=	standard deviation
SDS	=	sodium dodecyl sulfate
S.E.M.	=	standard error of the mean
SER	=	smooth endoplasmic reticulum
SGOT	=	serum glutamic oxaloacetic transaminase
SGPT	=	serum glutamic pyruvic transaminase
TCDD	=	tetrachlorodibenzodioxan
Tm	=	transport maximum
UDPG	=	uridine diphosphate glucose
UDPGA	=	uridine diphosphate glucuronic acid
UDPGT	=	uridine diphosphate glucuronyl transferase

HOMMAGE AU PROFESSEUR MARCEL LELONG
(1892–1973)

De 1928, où il était jeune chef de clinique de Lereboullet, jusqu'à 1963, où il quittait l'hôpital, Marcel Lelong a animé le vieil établissement parisien des 'Enfants Trouvés', devenu sous son impulsion le grand centre pédiatrique moderne qu'est encore l'hôpital Saint-Vincent-de-Paul. Pendant cette longue carrière vécue tout entière dans le même lieu, Marcel Lelong est devenu l'un des grands maîtres de la pédiatrie française, à la tête de la Clinique de Pédiatrie et de Puériculture, qui fut créée pour lui, au lendemain de la deuxième guerre mondiale.

Pendant les dix dernières années de sa vie hospitalière, il a su grouper autour de lui tout le prestige technique et humain que lui avait légué son maître Robert Debré dont il avait été le premier élève et dont il sut maintenir l'Ecole au niveau d'une remarquable activité dans le domaine de la connaissance, des soins et de la prévention des maladies de l'enfant. Ce que lui doit la médecine prénatale et périnatale de notre pays peut être mieux mesuré aujourd'hui où la néonatologie est enfin un secteur autonome de la pédiatrie.

La création de l'Ecole de Puériculture lui a permis d'implanter, en France et en Europe, les structures et les techniques qui ont longtemps servi de centre pilote dans ce domaine.

Son action médicale et sociale en faveur des enfants abandonnés lui a permis d'inspirer, à l'administration de l'Assistance Publique puis à l'Aide Sociale à l'Enfance, les solutions les meilleures pour le développement physique, mental et moral de ces enfants. Un grand nombre d'affections de l'enfance lui sont redevables de progrès dûs à la fois à la clinique et à la biologie car il savait associer ses observations raffinées faites au lit du malade et les investigations du laboratoire. Il apporta des connaissances nouvelles dans le domaine des maladies virales et bactériennes, parasitaires, des erreurs innées du métabolisme, des malformations congénitales, des troubles de la croissance et du développement, grâce à l'exercice d'une médecine traditionnelle excellente et aux recherches les plus récemment entreprises.

Novateur, animateur, grand chef d'Ecole, pédiatre universellement re-nommé, savant et homme de coeur, sa mémoire mérite d'être honorée et son nom donné par la Josiah Macy Jr. Foundation à ce séminaire voué à la pathologie hépato-biliaire de l'enfant.

EXTRACELLULAR AND INTRACELLULAR
TRANSPORT OF BILIRUBIN

IRWIN M. ARIAS, M.D.

Bilirubin is an orange organic anion of molecular weight 584 which is exclusively derived from the catabolism of heme protein. It has limited aqueous solubility at physiologic pH and when found in tissues is largely, if not exclusively, bound to protein or dissolved in lipid. At least 85% of bilirubin formed in man is derived from the systematic degradation of mature circulating erythrocytes as a function of their age. Conversion of heme to bilirubin in the reticuloendothelial cells is quantitative and apparently limited by activity of the microsomal heme oxygenase system. Bilirubin is also derived from erythropoietic sources and degradation of heme proteins, particularly liver heme proteins such as cytochrome P-450 because of its abundance and relatively short half-life. Whether bilirubin derived from these various sources enters the same body pools and participates in similar transport mechanisms in the liver is unexplored.

Bilirubin does neither good nor harm with exception of the risk of kernicterus in neonates and rare situations of lifelong profound unconjugated hyperbilirubinemia in adolescents. In pediatrics, the major emphasis has been on understanding the metabolism and regulation of this potential brain toxin; however, one should recognize that such studies may be more important for the information they yield regarding the transport of other organic anions of greater physiologic importance than bilirubin... such as various drugs and metabolites. Many of the transport processes utilized by bilirubin in its transfer from plasma into the bile are shared by other substrates which often alter hyperbilirubinemia in various ways.

The underlying basis of jaundice in neonates is the 'physiologic' hyperbilirubinemia seen in virtually all newborn infants. During the past 20 years, studies of this entity have had as their premise that understanding of the rate-limiting step resulting in 'physiologic' jaundice will permit proper therapeutic approaches to reduce unconjugated bilirubin when it accumulates in excess in the plasma and tissues of neonates and increases the risk of kernicterus (1). Of necessity much of this work has involved laboratory animals which introduces interpretative difficulties when such results are applied to man. The numerous studies of neonatal jaundice have not identified the rate-limiting step and have only emphasized our limited knowledge of the complexity of the liver in the neonate. Numerous qualitative observations have been made but to date there is no quantitative assessment of these parameters in man.

Theoretically, 'physiologic' jaundice can result from one or more of the mechanisms: 1. increased bile pigment production from hemolysis or sources other than mature, circulating erythrocytes; 2. impaired transfer of bilirubin from plasma to the site of glucuronide formation; 3. impaired formation of bilirubin glucuronide due to deficient or inhibited UDPGA formation or UDPGT activity; and 4. increased intestinal absorption of bilirubin after biliary excretion and hydrolysis of bilirubin glucuronide.

At present, the pathophysiology of 'physiologic' jaundice is considered to involve transient developmental deficiency of UDPGT. Increased production or intestinal reabsorption of bilirubin may be associated phenomena but are not capable of producing jaundice alone. The following summarizes evidence in support of this hypothesis (1):

1. In several animals, including primates, UDPGA formation and UDPGT activity are virtually absent in fetal liver and attain adult levels between the second and tenth day of life.

2. UDPGT is associated with the microsomal fraction of liver homogenates and electron microscopic studies of developing mouse liver reveal sparse endoplasmic reticulum with morphologic development during the first week of life.

3. Bilirubin glucuronide formation is virtually absent in liver slices and homogenates obtained from human fetuses in late stages as well as from neonates who died of various causes within the first 3 days of life.

4. Phenobarbital and several other drugs increase liver UDPGT activity, enhance microsomal protein synthesis, cause proliferation of smooth endoplasmic reticulum membranes, and reduce serum unconjugated bilirubin concentrations in newborn infants.

5. Lifelong deficiency of UDPGT is associated with permanent nonhemolytic acholuric unconjugated hyperbilirubinemia in man and rats (Gunn strain).

The following summarizes evidence against this hypothesis (1):

1. UDPGT activity is relatively unstable and the enzyme has not been isolated, purified and characterized. The enzyme is a lipoprotein and specifically requires lecithin for activation after it has been delipidated (14).

Heterogeneity of UDPGT involved in N-glucuronide formation as compared with acyl and ethereal glucuronide formation seems well established. With regard to the latter, the situation remains confusing and multiplicity of UDPGT is suggested by varied effects of hypohysectomy and thyroidectomy, ions, pH and other factors on acyl and ethereal glucuronide formation. However, it remains uncertain as to whether these and kinetic differences with different substrates represent different enzymes or altered affinity for these substrates by a single UDPGT.

2. The pattern of development of UDPGT varies greatly with species and substrates. For example, UDPGT in newborn rat liver exceeds the enzyme activity found in adult rat liver (9). There has not been a systematic study performed in man or primate manifesting 'physiologic' jaundice using bilirubin as a substrate. Di Toro et al. studied the development of 4-methyl unbelliferone glucuronide formation in human liver biopsy specimens and observed little increase in UDPGT activity until the fourth week of life (6).

3. UDPGT activity levels may be misleading when interpreted physiologically (particularly after activation of the enzyme with detergents). For example, delayed development of hepatic UDPG dehydrogenase and UDPGT activities is observed in vitro in guinea pigs; however, studies based upon bilirubin infusion in vivo indicate that hepatic excretion of conjugated bilirubin is rate-limiting at all ages in the transfer of bilirubin from blood to bile in this species (10). Bilirubin glucuronide accumulates in the liver and plasma in guinea pigs less than 2 days old and hepatic excretory function does not attain adult levels until the third week of life. Guinea pigs do not manifest 'physiologic' jaundice... perhaps because their excretory limitation is physiologically more severe than the observed deficiency in UDPG dehydrogenase and UDPGT activities.

Dr. Lawrence Gartner at the Albert Einstein College of Medicine has pursued this problem by performing bilirubin infusion studies in Rhesus monkeys 1 hour to 18 days of age (11). These studies reveal the following important facts:

1. The newborn Rhesus monkey has 'physiologic' jaundice with rapid rise of serum unconjugated bilirubin concentrations from less than 1 mgm% at birth to 4.5 mgm% within 24 hours (phase I). A rapid decline to 2 mgm% occurs in the second day of life; the serum bilirubin concentration remains at this level for approximately 4 days (phase II) and then declines to 0.1 mgm% by the fifth day.

2. Mean endogenous excretion of bilirubin in bile rises during the first

48 hours of life to 500% greater than adult levels, and remains significantly elevated for the first 18 days of life.

3. Mean cumulative hepatic uptake of bilirubin is approximately 30% of adult values at birth and slowly reaches adult levels by the fifth day of life.

4. Hepatic UDPGT (bilirubin) activity is almost zero at birth but rises rapidly at 24 hours and attains adult levels by the third day of life.

5. Hepatic excretion of conjugated bilirubin becomes rate-limiting during the late newborn period as manifested by exceeding the biliary Tm for bilirubin with accumulation of conjugated bilirubin in the plasma and liver.

6. Mathematical analysis suggests that the hepatic conjugating ability during the first 24 hours of life is less than the load of bilirubin presented to the liver. If the bilirubin load (endogenous bile pigment production) were not 7 times that observed in adults, available UDPGT would be sufficient to prevent unconjugated hyperbilirubinemia. In stage II, relative deficiency in hepatic uptake is the major factor responsible for hyperbilirubinemia inasmuch as UDPGT activity is virtually normal. These studies suggest that 'physiologic' jaundice of the newborn Rhesus monkey and, probably human newborns, does not result from a single enzymatic defect in bilirubin conjugation but represents a complex interaction of many functional disabilities, each of which is probably subjected to various controls which are currently neither recognized nor appreciated.

A critical limitation in our knowledge concerns the mechanism whereby bilirubin is transferred from plasma into the liver. For at least four decades it has been known that following injection of 'physiologic' amounts of bilirubin and other organic anions, a large proportion of the injected dose is recovered within the liver within a matter of minutes. The mechanism responsible for this rapid and seemingly selective transfer from plasma into the liver remains unknown; however, several hypotheses have been studied experimentally:

1. Bilirubin is noncovalently bound to serum albumin and may enter the liver cell by pinocytosis as a pigment: albumin complex. This hypothesis is unlikely because when ^{131}I albumin and ^{14}C bilirubin were injected simultaneously into a rat, the bile pigment entered the liver at a rate many times faster than did albumin.

2. An active transport system may exist in the plasma membrane of the parenchymal liver cell. This is unlikely because hepatic uptake takes place despite inhibitors of energy metabolism, and 'throughput' studies by Goresky and others reveal bidirectional bilirubin flux consistent with a passive process.

3. Hepatic bilirubin uptake may be determined by hepatic blood flow and a high extraction ratio for bile pigment. Although hepatic blood must influence perfusion of hepatic lobules, definitive studies of this parameter have not been performed with respect to bilirubin. Up to 25% increase or decrease in hepatic arterial flow do not alter net hepatic uptake of bilirubin per unit time.

4. 'Unbound' bilirubin in plasma may be transferred across the plasma membrane of the liver cell by simple or facilitated diffusion. Net flux may be determined by either intracellular binding of bilirubin, subsequent metabolism or excretion, or by a plasma membrane carrier system. Kinetic 'throughput' studies by Goresky, Paumgartner and others indicate that the uptake process is saturable. This precludes the existence of simple passive non-carrier mediated diffusion as the mechanism of bilirubin entry into liver cells. If the transfer were simple passive diffusion, the uptake mechanism should not be saturable. These studies do not reveal the nature or site of the carrier mechanism. In theory, such facilitated diffusion could result from specific membrane molecules or pores, and/or cytoplasmic proteins having high affinity for bilirubin which enters the plasma membrane by virtue of its lipid solubility.

My colleagues and I have been studying the role of hepatic cytoplasmic proteins in facilitating the net flux of bilirubin and other organic anions from plasma into the liver. These studies have resulted in identification, purification and partial characterization of ligandin (Y protein) and Z, two organic anion binding proteins in liver, as well as studies regarding their function. Our hypothesis is that these proteins, particularly ligandin, influence the net uptake of organic anions into the liver specifically by regulating efflux from the cell into the plasma. It seems obvious that there is no way in which a substance in plasma can know what is in the liver and, therefore, influx must be independent of cytoplasmic binding proteins. By-products of these studies have been immunologic methods for quantitating ligandin and Z protein, immunofluorescent methods for studying cell localization, and detailed binding studies using circular dichroism and equilibrium dialysis.

In 1968, we determined that approximately 80% of intrahepatic bilirubin is associated with the $100,000 \times g$ supernatant fraction of liver after radioactive bilirubin was injected into a rat (24). Fractionation by gel filtration revealed that radiobilirubin was found in two nonalbumin containing peaks called Y and Z. In subsequent years, a specific Y and a specific Z protein were purified and shown to account for at least 85% of the bilirubin binding in their respective fractions. Noncovalent binding of a large number of organic ligandin has been demonstrated to ligandin whether they were added in vitro or injected in vivo prior to gel chromatography (table 1) (2, 23, 31).

Table 1. Compounds bound to ligandin (Y protein) in vivo and in vitro.

I. Covalently bound
    azodye carcinogen
    methylcholanthrene metabolite
II. Noncovalently bound
    azodye GSH conjugate
    corticosteroids and metabolites
    bilirubin
    bilirubin glucuronide
    BSP, ICG, Rose Bengal, DBSP
    BSP glutathione
    glutathione
    hematin, heme
    phylloerythrin
    cholecystographic agents
    tri- and tetra-iodo thyronine
    methyl cholanthrene
    various sulfonamides
    various fatty acids
    probenecid
    penicillin
    vasoflavine
    cephalothin
    cephflex
    tetracyclines
    nitrofurantin
    ethacrynic acid
    gastrin

LIGANDIN

Ligandin [Y protein, azo carcinogen binding protein (Ketterer) (21), cortisol metabolite binding protein II (Litwack) (33), GSH Transferase B (Jakoby) (13)] was purified from rat liver and kidney by TEAE ion exchange chromatography, Sephadex G-100 gel filtration and QAE-A-50 chromatography (7, 23, 30). Purity was established by isoelectric focusing in ampholyte and gels; electrophoresis on acrylamide with and without added SDS, repeated amino acid analysis and the ability to produce monospecific precipitating antibody.

Identity between Y protein and the Ketterer, Litwack and Jakoby proteins was established by immunoelectrophoresis, -diffusion and -precipitation as well as comparison of physical-chemical features. Ligandin is a basic protein (pI 9.0) of 46,000 daltons consisting of two apparently identical monomeric subunits. Circular dichroism studies reveal an ordered structure with a high degree of α helix conformation. The protein from rat kidney gives identical structural and cross-immunologic responses.

By sensitive immunoquantitation (Mancini immunodiffusion and radioimmunoassay), this single protein constitutes 5% of rat liver, 2% of kidney and 2% of small intestinal mucosal supernatant protein; it was not detected in any other body tissue or fluid (7). Direct immunofluorescent studies confirmed this organ localization and revealed the protein to be restricted to all parenchymal liver cells, proximal tubular cells and non-goblet small intestinal mucosal cells. By virtue of the fact that proximal tubular cells of the kidney constitute approximately 40% of total kidney cells, the protein concentration in the proximal tubular cells approximates that found in rat liver cells.

A seemingly identical protein was isolated and purified by similar methods from human and primate liver. In these species, ligandin is also highly basic (pH 9.0) and has a molecular weight for the dimer of 44,000; the two monomers appear to have identical molecular weights. Immunologic studies (diffusion, electrophoresis, Mancini, radioassay and fluorescence) reveal similar tissue and cellular localization to that found in rats. The concentration in human liver is approximately 2% of supernatant protein (18 μg/mgm supernatant protein). Using these methods, the protein is absent from normal serum, urine and bile and does not appear in serum during acute liver injury.

The control of the protein in rat liver has been partially characterized (3, 7, 23, 35, 36). Following pulse-labeling with C^{14}-guanidino-arginine and immuno-precipitation, the half life for ligandin is 2.3 days. Dose response studies indicate that a new steady-state of approximately 220% of basal concentrations is reached following administration of phenobarbital, DDT, dieldrin, 16α-pregnenecarbonitrile, TCDD, methyl cholanthrene and benzpyrene. Double isotope studies reveal that this change results entirely from synthesis of new protein (induction). In mice and rats deprived of pituitary of thyroid glands, hepatic ligandin concentration is increased by an average of 60% over basal levels. Double isotope studies reveal that this is largely due to reduced degradation (stabilization) of the protein. In many hormonal replacement studies, only thyroxine in physiological doses restores hepatic ligandin concentration to normal. Administration of phenobarbital to thyroidectomized rats results in this single protein accounting for approximately 18% of liver supernatant protein. This dramatic change results from the combination of increased synthesis and reduced degradation. The renal and intestinal mucosal concentrations of ligandin are unaffected by administration of the above-stated drugs with exception of induction of the protein in the renal proximal tubules following administration of TCDD (23).

Ligandin is responsible for at least 80% of the organic anion binding by Y fraction from rat kidney or liver, or human liver (7, 23). This was proven by quantitation of bilirubin or BSP binding to Y fraction before and after addition of monospecific anti-ligandin IgG with nonspecific IgG serving as control.

Possible association of ligandin and S-aryl GSH transferase was suggested by Kaplowitz et al. (20). Identity of the protein in rat liver and kidney with GSH transferase B was demonstrated primarily by immunologic methods as well as the selective induction of this GSH transferase by phenobarbital administration (13). Monospecific precipitating antibody prepared against human ligandin reacts with each of four basic GSH transferases isolated from human liver; these have virtually identical amino acid analysis. We have studied induction of each basic GSH transferase in a Rhesus monkey following administration of TCDD; the results support the view that ligandin in human liver may be a single gene product. Kinetic studies reveal that several ligands (bilirubin, p-aminohippurate, etc.) are competitive inhibitors of the GSH transferase B catalytic activity of rat ligandin whereas other ligands (cholecystographic and renographic agents) are noncompetitive inhibitors; however, none of these ligands form GSH adducts as determined by various thin layer chromatographic procedures (12).

We have been unable to identify ligandin in liver cell plasma membranes and other organelles using immunologic technniques.

The following studies support the hypothesis that ligandin may influence the net flux specifically by reducing organic anion efflux from liver into the plasma.

1. Phylogenetic study revealed absence of ligandin by gel filtration of liver supernatants in the presence of added BSP or bilirubin in teleosts, elasmobranchs and several species of amphibia prior to metamorphosis. These species also have markedly delayed plasma disappearance of injected BSP and/or bilirubin with reduced hepatic uptake. By contrast, post-metamorphosis amphibia, reptiles, birds and mammals have abundant ligandin in their livers and manifest selective hepatic uptake of BSP and/or bilirubin in vivo (27).

2. Ontogenetic studies in newborn guinea pig, rat, monkey and man reveal impaired plasma disappearance and/or reduced hepatic content of BSP and/ or bilirubin and other organic anions. This process matures during the first ten days of life. Immunoquantitation of ligandin in these species reveals virtual absence of the protein in fetal liver, appearance shortly before or after birth, and maturation to adult concentrations within the first week of life in correlation with maturation of hepatic uptake (8, 25, 26).

3. Induction of hepatic ligandin following administration of phenobarbital or DDT is associated with increased plasma disappearance of organic anions (bilirubin, BSP, indocyanine green) and increased hepatic content of these organic anions 5 minutes after their intravenous injection. From 65-80% of intrahepatic exogenous organic anions were in the 100,000 × g supernatant fraction bound to the ligandin peak after gel filtration. In addition, kinetic studies of relative storage capacity and biliary Tm for BSP in rats treated with phenobarbital for 3 days revealed a significant increase in the former without change in the latter (35, 36).

4. Measurement of the influx and efflux rate constants, K_1 and K_2, was performed in dogs with and without phenobarbital administration using a multiple indicator technique and analysis with bilirubin as the test ligand. Phenobarbital administration for 6 days did not alter K_1 but significantly reduced K_2. This finding is consistent with observed induction of ligandin in the liver and reduced efflux of bilirubin from liver into the plasma (4).

5. Association constants derived from circular dichroism studies of various organic anions and rat liver ligandin were used to design experiments testing whether or not competition occurs for net transfer of these organic anions from plasma into the liver. For example, tri-iodothyronine binds to ligandin with an association constant of 10^6 M^{-1}. Bilirubin in the liver bound to ligandin in UDP glucuronyl transferase deficient (Gunn) rats... or after intravenous administration of unconjugated bilirubin to normal rats... reduced the transfer of I^{131}-triiodothyronine from plasma into the liver (28).

6. Induction of renal ligandin in the rat following administration of TCDD results in increased rate of removal of ^{14}C-penicillin from plasma and increased renal content and excretion of the antibiotic. Similar observations were made with respect to p-aminohippurate in the rat. In addition, BSP and probenecid bind to ligandin with greater affinity than does penicillin and their administration reduces renal uptake, excretion and ligandin-binding of ^{14}C-penicillin (23).

Because ligandin binds various ligands and also has catalytic activity, it has been proposed that this abundant protein may function both enzymatically and in influencing net organic anion flux across the plasma membrane of liver cells. The Kinetic studies reveal that ligandin serves as well as albumin with respect to various biotransformation reactions found in microsomal membranes in vitro. The protein may function as a form of 'intracellular albumin'. Ketterer et al. have suggested that ligandin may facilitate the transfer of heme from mitochondria to apocytochrome P-450 in the endoplasmic reticulum (22).

Ligandin may also protect cellular elements against 'toxic' injury. For example, bilirubin uncouples oxidative phosphorylation in isolated rat liver mitochondria. Such effects are not seen in liver in vivo even after administration of large amounts of bilirubin; however, uncoupling is observed in brain tissue. The central nervous system lacks ligandin as measured immunologically. Kinetic studies reveal that ligandin is equally as effective as serum albumin in protecting isolated liver mitochondria from uncoupling effects of bilirubin (15).

These studies provide qualitative, or associative information which support the role of ligandin in hepatic uptake of various ligands for binding (ex: bilirubin) or substrates for the catalytic activity (ex: BSP, ethacrynic acid). Quantitative evaluation of binding sites, affinities and kinetics is required for further evaluation of our hypothesis as well as the general problem of organic anion interaction with albumin, ligandin and Z protein.

Methods for characterizing ligand-protein interactions such as dialysis, ultrafiltration and gel filtration involve physical separation of the small free ligand molecules from the larger particles of protein and ligand-protein complexes, and are often limited by ligand binding to the supporting gel or membrane, inability to estimate rapid rates of ligand-unbinding, and difficulties in determining whether ligands compete at the same or different sites on the protein. Spectroscopic techniques, such as ultraviolet, visible absorption and fluorescence spectroscopy, optical rotatory dispersion and CD, and nuclear magnetic and electron spin resonance have the advantage of measuring the amount of bound and free ligand as well as providing important information on the nature of the ligand-protein interaction. The number of sites, relative affinities and competition between various ligands can be rapidly investigated without artificial membranes or gels, and specific groups on the ligand and protein can be studied in terms of three dimensional structure. These considerations are important in studying the interaction between bilirubin and other ligands with respect to serum albumin, ligandin and Z protein from various species including man.

We have studied the three dimensional structure of these proteins and their ligand complexes primarily using CD (29, 16-19). This method permits rapid and economical study of the site and affinity of bilirubin binding, specificity of interaction with competing organic anions, competitive binding of organic anions, as well as the transfer of bilirubin between albumin and ligandin.

Blauer and King have published CD studies of bilirubin binding to BSA and HSA (5). We have obtained similar results and, in addition, have studied the competition between various organic anions for binding of bilirubin by albumin preparations (16). Using CD, we analyzed competitive binding studies to determine the extent and manner in which various organic anions interact with BSA and HSA. Because the primary bilirubin binding sites are of very high affinity and relatively high protein concentrations (10^{-5}-10^{-6}M) were required for the spectropolarimetric experiments, bilirubin association constants were too large to be estimated directly from the CD studies. We utilized published K_B values for the primary bilirubin binding site of HSA to calculate relative affinity constants of competitive organic anions according to the f llowing relationship:

$$\bar{v}_B = \frac{K_B\ (B)}{1 + K_B\ (B) + K_A\ (A)}$$

Where $\bar{v}_B$ is the average number of moles bilirubin bound, K_A is the association constant for the competing anion, and $K_B = 1.4 \times 10^8$ for the HSA bilirubin complex (A) is the molar concentration of free organic anion assuming that the amount of bilirubin displaced reflects the amount of competing organic anion bound to the protein, and (B) is the concentration of bilirubin displaced by the organic anion A. Certain speculations are inherent in this approach, including the assumption that competitive binding occurs at the bilirubin site exclusively, and that neither complex binding nor cooperative effects occur.

The ellipticity pattern of the HSA-bilirubin complex was distinct from that of the BSA complex and was characterized by a positive peak at 460nm, a negative band of 405nm, and a crossover point at 438nm. An almost linear increase in ellipticity magnitude of both bands was observed after addition of bilirubin up to a molar ratio of 2:1. Between a molar ratio of 2 and 3:1, the slope of ellipticity increase became much shallower and above a molar ratio of 3:1, no further increase in optical activity resulted.

Addition of up to 6 moles of BSP or 9 moles of rose bengal per mole of a 1:1 HSA-bilirubin complex had little effect on optical activity generated by the complex. Several ligands studied decreased ellipticity magnitudes of HSA-bilirubin CD bands. In bilirubin-HSA 1:1 system, vasoflavine was the most effective competitor on a molar basis. Affinity constants (K) were estimated based on the effectiveness of the organic anions in displacing bilirubin from the primary binding site on HSA. The K values obtained were estimated as 2.5×10^7 M^{-1} for vasoflavine, 2.3×10^7 M^{-1} for ICG and iodipamide, 7.5×10^6 M^{-1} bilirubin glucuronide, 6×10^5 M^{-1} for flavaspidic acid, 2×10^5 M^{-1} for phenol red, and 5×10^5 M^{-1} for rose bengal. Under these conditions, the competing anions had no effect on the overall conformation of the proteins as determined from peptide ellipticity bands at 222nm and 208nm. These apparent affinity constants are first approximations because some of the competing anions may displace bilirubin from the primary binding site and the released bilirubin may form a complex at the second binding site. Since the ellipticity values associated with the second site are of the same sign and indistinguishable by CD from those of the first site, the resultant ellipticities after addition of the competing anions reflect both displacement of bilirubin and shifts to a second site. If this occurs, the anion would appear less effective in displacing bilirubin from the primary site.

The CD spectrum of rat liver ligandin reveals a pattern in the peptide absorption region (190-250nm) which is typical for a protein with highly ordered structure and helical content (17, 18, 29). Computer analysis relative to poly-peptides of known secondary structure reveals that this CD spectrum and 35% random coil. In the 250-300nm region, six bands are evident; and there is no ellipticity above 300nm. On addition of bilirubin, a large increase in ellipticity near 255nm is observed and three new ellipticity extrema appear in the region of bilirubin absorption. These bands are centered at 405, 455 and 515nm. If one plots ellipticity magnitude as a function of amount of bilirubin added, the 405nm band reaches maximum magnitude after addition of 1 mole of bilirubin, and the 455nm band attains about 80% of saturation values after addition of 1 mole. Thus, a 1:1 stoichimetry is reflected in the 405 and 455nm bands. Observations in the 515 and 255 regions indicate that an additional site(s) is involved after bilirubin is bound to ligandin in excess of 1:1 molar ratio; however, binding to this site(s) generates optically active bands distinct from that associated with the primary site.

Because up to a 1:1 molar ratio, no detectable unbound bilirubin is evident at protein concentrations of 10^{-5}M, the affinity of bilirubin for ligandin has an association constant of greater than 10^6 M^{-1} associated with the primary binding site.

ICG, BSP, iodipamide, and flavaspidic acid compete with bilirubin for hepatic uptake in vivo and exhibit competitive effects for a bilirubin binding site on ligandin. No Cotton effects are generated when these anions are bound to ligandin. The relative effectiveness of the competing anions and preferential binding to ligandin were monitored by their individual effects on the three observed bilirubin ellipticity bands. Based on the 455nm band, BSP and ICG have similar inhibitory effects, flavaspidic acid has an intermediary effect and iodipamide has a small effect. Association constants in the order of 10^6 M^{-1} for BSP and ICG, about 10^5 M^{-1} for flavaspidic acid, and less for iodipamide are estimated for the primary binding site.

The CD spectra of bilirubin-RSA complexes have positive ellipticity extrema at 455 nm and negative bands at 405 nm. This spectrum is virtually the mirror image of the CD spectrum associated with the ligandin-bilirubin complex and permits study of the transfer of bilirubin from ligandin to RSA directly without a need for artificial membranes or supporting gels. The relative affinity of the two proteins for binding bilirubin is readily derived from these CD experiments. If both proteins are present in equimolar amounts, over 90% of the bilirubin is bound to RSA. An isobestic point is also observed in the CD spectra indicating that the process is probably a 2 stage system involving transfer of bilirubin directly from ligandin to RSA. These results indicate that the association constant of RSA for bilirubin is approximately one order of magnitude greater than that of ligandin.

Despite the difference in association constants between albumin and ligandin, the latter may participate in hepatic organic anion uptake in vivo because: 1. the plasma membrane of the hepatocyte separates albumin and ligandin in vivo; 2. there is an abundance of ligandin within the cell which facilitates the concentration gradient for a specific ligand; and 3. binding to ligandin enhances the availability of most organic anions for subsequent biotransformation or excretion in the bile. Both mechanisms constitute 'pump'-like mechanisms.

Ketterer and colleagues (22) have reported higher affinity constants for bilirubin and heme binding to ligandin in native liver supernatant than with purified protein. Purification of ligandin appears to reduce its affinity substantially. The respective K values were 10^9 and 10^{10} respectively in cytosol and 10^6 and 10^7 respectively with purified ligandin. If these observations are correct, transfer of ligands from plasma into liver can proceed on the basis of facilitated diffusion with ligandin being a major factor in regulating this process.

Z PROTEIN

Z protein is an acidic cytoplasmic protein of 14,000 daltons present in the
small intestinal mucosa, liver, heart, kidney, skeletal muscle and fat cells
(31, 32, 34). It has an unusual binding affinity for long chain fatty acids and
their CoA derivatives in vitro. A role for Z in long-chain fatty acid transport
has been suggested; however, complete inhibition of hepatic oleate binding
in vivo by competition with flavaspidic acid did not reduce plasma t $\frac{1}{2}$, hepatic
uptake or rate of esterification of oleate (32). Z also has high affinity for
cholecystographic but not renographic agents. Other organic anions bind
to Z with high affinity in vitro (i.e.: flavaspidic acid, bunamiodyl) and inhibit
hepatic uptake of other less tightly bound organic anions (i.e.: bilirubin,
BSP, etc.) in vivo. Z develops phylogenetically in parallel with ligandin.
Ontogenetic development in guinea pigs, monkeys, and man is rapid in fetal
life and adult concentrations are present in the liver at birth. Drugs and
chemicals which induce ligandin have no apparent effect on Z. Clofibrate
and nafenopen, which are hypolipidemic drugs, increase the concentration
of Z protein in the liver. Z protein has no known enzymatic activity and its
functional interrelationship with ligandin has not been explored as yet.

SUMMARY

Evidence supporting as well as challenging the hypothesis that 'physiologic'
jaundice of the newborn results from delayed maturation of UDPGT is
summarized. Bilirubin infusion studies in newborn Rhesus monkeys suggest
that this syndrome does not result from a single enzymatic defect in bilirubin
conjugation but represents a complex interaction of functional disabilities
which are probably subjected to controls which are currently unknown.

   The transfer of bilirubin from plasma into the liver is saturable, non-
energy dependent, and manifests characteristics of carrier-mediated transport. The nature and site of the 'carrier' are unknown but could represent
membrane structures (proteins, pores) or cytoplasmic binding proteins.
Ligandin (Y protein, GSH transferase B) and Z protein are two such
relatively abundant hepatic cytoplasmic organic anion binding proteins.
Phylogenetic, ontogenetic, induction, immunofluorescent, competition and
kinetic studies suggest that ligandin is an important determinant of net flux
of bilirubin and other organic anions from plasma into the liver.

   Ligandin constitutes 2-5% of soluble protein in rat and human liver and is subject to remarkable control: it has a half-life of 2.3 days, is induced by many drugs and chemicals, and is stabilized in the absence of thyroid hormone.

In animal and human neonates, ligandin is virtually absent from liver and develops during the first week of life. Ligandin and albumin equally protect isolated liver mitochondria against bilirubin-produced uncoupling of oxidative phosphorylation.

Circular dichroism studies of serum albumin and ligandin reveal ordered structure and, in the presence of bilirubin, mirror-image chiralities which permit direct study of bilirubin transfer from one protein to another. The results indicate that bilirubin binds to purified ligandin with an association constant one order of magnitude less than that for the binding of bilirubin to serum albumin.

Studies by Meuwissen et al. suggest that the association constant of bilirubin to native ligandin (i.e.: within liver supernatant) is higher than that of bilirubin to albumin. If this is confirmed, bidirectional organic anion flux across the plasma membrane of the liver cell can be mathematically modelled in terms of binding to ligandin and serum albumin. Ligandin's catalytic activity (GSH transferase B) is inhibited by many ligands (e.g. bilirubin) which do not form GSH adducts.

REFERENCES

1. Arias, I. M., Pathogenesis of 'Physiologic' jaundice of the newborn: A reevaluation. *Birth Defects. Original Art. Ser. 6*: 55-59 (1970).
2. Arias, I. M., Transfer of bilirubin from blood to bile. *Semin. Hemat. 9*: 55-70 (1970).
3. Arias, I. M., G. Fleischner, R. Kirsch, S. Mishkin and Z. Gaitmaitan, On the structure, regulation, and function of ligandin. In: *Glutathione: metabolism and function*. I. M. Arias and W. B. Jakoby (eds.). Raven Press, New York 1976.
4. Arias, I. M. Unpublished data.
5. Blauer, G. and T. E. King, Interactions of bilirubin with bovine serum albumin in aqueous solution. *J. biol. Chem. 245*: 372-382 (1970).
6. Di Toro, R., L. Lupi and V. Ansanelli, Glucuronation of the liver in premature babies. *Nature 219*: 265-267 (1968).
7. Fleischner, G., J. Robbins and I. M. Arias, Immunological studies of Y protein: A major cytoplasmic organic anion binding protein in rat liver. *J. clin. Invest. 51*: 677-684 (1972).
8. Fleischner, G., K. Kamisaka, Z. Gaitmaitan and I. M. Arias, Immunologic studies of rat and human ligandin. In: *Glutathione: metabolism and function*. I. M. Arias and W. B. Jakoby (eds.). Raven Press, New York 1976.
9. Gartner, L. M. and I. M. Arias, Developmental pattern of glucuronide formation in rat and guinea pig liver. *Amer. J. Physiol. 205*: 663-666 (1963).
10. Gartner, L. M. and I. M. Arias, The transfer of bilirubin from blood to bile in the neonatal guinea pig. *Pediat. Res. 3*: 171-180 (1969).

11. Gartner, L. M., The functional basis of physiologic jaundice of the newborn. In: *Jaundice*. C. A. Goresky and M. M. Fisher (eds.), pp.257-266 (Plenum Press, New York 1975).

12. Goldstein, E. and I. M. Arias, Ligandin: Interaction with radiographic contrast media. *Invest. Radiol.* (in press).

13. Habig, W., M. Pabst, G. Fleischner, Z. Gatmaitan, I. M. Arias and W. Jakoby, The identity of glutathione transferase B with ligandin, a major binding protein of liver. *Proc. Nat. Acad. Sci. (Wash.) 71*: 3879-3882 (1974).

14. Jansen, P. and I. M. Arias, Delipidation and reactivation of UDP glucuronyl-transferase from rat liver. *Biochim. biophys. Acta 391*: 288-38 (1975).

15. Kamisaka, K., Z. Gatmaitan, C. Moore and I. M. Arias, Ligandin reverses bilirubin inhibition of liver mitochondrial respiration in vitro. *Pediat. Res. 9*: 903-905 (1975).

16. Kamisaka, K., I. Listowsky, J. Betheil and I. M. Arias, Competitive binding of bilirubin, sulfobromophthalein, indocyanine green and other organic anions to human and bovine serum albumin. *Biochem. biophys. Acta 365*: 169-180 (1974).

17. Kamisaka, K., I. Listowsky, G. Fleischner, Z. Gatmaitan and I. M. Arias, Studies of the binding of bilirubin and other organic anions to serum albumin and ligandin (Y protein). *Birth defects: Original Art. Ser.* (1974). In press.

18. Kamisaka, K., I. Listowsky, Z. Gatmaitan and I. M. Arias, Interactions of bilirubin and other ligands with ligandin. *Biochemistry* (Wash.) *14*: 2175-2180 (1975).

19. Kamisaka, K., I. Listowsky, Z. Gatmaitan and I. M. Arias, Circular dichroism analysis of the secondary structure of Z protein and its complexes with bilirubin and other organic anions. *Biochem. biophys. Acta 393*: 24-30 (1975).

20. Kaplowitz, N., I. W. Percy-Robb and N. B. Javitt, Role of hepatic anion-binding protein in bromsulphthalein conjugation. *J. exp. Med. 138*: 483-487 (1973).

21. Ketterer, B., P. Ross-Mansell and J. K. Whitehead, The isolation of carcinogen-binding protein from livers of rats given 4-dimethyl-aminoazobenzene. *Biochem. J. 103*: 316-324 (1967).

22. Ketterer, B., E. Tipping, D. Beale and J. A. T. P. Meuwissen, Ligandin, glutathione, and carcinogen binding. In: *Glutathione: metabolism and function*. I. M. Arias and W. B. Jakoby (eds.). Raven Press, New York 1976.

23. Kirsch, R., K. Kamisaka, G. Fleischner and I. M. Arias, Structural and functional studies of ligandin, a major renal organic anion binding protein. *J. clin. Invest. 55*: 1009-1019 (1975).

24. Levi, A. J., Z. Gatmaitan and I. M. Arias, The role of two hepatic cytoplasmic proteins (Y and Z) in the transfer of sulfobromophthalein (BSP) and bilirubin from plasma into the liver. *J. clin. Invest. 48*: 2156-2167 (1969).

25. Levi, A. J., Z. Gatmaitan and I. M. Arias, Deficiency of hepatic organic anion binding protein: A possible cause of 'physiologic' jaundice in the newborn. *Lancet 2*: 139-140 (1969).

26. Levi, A. J., Z. Gatmaitan and I. M. Arias, Deficiency of hepatic anion binding protein impaired organic anion uptake by liver and 'physiologic' jaundice in newborn monkeys. *New Engl. J. Med. 283*: 1136-1139 (1970).

27. Levine, R. J., H. Reyes, A. J. Levi, Z. Gatmaitan and I. M. Arias, Phylogenetic study of hepatic organic anion uptake mechanisms. *Nature 231*: 277-279 (1971).

28. Lichter, M., G. Fleischner, R. Kirsch, A. J. Levi, K. Kamisaka and I. M. Arias, The role of ligandin and Z protein in the transfer of thyroid hormones from plasma into the liver. *Amer. J. Physiol.* (1975). In press.

29. Listowsky, I., K. Kamisaka and I. M. Arias, Circular dichroism studies of Y protein (Ligandin), a major organic anion binding protein in liver, kidney and small intestine. *Ann. N.Y. Acad. Sci. 226*: 148-153 (1973).

30. Litwack, G., B. Ketterer and I. M. Arias, Ligandin: An abundant liver protein which binds steroids, bilirubin, carcinogens and a number of exogenous anions. *Nature 234*: 466-467 (1971).
31. Mishkin, S., L. Stein, Z. Gatmaitan and I. M. Arias, The binding of fatty acids to cytoplasmic proteins: Binding to Z protein in liver and other tissues of the rat. *Biochem. Biophys. Res. Commun. 47*: 997-1003 (1972).
32. Mishkin, S., L. Stein, G. Fleischner, Z. Gaitmaitan and I. M. Arias, Z protein in hepatic uptake and esterification of long-chain fatty acids. *Amer. J. Physiol. 228*: 1634-1640 (1975).
33. Morey, K. S. and G. Litwack, Isolation and properties of cortisol metabolite binding proteins of rat liver cytosol. *Biochemistry* (Wash.) *8*: 4813-4821 (1969).
34. Ockner, R. K., Fatty acid-binding protein in small intestine. Identification, isolation, and evidence for its role in cellular fatty acid transport. *J. clin. Invest. 54*: 326-338 (1974).
35. Reyes, H., A. J. Levi, Z. Gatmaitan and I. M. Arias, Organic anion-binding protein in rat liver: Drug induction and its physiologic consequence. *Proc. Nat. Acad. Sci. (Wash.) 64*: 168-170 (1969).
36. Reyes, H., A. J. Levi and I. M. Arias, Studies of Y and Z: Two hepatic cytoplasmic organic anion-binding proteins: Effect of drugs, chemicals, hormones and cholestasis. *J. clin. Invest. 50*: 2242-2252 (1971).

DETECTION OF FREE BILIRUBIN:
A CRITERION FOR EXCHANGE TRANSFUSION

R. BRODERSEN, PH.D.

Kernicterus in the newborn continues to be a major concern in neonatology, in spite of important therapeutic progress and improved prevention. Exchange transfusion remains the ultimate treatment. During the latest 20 years a very high number of exchange transfusions have been given and Diamond (5) estimated that in the United States alone more than 100,000 children have been saved from death or physical and mental impairment by this therapy. Exchange transfusion thus ranks among the more important resources of modern medicine.

The problem of indications for exchange transfusion, however, has not been fully solved. It was originally thought that serum bilirubin levels above a certain limit could serve as a criterion. Exchange transfusion is often given when serum bilirubin exceeds 18 or 20 mg per 100 ml (300 to 340 μM).* It has been shown, on the other hand, that kernicterus may occur at much lower serum bilirubin levels (7) and, at the other extreme, children with 30 or even 40 mg per 100 ml have escaped without obvious harm. This is understood if we consider the mechanism of kernicterus.

According to Odell (26) an equilibrium of binding of bilirubin to serum albumin leaves a small concentration of unbound or free bilirubin. The free pigment is capable of entering the central nervous system while the albumin bound fraction is not.

$$\text{Brb-Alb} \rightleftharpoons \text{Free bilirubin} \rightleftharpoons \boxed{\text{CNS}}$$
$$+ \text{ albumin}$$

Other conditions, anoxia, acidosis, and immaturity, favour uptake of bilirubin by the nerve cells, but the presence of free bilirubin in a certain concentration seems to be necessary for establishment of kernicterus. If a displacing drug is given, such as sulfisoxazole, or if an endogenous metabolite

* μM micromoles per litre. 1 μM bilirubin is 0.058 mg per 100 ml.

occupies the bilirubin binding site on albumin, the free bilirubin concentration goes up and bilirubin leaves the blood stream to be taken up by other receptors. The binding proteins of the liver, discovered by Arias and co-workers (6) seem to be important reservoirs. The danger of kernicterus is increased under these circumstances, in spite of a lowered serum bilirubin. Indeed, after giving a displacing drug the first alarming sign of danger is a decreasing serum bilirubin level. It is obvious that a high serum bilirubin is not an indication for exchange transfusion in this case.

The actual neurotoxicity of the blood plasma is not determined by the concentration of bilirubin but rather by the free bilirubin. Considerable efforts have accordingly been directed towards determination of free bilirubin in blood plasma. In recent years many publications have appeared on this subject from several laboratories, including the author's. A final solution has, as far as I know, not yet been found, due to extraordinary analytical difficulties. It is possible in model systems with purified albumin and bilirubin to determine free bilirubin indirectly by studies of the rate of oxidation with hydrogen peroxide and peroxidase. This principle has been utilized for determination of free bilirubin in diluted samples of blood serum (14). No other method is available for quantitative determination of free bilirubin.

Direct determination of free bilirubin by spectroscopy or similar means is not possible due to its very low concentration and the presence of bound pigment in much larger amounts. In a solution of pure albumin and bilirubin in concentrations as in blood plasma of an icteric neonate, 400 and 300 μM respectively, the free bilirubin concentration can be calculated from the law of mass action since the binding constant is known (12). Free bilirubin concentration is 0.04 μM, or about 10,000 times less than the bound concentration. It would be reasonable to guess that the concentration in blood plasma would be of a magnitude similar to the levels of albumin and bilirubin. A concentration of this order probably indicates the lower limit of neurotoxic levels of free bilirubin. It is obviously not possible to determine this by spectrophotometry.

Bound bilirubin gives a fluorescence which is not shown by the free pigment. Determination of the bound pigment may thus be based on fluorescence and the total, free plus bound, can be determined by known methods. It is, however, not possible to determine the free fraction as total minus bound, again because of its low value relative to the total.

Several authors have tried to circumvent the problem by determining the residual binding capacity of albumin, and this seems to be somewhat easier. Clinically, it may be equally useful to know how much bilirubin can still be bound to available sites on albumin before a dangerous level of neurotoxicity develops.

It is not possible in this paper to go into details concerning the many methods which have been proposed for determination of free bilirubin or residual binding capacity. Some of the more important approaches are listed in table 1.

Table 1. Some methodological studies of free bilirubin concentration, residual bilirubin-binding capacity of albumin, loosely bound bilirubin, albumin titrable bilirubin, etc. in neonatal blood plasma.

Waters and Porter, 1961 (34)
Watson, 1964 (36)
Waters and Porter, 1964 (35)
Waters, 1967 (33)
Jirsová, Jirsa, Koldovsky and Weirichova, 1967 (15)
Kaufmann, Simcha and Blondheim, 1967 (19)
Rutkowski, 1967 (30)
Odell, Storey and Rosenberg, 1968 (28)
Odell, Cohen and Kelly, 1969 (27)
Hertz, 1969 (8)
Keenan, Arnold and Sutherland, 1969 (21)
Csögör, Csutak and Pressler, 1968 (4)
Kaufmann, Kapitulnik and Blondheim, 1969 (17)
Jacobsen and Fedders, 1970 (13)
Zamet and Chunga, 1971 (37)
Howorth, 1971 (11)
Chunga and Lardinois, 1971 (3)
Schiff, Chan and Stern, 1972 (31)
Krasner, Giacoia and Yaffe, 1973 (22)
Bratlid, 1973 (2)
Kaufmann, Kapitulnik and Blondheim, 1973 (18)
McCluskey, More, Storey and O'Sullivan, 1973 (24)
McCluskey, Storey, Brown, More and O'Sullivan, 1974 (25)
Kapitulnik, Valaes, Kaufmann and Blondheim, 1974 (20)
Jacobsen and Wennberg, 1974 (14)
Athanassiadis, Chopra, Fischer and McKenna, 1974 (1)
Kapitulnik, Horner-Mibashan, Blondheim, Kaufmann and Russell, 1975 (16)
Pays and Beljean, 1975 (29)
Valaes, Kapitulnik, Kaufmann and Blondheim, 1975 (32)
Lee, Gartner and Zarafu, 1975 (23)
Hertz, 1975 (9, 10)

The Sephadex method is widely used. It was originally proposed by Jirsova et al. (15), was further developed in several places, and can be executed by use of a commercial kit. A sample of serum, usually diluted, is passed through a small column of Sephadex G-25. In some cases a yellow pigment is bound to the Sephadex. The amount of this is higher than the expected amount of free bilirubin. It is unfortunate that this pigment has been named 'free bilirubin'. A better term is 'loosely bound bilirubin', as used by Valaes et al. (32). The exact chemical identity of the yellow pigment, or mixture of pigments, remains to be determined by mass spectroscopy or other means. It is possible, however, that the amount of yellow pigment bound to Sephadex is related to the concentration of free bilirubin; the prospect of this method seems promising, since practical experience appears to support its clinical value.

In certain modifications of the Sephadex method, and indeed in most of the other proposed techniques, the serum sample is diluted, from eight to one hundred-fold or more. It seems important to note that any effect of a displacing drug in the sample is likely to be missed after dilution. The displacing effect is proportional to the unbound concentration of the drug and is in most cases reduced to insignificant levels by tenfold dilution. A recent modification of the Sephadex method (29) avoids dilution and would appear preferable to other related procedures.

Methods for determination of residual binding capacity usually are based on addition of a dye which is bound to available sites on albumin and thereby undergo a shift of light absorption spectrum. Para-hydroxybenzeneazobenzoic acid has been much used (35). A recent procedure, developed by Hertz (9, 10), using bromphenol blue, has shown promising results.

An interesting approach has also been made by McCluskey et al. (24, 25), determining 'loosely bound bilirubin' by titration with albumin to an endpoint monitored by fluorescence.

Several workers have used addition of bilirubin for determination of the binding capacity. The point of saturation is determined by the Sephadex technique (20), by fluorescence (22), or by other means. Bilirubin is likely under these circumstances to displace any competing substances, such as sulfonamides, entirely. The result is therefore a determination of the total bilirubin binding capacity, disregarding any displacers with lower affinity. For a meaningful determination of the actual amount of vacant sites on albumin it is necessary to use a 'soft' ligand, binding with moderate affinity, and to avoid dilution. Such a technique remains to be developed.

Current methods, using high dilutions or using added bilirubin for determination of residual binding capacity, might, as we have seen, be expected to determine the amount of albumin not occupied by bilirubin. Since each albumin molecule probably will carry no more than one molecule of bilirubin and since the free bilirubin concentration is low, this figure would be the same as the molar concentration of albumin minus that of bilirubin. It has been found by several investigators (22, 14, 16), however, that the actual results deviate from those obtained in model systems with purified adult serum albumin. This seems to indicate that albumin in certain newborns is different from adult albumin. The difference may be due to a tightly bound, displacing substance or to a different chemical structure of fetal albumin. The methods in question actually measure the competence of albumin for bilirubin transport, disregarding the effect of any displacing substances with less tight binding, such as sulfonamides.

In conclusion it appears that final selection of a suitable procedure must await further investigations. It would be desirable to establish an organized evaluation and comparison on equal conditions of the many principles proposed.

SUMMARY

It is generally recognized that indications for exchange transfusion in threatening kernicterus cannot be based upon serum bilirubin determination. The concentration of free bilirubin, not bound to albumin, would be a more reliable measure of the actual neurotoxicity of the blood plasma. This concentration is extremely low and the ultimate method for its determination in blood plasma remains to be developed. The much used Sephadex method does not give free bilirubin concentrations in the true sense but may prove to be of clinical value on an empirical basis. Determination of residual binding capacity of albumin is another possible solution. Current methods using high dilution of the sample and added bilirubin for capacity determination tend to nullify the effect of displacing substances, such as sulfonamides. These procedures seem to disclose a defect of bilirubin-transporting competence of albumin in certain neonates.

The need is stressed for theoretical evaluation and uniform testing of the many different procedures available.

REFERENCES

1. Athanassiadis, S., D. R. Chopra, M. A. Fischer and J. McKenna, An electrophoretic method for detection of unbound bilirubin and reserve bilirubin binding capacity in serum of newborns. *J. Lab. clin. Med. 83*: 968-976 (1974).
2. Bratlid, D., Reserve albumin binding capacity, salicylate saturation index, and red cell binding of bilirubin in neonatal jaundice. *Arch. Dis. Childh. 48*: 393-397 (1973).
3. Chunga, F. and R. Lardinois, Separation by gel filtration and microdetermination of unbound bilirubin. I. In vitro albumin and acidosis effects on albumin-bilirubin-binding. *Acta paediat. scand. 60*: 27-32 (1971).
4. Csögör, S., J. Csutak and A. Pressler, Modifications of albumin transport capacity in pregnant women and newborn infants. *Biol. Neonat.* (Basel) *13*: 211-218 (1968).
5. Diamond, L. K., A history of jaundice in the newborn. Birth defects. *Original art. ser. 6*: 3-6 (1970).
6. Fleischner, G., J. Robbins and I. M. Arias, Immunological studies of Y-protein. A major cytoplasmic organic anion-binding protein in rat liver. *J. clin. Invest. 51*: 677-685 (1972).
7. Harris, R. C., J. F. Lucey and J. R. Maclean, Kernicterus in premature infants associated with low concentrations of bilirubin in plasma. *Pediatrics 21*: 875-884 (1958).
8. Hertz, H., The measurement of the bilirubin binding capacity of serum albumin and its clinical significance. *Pediat. Res. 3*: 90 (1969).
9. Hertz, H., A direct spectrometric method for determination of the concentration of available bilirubin binding sites in serum using bromphenol blue. *Scand. J. clin. Lab. Invest. 35*: 545-559 (1975).
10. Hertz, H., Available bilirubin binding sites of serum from newborns determined by a direct spectrophotometric method using bromphenol blue. *Scand. J. clin. Lab. Invest. 35*: 561-568 (1975).
11. Howorth, P. J. N., Determination of serum albumin in neonatal jaundice. The albumin saturation index. *Clin. chim. Acta 32*: 271-278 (1971).
12. Jacobsen, J., Binding of bilirubin to human serum albumin. Determination of the dissociation constants. *FEBS Lett. 5*: 112-114 (1969).
13. Jacobsen, J. and O. Fedders, Determination of non-albumin-bound bilirubin in human serum. *Scand. J. clin. lab. Invest. 26*: 237-241 (1970).
14. Jacobsen, J. and Rich. P. Wennberg, Determination of unbound bilirubin in the serum of newborns. *Clin. Chem. 20*: 783-789 (1974).
15. Jirsová, V., M. Jirsa, O. Koldovsky and J. Weirichova, The use and possible diagnostic significance of Sephadex gel filtration of serum from icteric newborn. *Biol. Neonat.* (Basel) *11*: 204-208 (1967).
16. Kapitulnik, J., R. Horner-Mibashan, S. H. Blondheim, N. A. Kaufmann and A. Russell, Increase in bilirubin-binding affinity of serum with age of infant. *J. Pediat. 86*: 442-445 (1975).
17. Kaufmann, N. A., J. Kapitulnik and S. H. Blondheim, The adsorption of bilirubin by Sephadex and its relationship to the criteria for exchange transfusion. *Pediatrics 44*: 543-548 (1969).
18. Kaufmann, N. A., J. Kapitulnik and S. H. Blondheim, Bilirubin binding affinity of serum: Comparison of qualitative and quantitative Sephadex gel filtration methods. *Clin. Chem. 19*: 1276-1279 (1973).
19. Kaufmann, N. A., A. J. Simcha and S. H. Blondheim, The uptake of bilirubin by blood cells from plasma and its relationship to the criteria for exchange transfusion. *Clin. Sci. 33*: 201-208 (1967).
21. Keenan, W. J., J. E. Arnold and J. M. Sutherland, Serum bilirubin binding determined by Sephadex column chromatography. *J .Pediat. 74*: 813 (1969).

20. Kapitulnik, J., T. Valaes, N. A. Kaufmann and S. H. Blondheim, Clinical evaluation of Sephadex gel filtration in estimation of bilirubin binding in serum in neonatal jaundice. *Arch. Dis. Childh. 49*: 886-894 (1974).
22. Krasner, J., G. P. Giacoia and S. J. Yaffe, Drug-protein binding in the newborn infant. *Ann. N.Y. Acad. Sci. 226*: 101-114 (1973).
23. Lee, K., L. M. Gartner and J. Zarafu, Fluorescent dye method for determination of bilirubin-binding capacity of serum albumin. *J. Pediat. 86*: 280-285 (1975).
24. McCluskey, S., D. G. More, G. N. B. Storey and W. J. O'Sullivan, The use of fluorimetry to determine non-albumin bound bilirubin in the jaundiced neonate. *Med. Res.* 62-63 (1973).
25. McCluskey, S. B., G. N. B. Storey, G. K. Brown, D. C. More and W. J. O'Sullivan, Albumin titratable bilirubin. *Bilirubin Meeting*, Hemsedalen, Norway, September 1974, 75a-82a.
26. Odell, G. B., The dissociation of bilirubin from albumin and its clinical implications. *J. Pediat. 55*: 268-279 (1959).
27. Odell, G. B., S. N. Cohen and P. C. Kelly, Studies in kernicterus. II. The determination of the saturation of serum albumin with bilirubin. *J. Pediat. 74*: 214-230 (1969).
28. Odell, G. B., G. N. B. Storey and L. A. Rosenberg, The saturation of serum proteins with bilirubin during neonatal life and its relationship to brain damage at 5 years. In: *Amer. Pediat. Soc.* 78th Ann. meeting, Atlantic City, N.J., 1968.
29. Pays, M. and M. Beljean, Microdetermination of unbound bilirubin in sera. Application to the prevention of kernicterus by estimating the bilirubin-binding capacity of serum albumin. *Clin. chim. Acta 59*: 121-128 (1975).
30. Rutkowski, R. B., The determination of maximum bilirubin-binding capacity of human albumin and serum by a calcium carbonate adsorption technique. *Clin. chim. Acta 17*: 31-38 (1967).
31. Schiff, D., G. Chan and L. Stern, Sephadex G-25 quantitative estimation of free bilirubin potential in jaundiced newborn infant's sera: A guide to prevention of kernicterus. *J. Lab. clin. Med. 80*: 455-462 (1972).
32. Valaes, T., J. Kapitulnik, N. A. Kaufmann and S. H. Blondheim, Experience with Sephadex gel filtration in assessing the risk of bilirubin encephalopathy in neonatal jaundice. Birth defects: Original Art. Ser. (1975). In press.
33. Waters, W. J., The reserve albumin binding capacity as a criterion for exchange transfusion. *J. Pediat. 70*: 185-192 (1967).
34. Waters, W. J. and E. G. Porter, Dye-binding capacity of serum albumin in hemolytic disease of the newborn. *Amer. J. Dis. Child. 102*: 59-66 (1961).
35. Waters, W. J. and E. G. Porter, Indications for exchange transfusion based upon the role of albumin in the treatment of hemolytic disease of the newborn. *Pediatrics 33*: 749-757 (1964).
36. Watson, D., Bilirubin-binding-capacity of blood plasma in relation to foetal erythroblastosis. *Aust. N. Z. J. Obstet. Gynaec. 4*: 121-124 (1964).
37. Zamet, P. and F. Chunga, Separation by gel filtration and microdetermination of unbound bilirubin. 2 - Study of sera in icteric newborn infants. *Acta paediat. scand. 60*: 33-38 (1971).

NEONATAL HYPERBILIRUBINEMIA

M. MICHAEL THALER, M.D.

PERINATAL BILIRUBIN METABOLISM: DEVELOPMENTAL PATTERNS AND ADAPTIVE RESPONSES

Bilirubin accumulates in newborn infants during the first week after birth. Expressed in general terms, this universal phenomenon can be attributed to temporary imbalance between bilirubin production and clearance, created at birth by the abrupt termination of placental clearance functions. Prematurity accentuates the disparity between production and elimination of bilirubin. Accordingly, neonatal unconjugated hyperbilirubinemia ('physiologic jaundice') is an expression of maturational dysequilibrium between metabolic processes governing bilirubin formation and excretion after birth. Physiologic jaundice may reflect excessive *formation* of pigment from erythrocyte and tissue heme pools, immaturity of mechanisms responsible for pigment *removal*, or a *combination* of both. This type of jaundice may become pathologic when conditions which add to pigment load, or interfere with pigment clearance, intervene during the labile period of adjustment to extrauterine life (12). Inherited or acquired hemolytic disorders such as maternal-fetal blood group incompatibility, red cell enzymopathies (most commonly glucose-6-phosphatase deficiency) and hematoma due to trauma at delivery may elevate the body content of unconjugated bilirubin dangerously. Clinical evidence suggests that common metabolic problems of premature or ill newborns – hypoxia, hypoglycemia, caloric deficiency, acidosis, dehydration – may shift the input/output bilirubin ratio further toward sequestration of pigment.

Knowledge of postnatal metabolic capacities for bilirubin formation and removal, and of adaptive responses to exigencies after birth that place additional demands on these capacities, may clarify the manner in which 'physiologic' and 'pathologic' varieties of neonatal unconjugated hyperbilirubinemia develop. This paper compares the perinatal behavior in rats of pivotal microsomal enzyme systems responsible for bilirubin formation and clearance: heme oxygenase (HO), catalyzing the breakdown of heme to bilirubin, and bilirubin UDP-glucuronyltransferase (GT), active in conjugation of the pigment to an excretable derivative. In addition, the effects of acute hemolysis and fasting on the postnatal development of HO and GT will be analyzed. Thirdly, mechanisms are suggested whereby bilirubin-forming processes may be regulated in newborns.

PERINATAL DEVELOPMENT OF HO AND GT

The liver is of greatest importance for the physiologic expression of HO and GT activities (9). HO activity per g tissue is higher in spleen, but total activity per organ is considerably greater in newborn liver (13). Moreover, in contrast with splenic HO, hepatic HO increases in response to changing metabolic conditions. GT activity is present in non-hepatic tissues (e.g. kidney and intestine), but bilirubin conjugation in vivo is largely a function of

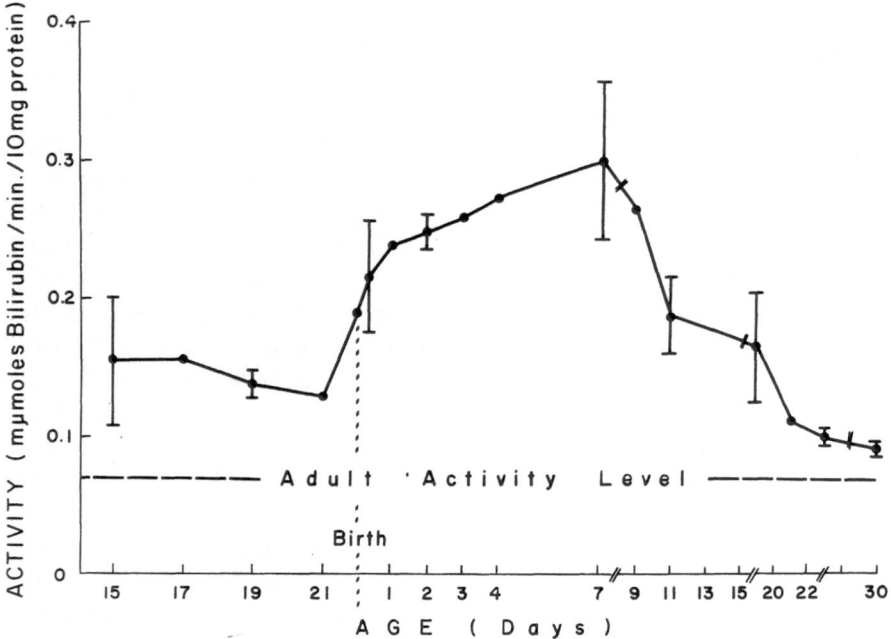

Fig. 1. Development of hepatic heme oxygenase activity during gestation and after birth. Brackets represent standard deviations from the mean.

liver GT. Microsomal HO converts heme to biliverdin, which is immediately reduced to bilirubin by a specific biliverdin reductase present in excess in most tissues of newborn and mature rats (10). Bilirubin, rather than biliverdin, is the final product of heme catabolism at all ages examined.

Hepatic HO is already highly developed in 15-day old fetuses, and ranges in activity between 100 to 150% of adult activity during the remainder of gestation (13). A rapid increase in hepatic HO activity to nearly 4 times adult activity occurs during the first week after birth (fig. 1). Splenic HO is relatively unchanged during the perinatal period, and does not exceed adult activity. Thus, the metabolic *capacity* for bilirubin formation is relatively greater in newborns compared with adults, and is further increased in the immediate postnatal period.

Bilirubin formed in the liver, spleen and other organs by microsomal HO is converted to its diglucuronide by GT located in the hepatic microsomal system. In contrast with hepatic HO, GT is relatively poorly developed in

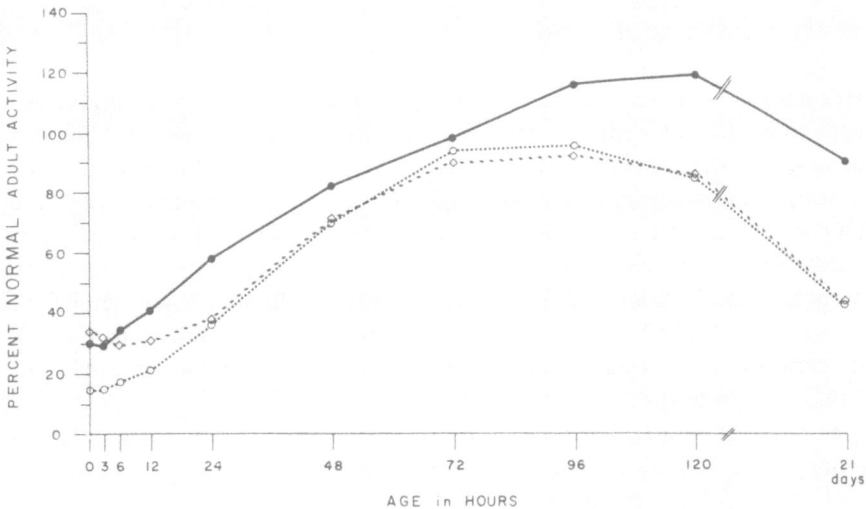

Fig. 2. Postnatal development of bilirubin UDP-glucuronyl transferase activity in rats. Solid dots, normal strains; diamonds, heterozygous Gunn rats, offspring of jaundiced females; open circles, heterozygous Gunn rats, offspring of anicteric females. Heterozygous newborn rats delivered by jaundiced females had normal activity at birth, whereas rats delivered by anicteric females had approximately 50% normal activity. Heterozygous animals developed nearly 100% of the activity seen in normal animals by the third day, whereas only 50% normal activity would be expected on a genetic basis. These findings are consistent with accelerated development of conjugating activity in the presence of bilirubin.

fetuses and newborns. Fetal GT is barely detectable at 17 days gestation in rats, and reaches approximately 20% of adult activity at birth (11). Adult activity levels are achieved between the second and fourth day after birth (fig. 2). These developmental patterns indicate that postnatal maturation of the mechanism for bilirubin conjugation lags behind maturation of the bilirubin-forming system in liver. These findings are of general biological interest, since they reflect selective differentiation of various functional components in membranes of hepatic smooth endoplasmic reticulum after birth.

Many enzymatic activities increase rapidly after birth, whereas the increase is more gradual in others. Substrate induction (7) hormonal induction (3) or a combination of these mechanisms may be responsible for the postnatal development of any given enzyme system. The effect of heme, (substrate for HO) and of bilirubin, (substrate for GT) on the perinatal development of HO and GT will be examined next.

EFFECTS OF HEMOLYSIS, HEME AND BILIRUBIN ON PERINATAL DEVELOPMENT OF HO AND GT

HO activity in liver, but not in spleen, of mature rats can be stimulated with injections of heme, (methemalbumin) or by experimentally induced hemolysis (9). Severe hemolysis induced in utero or postnatally with the hemolytic agent phenylhydrazine (1 mg/10 g body weight) increased hepatic HO activity consistently within 24 hours after treatment (5). Intraperitoneal injections of heme, administered as methemalbumin (4 μmoles/100 g) to pregnant rats 24 hours before delivery, or during the first 5 postnatal days caused a 50 to 100% increase in hepatic HO activity of offspring (fig. 3). In contrast, these treatments had no effect on HO activity in spleen of fetuses or newborns.

In contrast with their effects on HO activity, hemolysis or heme injection reduced GT activity in liver from fetuses and newborns to approximately 40% of control activity during the first 3 days after birth (fig. 3). GT became resistant to the inhibitory effects of hemolysis or heme between the 5th and 6th postnatal day. Thus, the early developmental difference between hepatic HO and GT is magnified in the presence of heme injected directly or derived from hemoglobin released in the course of hemolysis.

Bilirubin has no effect on hepatic HO activity in mature rats (9) or newborns (unpublished observations). In contrast, bilirubin stimulates development of GT activity in utero and after birth. The GT activities of newborn

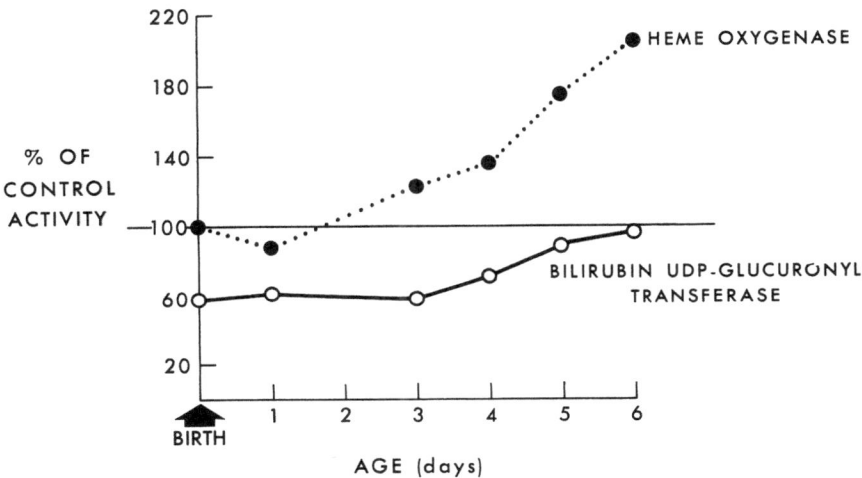

Fig. 3. Effect of hemolysis induced by phenylhydrazine on postnatal development of heme oxygenase and bilirubin UDP-glucuronyl transferase activity. Results expressed in terms of percent of activities in age-matched untreated newborns (control).

heterozygous offspring of mothers with unconjugated hyperbilirubinemia due to hereditary deficiency in GT (Gunn rats) are elevated into the normal homozygous range during exposure to maternal bilirubin in utero, whereas in heterozygote newborn offspring of heterozygous non-jaundiced Gunn rats mated with jaundiced homozygous males GT is at the expected 50% level of normal homozygous littermates (13) (fig. 2). GT activity develops more rapidly after birth in heterozygous, compared with homozygous normal rats, suggesting that bilirubin may stimulate maximal postnatal development of conjugating activity in partially GT-deficient newborns (fig. 2). In summary heme stimulates bilirubin-forming processes, and bilirubin triggers conjugating activity. Excessive heme released during hemolysis or from rapid turnover of non-erythrocyte hemoproteins tends to accentuate the disparity in relative rates of postnatal development of these processes (fig. 3), and may overwhelm the capacity of newborn liver for bilirubin conjugation. Neonatal hyperbilirubinemia develops in newborn rats with drug-induced hemolysis (5), reflecting increased bilirubin formation in the presence of reduced conjugating capacity. These experimental findings may explain the rapidity with which serum bilirubin concentrations often rise in newborn infants with severe hemolytic conditions such as erythroblastosis or glucose-6-phosphate dehydrogenase deficiency.

EFFECTS OF FASTING ON PERINATAL DEVELOPMENT OF HO AND GT

In newborn rats prevented from nursing, hepatic HO activity increased 50% in 3 hr and doubled within 6 hr when compared with fed controls (table 1) (13). Hepatic HO in starved newborns declined to control values

Table 1. Effects of fasting and refeeding on hepatic heme oxygenase in newborn rats.

Age, hour	No. of animals	Activity[1]		
		Normal	Fasted	Refed
0	12	0.23 ± 0.03		
3	6	0.29 ± 0.08	0.43 ± 0.18	
6	5	0.32 ± 0.12	0.65 ± 0.08	0.28 ± 0.07

1. Expressed as millimicromoles of bilirubin produced per minute per 10 mg protein ± standard deviation.

within 3 hrs after being allowed to feed. Similarly, fasting of pregnant rats during gestation and prior to delivery significantly increased hepatic HO in fetuses and newborn offspring ($p < 0.05$). Prenatal and postnatal fasting had no effect on splenic HO, suggesting that the liver was primarily responsible

Table 2. Effect of starvation on GT activity in normal newborn and adult rats.

Newborns (Age in hours)	GT activity (mg bilirubin conjugated/g liver/hr) Fed	Starved (24 hrs)	P value
0-24	3.19 ± 0.41*	1.14 ± 0.19	<0.001
25-48	4.00 ± 0.55	1.87 ± 0.27	<0.010
49-72	4.11 ± 0.14	3.21 ± 0.20	<0.025
Adults (Hours fasted)			
0	6.36 ± 0.26		<0.025
24	4.98 ± 0.32		<0.025
48	7.77 ± 0.87		N.S.**
72	6.85 ± 0.52		N.S.
96	7.75 ± 0.55		N.S.

* Mean ± SEM
** N.S. = not significant

for homeostatic adjustments in bilirubin-forming capacity during fasting. In marked contrast with the influence of fasting on HO activity, GT activity was strikingly reduced in newborn rats fasted for 24 hrs. As shown in table 2, GT activities during fasting declined 64% in 1-day old rats, 54% in 2-day old rats, and 22% in 3-day old rats. Fasting had little effect on GT in adult rats, although activities declined temporarily during the first day without food.

These results indicate that fasting reduces bilirubin conjugation during the immediate postnatal period, while capabilities for bilirubin formation are enhanced. Hyperbilirubinemia which is frequently observed in newborn infants who are hypoglycemic or from whom feeding is withheld for 24 hrs after birth (8, 4) may reflect these disparate effects of fasting on HO and GT activities during the first few postnatal days.

REGULATION OF PERINATAL BILIRUBIN METABOLISM BY GLUCAGON

Many hepatic enzymes are activated at birth by hormones responsive to hypoglycemia and fasting (3). Because the newborn liver is depleted of glycogen, hypoglycemia develops rapidly when maternal supplies of glucose are interrupted. Moreover, hypoglycemia, glucagon and epinephrine were shown to enhance hepatic HO activity in adult rats whereas splenic activity remained unresponsive (1). Similar enhancement of HO was produced in liver of congenitally jaundiced newborn rats treated with glucagon (2). The increase in HO activity was accompanied by a rise in hepatic bilirubin content, and accelerated formation of radioactive bilirubin from hepatic hemes and hemoproteins which had been prelabeled in vivo with ^{14}C-delta amino-levulinic acid (fig. 4). These findings indicate conclusively that bilirubin formation in newborn rats is accelerated by glucagon, the hormone released in response to hypoglycemia. Thus, neonatal hyperbilirubinemia observed in infants prone to hypoglycemia, such as prematures and infants of diabetic mothers, in malnourished or unfed newborns, and in infants with caloric deficiency due to upper intestinal obstruction, may be due to glucagon-stimulated conversion of non-erythrocyte hemes to bilirubin.

The experimental findings reviewed above suggest that the capacity for bilirubin formation is fully developed in utero, and exceeds adult capacity at birth. In contrast, development of bilirubin conjugation is more gradual, and appears accelerated after birth by pigment which accumulates because it is no longer cleared by the placenta. The developmental lag between bili-

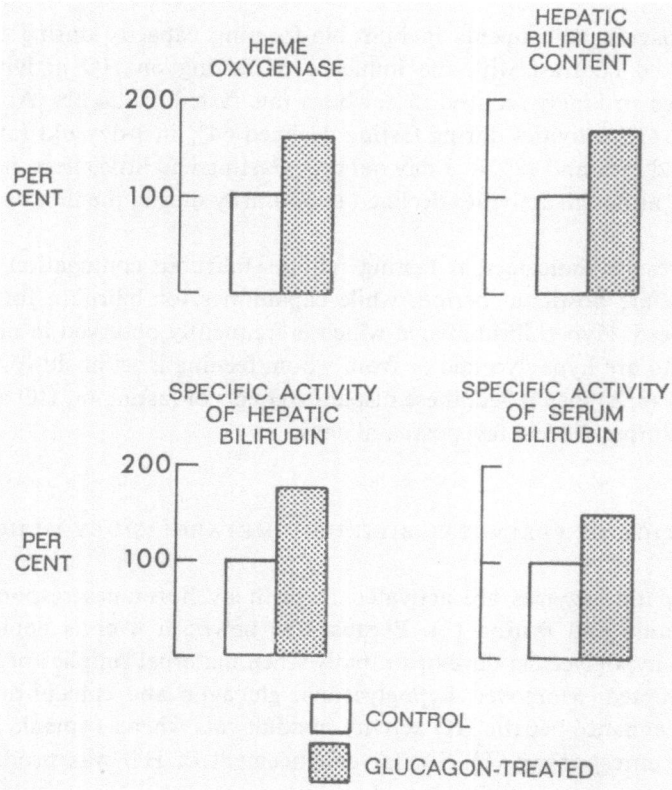

Fig. 4. Correlations between the effects of glucagon on hepatic heme oxygenase, bilirubin concentration and specific activity, and serum bilirubin concentration in newborn rats.

rubin-forming and bilirubin-clearing mechanisms may explain the phenomenon of 'physiologic jaundice'. Disorders associated with moderate or severe unconjugated hyperbilirubinemia in newborns, such as hemolysis and caloric insufficiency, further contribute to the disparity between these processes. Under these conditions, bilirubin can accumulate rapidly, and the jaundice may become 'pathologic'. Heme and glucagon stimulate the enzyme which catabolizes heme in newborns and adult rats. Glucagon has been recently shown to enhance hepatic bilirubin formation in newborn rats. Thus, substrate induction (heme) and hormonal activation (glucagon) may be responsible for the tendency to overproduction of bilirubin in newborns, compared with adults (6).

REFERENCES

1. Bakken, A. F., M. M. Thaler and R. Schmid, Metabolic regulation of heme catabolism and bilirubin production. I. Hormonal control of hepatic heme oxygenase activity. *J. Clin. Invest. 51*: 530-536 (1972).
2. Dawber, N. H. and M. M. Thaler, Glucagon stimulates bilirubin production. *Clin. Res. 21*: 313 (1973).
3. Greengard, O., Enzymatic differentiation in mammalian liver. *Science 163*: 891-895 (1969).
4. Hubbell, J. P., J. E. Drorbaugh, A. J. Rudolph, P. A. M. Auld, R. B. Cherry and C. A. Smith, 'Early' versus 'late' feeding of infants of diabetic mothers. *New Engl. J. Med. 265*: 835-837 (1961).
5. Kerner, J. A., D. L. Gemes, N. H. Dawber and M. M. Thaler, Perinatal bilirubin metabolism: effects of hemolysis. *Pediat. Res. 6*: 405 (1972).
6. Maisels, M. J., A. Pathak, N. M. Nelson, D. G. Nathan and C. A. Smith, Endogenous production of carbon monoxide in normal and erythroblastotic human infants. *J. clin. Invest. 50*: 1-8 (1971).
7. Nemeth, A. M., Initiation of enzyme formation by birth. *Ann. N.Y. Acad. Sci. 111*: 199-202 (1963).
8. Stimmler, L., J. V. Brazie and D. O'Brien, Plasma-insulin levels in the newborn infants of normal and diabetic mothers. *Lancet 1*: 137-138 (1964).
9. Tenhunen, R., H. S. Marver and R. Schmid, The enzymatic catabolism of hemoglobin: stimulation of microsomal heme oxygenase by hemin. *J. Lab. clin. Med. 75*: 410-421 (1970).
10. Tenhunen, R., M. E. Ross, H. S. Marver and R. Schmid, Reduced NADP-dependent biliverdin reductase: partial purification and characterization. *Biochemistry (Wash.) 9*: 298-303 (1970).
11. Thaler, M. M., Substrate-induced conjugation of bilirubin in genetically deficient newborn rats. *Science 170*: 555-556 (1970).
12. Thaler, M. M., Neonatal hyperbilirubinemia. *Semin. Hemat. 9*: 107-112 (1972).
13. Thaler, M. M., D. L. Gemes and A. F. Bakken, Enzymatic conversion of heme to bilirubin in normal and starved fetuses and newborn rats. *Pediat. Res. 6*: 197-201 (1972).

BREAST-FEEDING AND NEONATAL HYPERBILIRUBINEMIA

MICHEL ODIÈVRE, M.D.

A variety of prolonged neonatal jaundice has been observed in certain infants fed with maternal milk (2, 10) and has since been confirmed in several reports. A causal relationship between breast-feeding and jaundice was inferred from the inhibitory effect of milk on human liver slices and homogenates using bilirubin and o-aminophenol as substrates for conjugation (2); rapid disappearance of hyperbilirubinemia after cessation of breast-feeding also supported such a relation (2).

The hyperbilirubinemia was attributed to the transmission from mother to infant of an isomer of a natural steroid, the 3-alpha-20-beta-pregnane-diol, present in breast-milk (2); this steroid was present in inhibitory human milk and was demonstrated to inhibit the o-aminophenol conjugation by guinea pig liver microsomes. However, bilirubin conjugation by slices from two human livers and soluble enzyme from one was not inhibited by 3-alpha-20-beta-pregnane-diol, even at high concentrations (1) and doubt has been cast on the role of this steroid in the etiology of jaundice.

More recently, it was found that free fatty acids also have an inhibitory effect on bilirubin conjugation in vitro (3, 6, 7). The relative inhibitory strength of the saturated fatty acids is, in decreasing order, capric acid > lauric acid > myristic acid > palmitic acid > stearic acid. The relative inhibitory strength of the C18 unsaturated fatty acids is, in decreasing order, linolenic acid > linoleic acid > oleic acid. Fresh milk samples from mothers of jaundiced infants had an increased lipoprotein lipase activity (9) and a low concentration of free fatty acids; progressive release of free fatty acids above 1 mEq/liter/day was observed when these milks were stored at $+4°$ C for 3-5 days at which time bilirubin conjugation in vitro is inhibited by 50% or more. Preheating at $+56°$ C for 15 minutes prevented such a release (8).

Additional evidence for a relation between the inhibitory effect of free fatty acids and prolonged neonatal jaundice was obtained by the rapid disappearance of hyperbilirubinemia after substitution with pre-heated milk (8).

The milks from mothers of jaundiced infants also inhibited BSP binding to cytoplasmic Z protein when stored at $+4°$ C for 4 days and were without effect on BSP binding to Y protein (5). No inhibitory effect was found with fresh milk samples or with preheated milk at $+56°$ C. The inhibitory effect of free fatty acids has also been documented (5).

The mechanism by which an increased concentration of free fatty acids in certain human milks can interfere in vivo with bilirubin conjugation, and eventually with bilirubin transport into the hepatocyte when the capacity of Y protein is still reduced, remains unclear.

Additional difficulties in understanding came from several reports when occasional inhibition was also observed in milk from mothers of unjaundiced infants. Twelve specimens of milk from 5 mothers of normal infants inhibited glucuronyl transferase activity in vitro in excess of 20% (2). Considerable inhibitory activity was also observed in maternal milks studied as soon as possible after collection on the 6th day post partum in an unselected series of breast-fed infants (4).

The present study was undertaken so as to determine the frequency of inhibitory activity in milk from mothers whose infants had no prolonged neonatal jaundice.

MATERIAL AND METHODS

Milk was obtained by expression from 27 randomized mothers, whose infants had no prolonged neonatal jaundice. At no time during pregnancy, labor or lactation did any mother receive steroids or hormonal medication. In all cases, one milk sample was collected on days 3, 6, 10, 20 and 30 post partum and was stored at $+4°$ C for 3-4 days. Milk samples from eight mothers of jaundiced infants were used as controls.

Free fatty acid concentration was measured in each sample on the first day and at the end of the storage period; the difference between the two values was considered as the amount released during storage and was expressed as mEq/liter/day.

Lipoprotein lipase activity was measured in all fresh milk samples.

Inhibitory effect on bilirubin conjugation by rat liver microsomes was occasionally studied in order to confirm the previously established relation between the inhibition of bilirubin conjugation and the amount of free fatty acid in the incubation milieus.

All the methods used have been previously described (7, 8, 9).

RESULTS

The relation between the inhibitory activity of milk and its free fatty acid concentration is shown in figure 1: bilirubin conjugation in vitro is inhibited 50% or more when free fatty acid concentration is above 4 mEq/liter, corresponding to a daily release of about 1 mEq/liter.

The amount of free fatty acids released after storage is shown in figure 2 and the percentage of milk samples containing a large amount of free fatty acids in figure 3. Lipoprotein lipase activity is shown in figure 4.

The results show that the concentration of free fatty acids and the amount of inhibitory activity do not differ in many milk samples from those observed from mothers whose infants have a prolonged neonatal jaundice. The in vitro

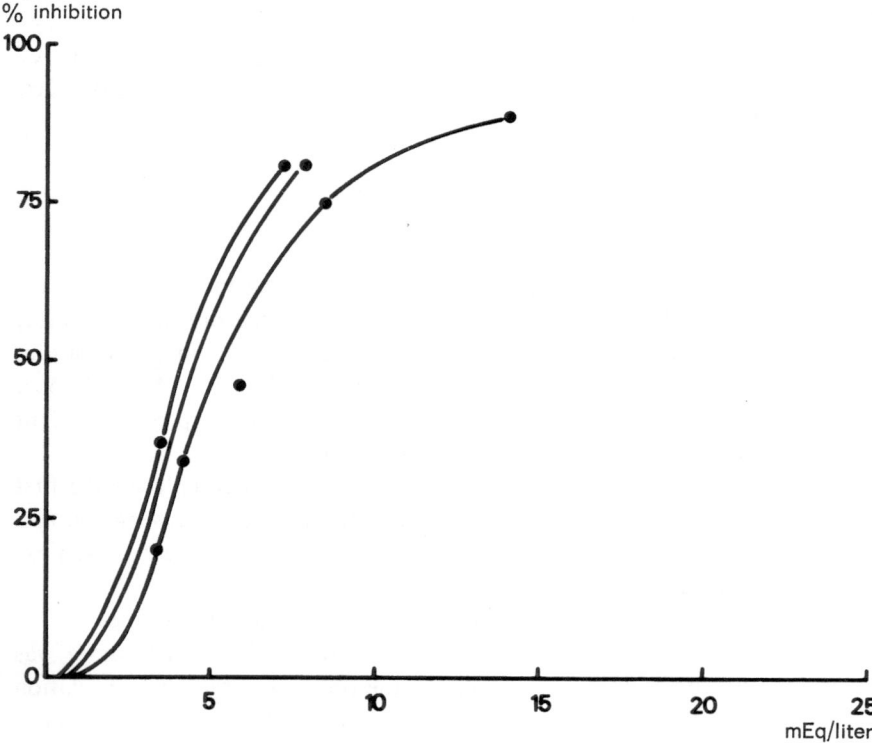

Fig. 1. Relation between the inhibitory activity of in vitro bilirubin conjugation and free fatty acid concentration.

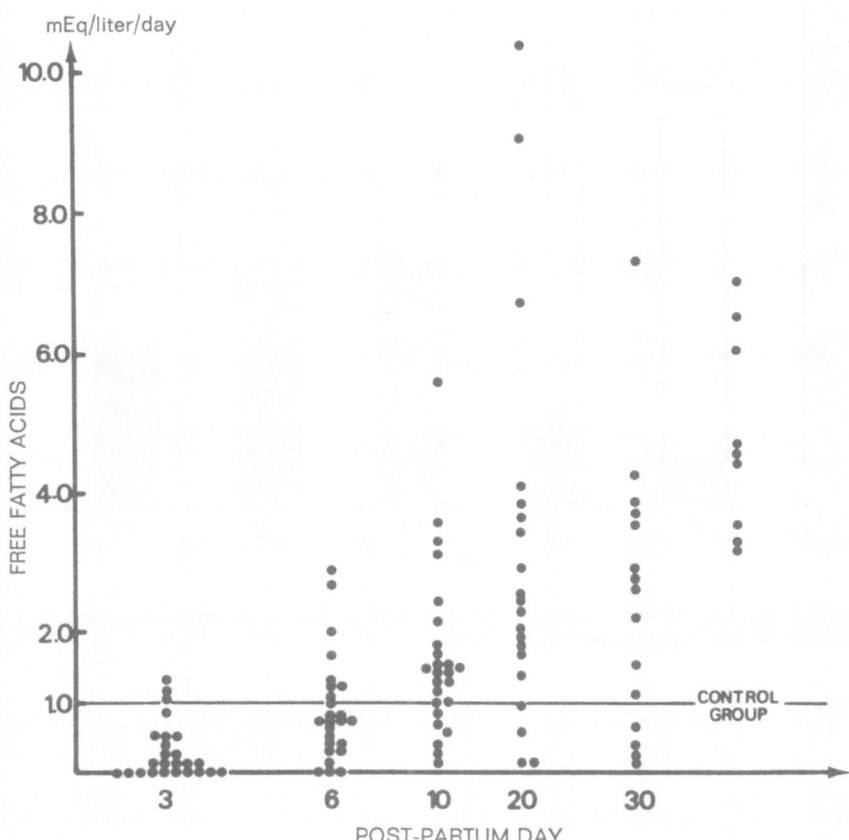

Fig. 2. Amount of free fatty acids released after storage in maternal milk collected at different days post-partum. (Control group: milk samples from 8 mothers of infants with prolonged neonatal jaundice.)

inhibition develops from the 6th day post partum and becomes more frequent on subsequent days. Lipoprotein lipase activity also develops from the 6th day post partum.

Jaundice was minimal during the first 5-6 days of life in 13 infants and attributed to physiologic hyperbilirubinemia; it persisted until 10 days post partum in 3 other infants and subsequently disappeared while breast-feeding continued.

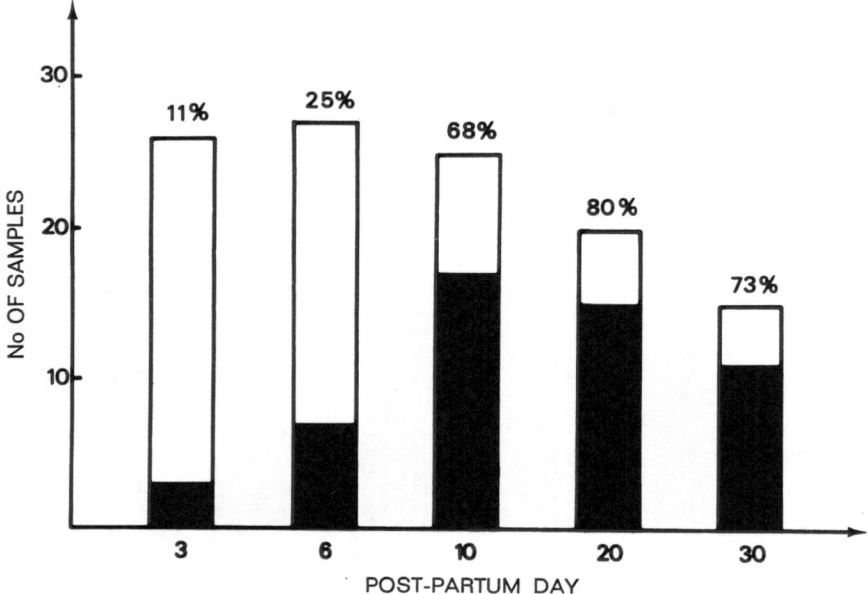

Fig. 3. Percentage of milk samples collected at different days post-partum and containing large amounts of free fatty acid.

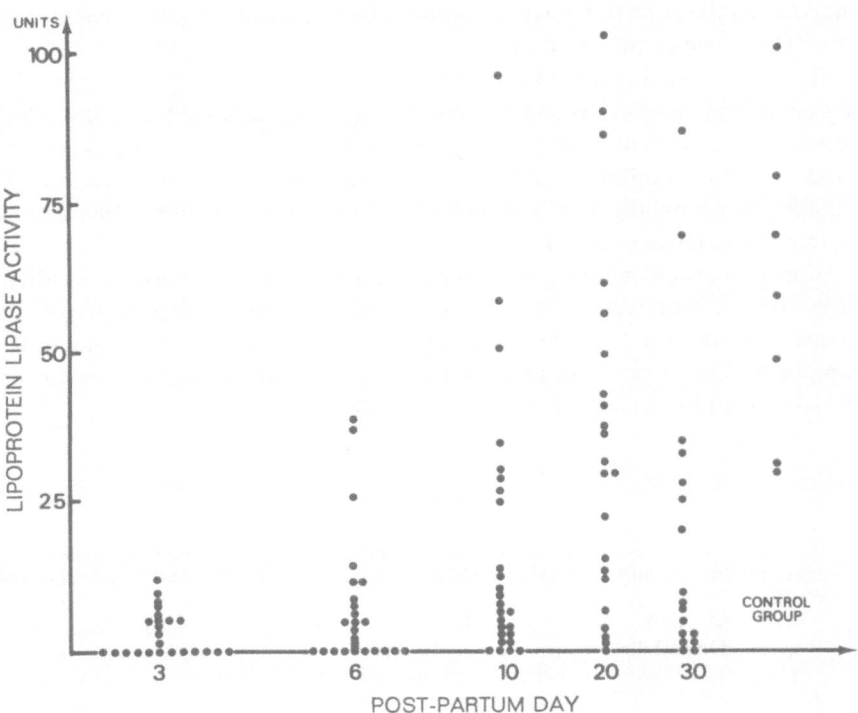

Fig. 4. Lipoprotein lipase activity in fresh milk samples collected on different post-partum days. (Control group: milk samples from 8 mothers of infants with prolonged neonatal jaundice.)

DISCUSSION

The development of neonatal jaundice in breast fed infants is probably the result of the interaction of several factors: whether prolonged hyperbiliru-binemia is due to decreased activity of liver glucuronyl transferase, decrease of bilirubin transport within the hepatocyte or increased amount of inhibitory substance cannot be answered. The possibility that 3-alpha-20-beta-pregnane-diol is the inhibitory substance was not consistently supported (1, 11); the failure to observe inhibitory activity in fresh milk samples supports the con-clusion that this steroid is unlikely to be the causative agent of the in vitro inhibition of bilirubin conjugation. The development of inhibitory activity during storage and its prevention by pre-heating at +56° C suggest that the enzymatic release of free fatty acids could be responsible for in vitro inhibition of bilirubin conjugation (8).

The results obtained in the present study show that a similar enzymatic release of free fatty acids can be observed in many milks from mothers of non-jaundiced infants. Whether the failure of infants to develop jaundice when ingesting inhibitory milk may be attributed to the maturation of hepatic glucuronyl transferase or delayed appearance of the inhibitory activity remains to be determined.

Some other implications result from our findings: they concern the validity of in vitro measurements of inhibitory activity in supporting a diagnosis of breast feeding jaundice, the necessity to test all presumed normal milk samples before using them as controls for in vitro inhibitory studies or as in vivo substitutes to pathologic maternal milk.

REFERENCES

1. Adlard, B. P. F. and G. H. Lathe, Breast milk jaundice: effect of 3-alpha-20-beta-pregnanediol on bilirubin conjugation by human liver. *Arch. Dis. Childh. 45*: 186-189 (1970).
2. Arias, I. M., L. M. Gartner, S. Seifter and M. Furman, Prolonged neonatal unconjugated hyperbilirubinemia associated with breast feeding and a steroid, pregnane-3 (alpha), 20 (beta)-diol, in maternal milk that inhibits glucuronide formation in vitro. *J. clin. Invest. 43*: 2037-2047 (1964).
3. Bevan, B. R. and J. B. Holton, Inhibition of bilirubin conjugation in rat liver slices by free fatty acids, with relevance to the problem of breast milk jaundice. *Clin. chim. Acta 14*: 101-107 (1972).
4. Cole, A. P. and T. Hargreaves, Conjugation inhibitors and early neonatal hyperbilirubinemia. *Arch. Dis. Childh. 47*: 415-418 (1972).
5. Foliot, A., J. P. Ploussard, E. Housset, B. Christoforov, R. Luzeau and M. Odièvre, Breast-milk jaundice. In vitro inhibition of rat liver bilirubin-UDP-glucuronyl transferase activity and Z protein-BSP binding by human breast-milk. *Pediat. Res.* In press.
6. Hargreaves, T., Effect of fatty acids on bilirubin conjugation. *Arch. Dis. Childh. 48*: 446-450 (1973).
7. Levillain, P., M. Odièvre, R. Luzeau et A. Lemonnier, Possibilités d'inhibition de la glucuro-conjugaison de la bilirubine en fonction de la teneur en acides gras libres du lait maternel. *Biochim. biophys. Acta* (Amst.) *264*: 538-547 (1972).
8. Luzeau, R., P. Levillain, M. Odièvre and A. Lemonnier, Demonstration of a lipolytic activity in human milk that inhibits the glucuro-conjugation of bilirubin. *Biomedicine 21*: 258-262 (1974).
9. Luzeau, R., M. Odièvre, P. Levillain et A. Lemonnier, Activité de la lipoprotéine lipase dans les laits de femme inhibiteurs in vitro de la conjugaison de la bilirubine. *Clin. chim. Acta 59*: 133-138 (1975).
10. Newman, A. J. and S. Gross, Hyperbilirubinemia in breast-fed infants. *Pediatrics 32*: 995-1001 (1963).
11. Ramos, A., M. Silverberg and L. Stern, Pregnanediols and neonatal hyperbilirubinemia. *Amer. J. Dis. Child. 111*: 353-356 (1966).

CLINICAL ASPECTS OF LIVER DISEASE IN CHILDREN WITH α-1 ANTITRYPSIN DEFICIENCY

THOMAS SVEGER, M.D. AND ØYSTEIN AAGENAES, M.D.

Since Sharp first showed the relationship between α-1 antitrypsin deficiency and cholestasis in infancy and cirrhosis in childhood in 1969 (5), a substantial number of reports have appeared from different parts of the world, all confirming Sharp's work. In many parts of the world this is now one of the major causes of intrahepatic cholestasis in infancy. Depending on the frequency of the Pi Z gene, the frequency of Pi ZZ infants in children with neonatal intrahepatic cholestasis will be around 15-30%, and the other way round, between 10 and 15% of children with Pi type ZZ seem to develop liver disease in infancy (4).

This presentation is based on the clinical material of patients with neonatal cholestasis and α-1 antitrypsin deficiency, who have been investigated at the Department of Pediatrics, University Hospital, Rikshospitalet in Oslo, and reported in (1), and on the data from a screening study of 200,000 newborn infants in Sweden, where 118 Pi ZZ infants have been found and followed prospectively through the first year of life. The data from this study are described in (6).

The Oslo material consists of 7 children, of whom 6 are living, between 1 and 18 years of age.

The birth weights of the infants were lower than normal, averaging 3,123 g. Small birth weights were also confirmed by Sveger's (6) data, 7 of 14 infants with neonatal obstructive jaundice being small for gestational age.

Of a total of 16 children with clinical obstructive jaundice, all were diagnosed before 6 weeks of age, most often in the first weeks of age. Light stools and dark urine were also found in all infants in this period (table 1). In 2 of the 7 Norwegian children and in 1 of 22 of the Swedish children with proven or probable liver disease, umbilical bleeding was the first sign of liver disease.

Of other clinical findings hepatomegaly was found in 4 of 6 of the Norwegian infants and 5 of 9 of the Swedish with clinical obstructive jaundice, splenomegaly in 3 of the 6 Norwegian and 4 of the 9 Swedish at diagnosis.

Table 1. α_1-Deficiency + cholestasis. Age at diagnosis of jaundice.

<4 weeks	7/7	(Aagenaes)
<6 weeks	9/9	(Sveger)

At follow-up hepatomegaly disappeared in some of the children, but spleno-megaly was found in 3 of the 4 children who are now over 5 years of age.

Growth was in the normal range in 4 of 5 Norwegian children.

Maximal serum bilirubins were in the same range in the Norwegian and the Swedish material with clinical cholestasis. In addition the Swedish material consists of a small group of 5 infants with subclinical cholestasis where maximal serum bilirubin was 2-4 mg% (table 2).

Table 2. α_1-Deficiency + cholestasis. Maximal serum bilirubin.

6 -15 mg%	(Aagenaes)
4,7-12 mg%	(Sveger - group I A)
2 - 4 mg%	(Sveger - Group I B)

Group I A = clinical cholestasis
Group I B = subclinical cholestasis

Laboratory examinations did not differ from other patients with intra-hepatic cholestasis in infancy; the serum transaminases, alkaline phospha-tases and γ-glutamyltranspeptidase were moderately increased. Those who were studied during the phase of cholestasis also showed hyperlipidemia, of a relatively moderate degree.

The radio active Rose-Bengal excretion in 3 days was in a range of 10-20% in all 3 infants studied, pointing to an intrahepatic cholestasis.

In 14 of 15 infants with cholestasis, the cholestasis subsided before 4 months of age. In one child the cholestasis lasted about 1 year.

The screening study findings indicate that the clinical obstructive jaun-dice is only the top of an iceberg in infants with α-1 antitrypsin deficiency. Of 200,000 newborn infants in Sweden, screened for α-1 antitrypsin deficiency, 118 were found to have Pi type ZZ. Followed prospectively, ten per cent of them showed obstructive jaundice, 7% clinical jaundice and 3% subclinical jaundice. On clinical examination another 8 infants (6%) gave evidence of liver disease: hepatomegaly, splenomegaly, umbilical bleeding etc.

Examined at 3 months and 6 months of age another 55 of the infants, 41%, showed biochemical evidence of liver disease, with an increase in one or more of the liver enzymes. Serum levels of alkaline phosphatase above twice the upper normal limit for children 2-6 months of age has been taken as abnormal. Alanin aminotransferase 50% above the upper normal limit for age was also considered abnormal, and a level above 150 units was declared as abnormal for γ-glutamyltranspeptidase, upper normal limits being 120 units. Because of these strict criteria, the number with increased liver enzymes is probably even higher. These findings confirm earlier clinical suspicion from the Oslo material in 'normal' ZZ-individuals (1).

In neither the Norwegian nor the Swedish material have there been clinical clues to other pathogenic factors. Viral studies, including Australia antigen, were negative in all patients with obstructive jaundice. Neither the frequency of asphyxia nor intrauterine injury of any sort, was increased.

Two of the Swedish children with obstructive jaundice had had siblings with a similar disease. In none of the Norwegian children were there siblings with neonatal cholestasis, although there were quite a few siblings with Pi type ZZ. We are not able to say whether this number of affected siblings (2 siblings of 21 probands) is higher than should be expected, as we do not have a complete family study.

All the Swedish infants with obstructive jaundice were thriving and well at 6 months of age. One of the Norwegian infants died of pneumococcal/ pneumonia after a surgical exploration. One of the others has had two attacks of peritonitis. He also had a surgical exploration performed before the diagnosis was made. Portal hypertension was diagnosed at age 6 in our oldest child. He is now 18, and he has had no oesophageal bleeding thus far. As we have done no further splenoportography, we have no data on portal tension in the rest of our patients, but with 3 of 4 having splenomegaly, portal hypertension probably is present in most of them. Only one child is, and has always been, in relatively poor clinical condition. All the rest appear relatively normal, but with the development of portal hypertension, the prognosis is uncertain.

Some of the patients with subclinical obstructive jaundice probably also will develop cirrhosis, while most of the patients with increased liver enzymes but no other signs of liver disease, probably have a good liver prognosis. The basis for this statement, is the rarity of α-1 antitrypsin deficiency in young adult cirrhotics with no history of neonatal cholestasis (3).

In late adulthood, when emphysema has developed, the danger of developing liver cirrhosis and/or liver cancer is again about 10-15% (2).

As a conclusion we must state that our study has not revealed any additional pathogenic factor. From the data on birth weights we can conclude that the additional pathogenic factor must act before birth.

SUMMARY

The clinical picture of liver disease in α-1 antitrypsin deficiency in infancy is dominated by cholestasis. In some, the cholestasis is so severe that biliary atresia is suspected. In others a bleeding tendency and a suspicion of septicemia have been the reason for admission.

The cholestatic phase is, most often, of a few months duration; later the clinical picture is dominated by progressive cirrhosis. In some, ascites and oesophageal varices develop before school age, while others first develop symptoms of cirrhosis in young adulthood. Most, if not all of the cirrhotic α-1 antitrypsin deficient children seem to have had some cholestasis in infancy. Also, results from the screening of 200,000 newborns show that a temporary increase in liver enzymes, slightly prolonged conjugated hyperbilirubinemia and/or moderate hepatomegaly, are present in a substantial number of the Pi ZZ infants.

In later adult life, mainly described in emphysematous patients, cirrhosis and/or hepatoma may again develop.

In conclusion, about 10% of α-1 antitrypsin deficient infants develop cirrhosis in childhood; of the remainder about 10% develop cirrhosis later. In addition a temporary increase in liver enzymes is frequently found, mainly in infancy, but also later.

REFERENCES

1. Aagenaes, Ø., M. Fagerhol, K. Elgjo, E. Munthe and T. Hovig, Pathology and patho- genesis of liver disease in alpha-1-antitrypsin deficient individuals. *Postgrad. med. J. 50*: 365-375 (1974).
2. Eriksson, S. and I. Hägerstrand, Cirrhosis and malignant hepatoma in α_1-antitrypsin deficiency. *Acta med. scand. 195*: 451-458 (1974).
3. Fischer, R. L., L. Taylor, M. Maze and S. Sherlock, α-1-antitrypsin deficiency in liver disease: The extent of the problem. *Digestion 10*: 320-321 (1974).
4. Porter, C. A., A. P. Mowat, P. J. L. Cook, D. W. G. Haynes, K. B. Shilkin and R. Williams, α_1-antitrypsin deficiency and neonatal hepatitis. *Brit. med. J. 3*: 435-439 (1972).
5. Sharp, H. L., R. A. Bridges, W. Krivit and E. F. Freier, Cirrhosis associated with alpha-1-antitrypsin deficiency: A previously unrecognized inherited disorder. *J. Lab. clin. Med. 73*: 934-939 (1969).
6. Sveger, T., Mass-screening for α_1-antitrypsin deficiency: Liver disease during the first 6 months of life. *New Engl. J. Med.* 1976 (in press).

PATHOLOGIC LIVER CHANGES IN
ALPHA-1-ANTITRYPSIN DEFICIENT INFANTS
(Pi ZZ PHENOTYPE)

M. HADCHOUEL AND MARTHE GAUTIER

Since the first report of Freier, Sharp and Bridge in 1968, many authors have stressed the association of alpha-1-antitrypsin deficiency and liver disease in children. Aagenaes, in 1972, was the first to emphasize the frequency of prolonged neonatal cholestasis.

Alpha-1-antitrypsin-deficient adults usually present with pulmonary disorders. In some, liver involvement can be found, with or without clinical manifestations. Pulmonary emphysema usually appears during the third decade. Consequently, it may be difficult to obtain precise information about the neonatal period. Many of these adults are known to have clinically and biologically normal livers, and the relationship between alpha-1-antitrypsin deficiency and liver disease is still unknown.

Twenty-six Pi ZZ children have been studied retrospectively since 1970 (fig. 4). All children had been referred for liver disease: neonatal cholestasis, or cirrhosis. All cirrhotic patients had a history of neonatal cholestasis. This study concerns only the 17 patients on whom histological examination was performed during the initial neonatal cholestasis. Biopsies were repeated in most patients. The children in this study have been followed from 1 to 19 years; 7 of them for longer than 3 years.

We tried to compare the histologic findings with the biologic and clinical evolution in these 17 patients. It seems that a correlation could be established between the initial histologic pattern and the course of the disease.

ANALYTIC EXAMINATION

Constant features have been observed on the repeated biopsies:

1. In all cases amylase resistant, PAS+ globules were found in hepatocytes; their sizes ranged from 1 to >20 μ, the larger accompanying cirrhosis. They were then surrounded with a halo. They were always predominant in periportal areas, which were their only sites when not numerous.

The size and number of globules increase with ageing, whatever the importance (or even absence) of fibrosis.

Distinction between granules and lipofuscins is difficult during the first months of life, especially during cholestasis.

In some cases, PAS+ inclusions could be found in biliary epithelium.

Nuclear vacuolization was frequent in periportal areas. Sometimes, PAS+ intranuclear inclusions were observed, even when intracytoplasmic globules were absent.

2. Steatosis was also predominant in the periportal areas, and was not confined to hepatocytes loaded with PAS+ globules. It was always moderate and did not increase with age. It was less frequent in cases with cirrhosis.

3. Periportal intracellular iron deposits were constantly found on the first biopsies.

4. Inflammation, when present, was more often portal. It consisted of mononuclear cells.

5. Minimal necrosis was always present; however, it was not confined to hepatocytes containing globules.

Besides these constant features, 3 morphological patterns could be distinguished during the neonatal cholestatic period.

Moderate portal fibrosis: 7 cases (group I).

In 7 cases, portal fibrosis was moderate. Ductular proliferation was absent in 5, and slight in 2. Mononuclear infiltration was frequent and confined to the portal areas. Lobular architecture was disturbed by giant cells and pseudo-acinar rearrangement. Cholestasis was confined to liver cells. No bile plugs were observed in portal areas.

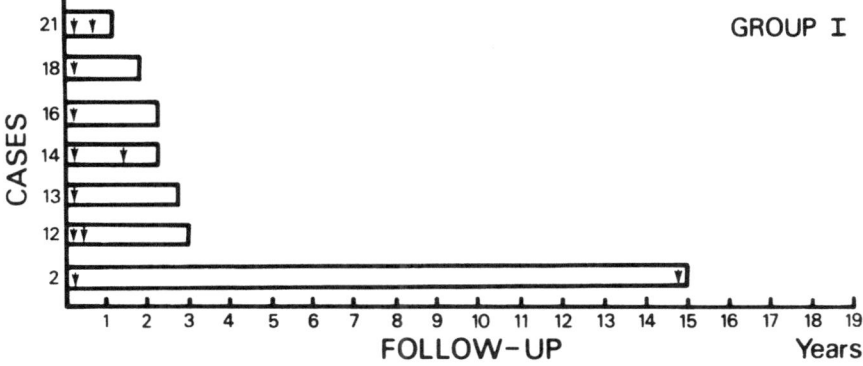

Fig. 1. Arrows indicate age at which biopsies were done.

Group I (7 cases)

Clinical course
Disappearance of jaundice before 6 months of age Progressive decrease of hepatomegaly No portal hypertension

Extensive portal fibrosis with ductular proliferation: 6 cases (group II).

In 6 cases, portal fibrosis was marked; it was annular in 5, and true cirrhosis was present in 2. Ductular proliferation was important. Cholestasis was always present and, in one case, a bile plug was observed in the portal area.

This morphological pattern could easily be mistaken for extrahepatic biliary obstruction, leading the patients to surgery. However, some cases have been reported as having both diseases.

Group II (6 cases)

Clinical course
Disappearance of jaundice before 6 months of age Liver enlargement Development of splenomegaly Portal hypertension (proven in 2 cases)

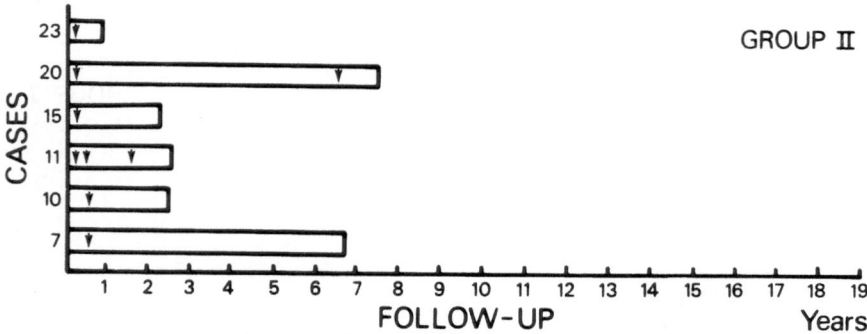

Fig. 2. Arrows indicate age at which biopsies were made.

Intrahepatic ductular hypoplasia: 4 cases (group III).

In 4 cases, paucity of inter-lobular biliary ducts was observed. Portal fibrosis was minimal or absent, without ductular proliferation. Important cholestasis was intra-lobular.

Group III (4 cases)

Clinical course

Persistent jaundice and pruritus
Hepatomegaly
Portal hypertension in 2 cases
Patent biologic cholestasis

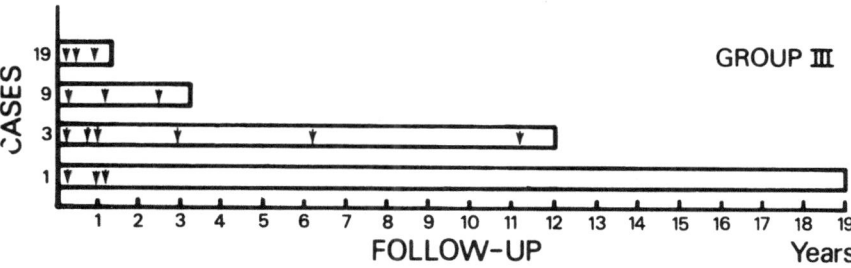

Fig. 3. Arrows = age when biopsies were done.

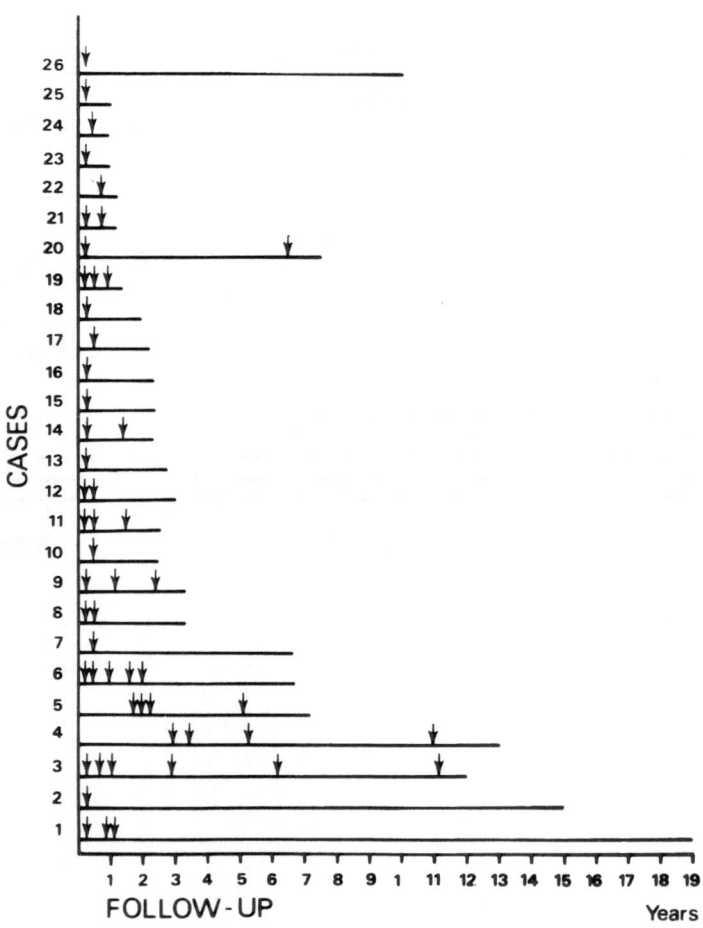

Fig. 4. Arrows = age when biopsies were done.

DISCUSSION

PAS+ globules diastase resistant were the only specific findings in the 17 cases studied. They may be small or few in number, during the 2 first months of life and they may be difficult to identify during cholestasis. Therefore, diagnosis cannot be assessed solely histologically.

Diagnosis requires the measurement of antitrypsic acitivity and Pi phenotype determination.

In group III, the paucity of inter-lobular biliary ducts has to be emphasized. One patient was considered as presenting with idiopathic intrahepatic biliary hypoplasia, since alpha-1-antitrypsin measurement. Moreover, PAS+ granules have been observed in the cells of biliary ducts in patients of groups I and II. On the other hand, Scotto et al. (2) studied 7 of these patients in electron microscopy, with special regard to ductular cells and Hering's junctions; dense polymorphic and vacuolar bodies were seen in 5 cases.

From these findings one may hypothesize that damage of biliary epithelium could explain the initial cholestatic stage of liver disease, in alpha-1-antitrypsin deficiency.

It seems that a correlation between the subsequent clinical course and the histologic features of the initial cholestatic stage could be established:

– When fibrosis is slight, all clinical manifestations will disappear.
– When fibrosis is extensive, cirrhosis with portal hypertension will develop early.
– In cases with intra-hepatic biliary hypoplasia, clinical cholestasis will persist, with possible evolution to portal fibrosis.

However, the follow-up period is still too short, in this study, to allow any definite conclusion.

REFERENCES

1. Aagenaes, Ø., A. Matlary, K. Elgjo, E. Munthe and M. Fagerhol, Neonatal cholestasis in alpha-1-antitrypsin deficient children. Clinical, genetic, histological and immuno-histochemical findings. *Acta paediat. scand. 61*: 632-642 (1972).
2. Scotto, J. M., H. G. Stalin et D. Alagille, Déficit en alpha-1-antitrypsine chez l'enfant. Ultrastructure du foie et spéculations. *Virchows Arch. Abt. A.* (1976, January issue).
3. Sharp, H., E. Freier and R. Bridges, Alpha-1-globulin deficiency in a familial infantile liver disease. *Pediat. Res. 2*: 298 (1968).

Editor's note: The following paper will be of interest to readers, since it discusses certain other aspects of some of the patients described above: Odièvre, M.; Martin, J. P.; Hadchouel, M. and Alagille, D.: Alpha$_1$-antitrypsin deficiency and liver disease in children: Phenotypes, manifestations and prognosis. *Pediatrics 57*: 226-231 (1976).

RELATIONSHIP BETWEEN ALPHA-1-ANTITRYPSIN DEFICIENCY AND LIVER DISEASE

HARVEY L. SHARP, M.D.

Alpha-1-antitrypsin (α1AT) is a glycoprotein synthesized by the liver (32, 18, 31, 1) which functions as an enzyme inhibitor. In vitro synthesis and release of α1AT has been demonstrated with the technique of short term liver cultures in the presence of radiolabeled amino acids (1). The quality and quantity of α1AT obtained from the culture media correlated with the genetic status of the patient from whom the liver was obtained.

α1AT is the predominant glycoprotein responsible for the α-1-globulin band on routine protein electrophoresis. Besides trypsin (20) it inhibits leukocyte proteases including elastase (23, 21, 29) and collagenase (9, 30), in addition to chymotrypsin (29, 33), plasmin (20, 6) and Hageman factor cofactor (6). Serum levels of α1AT increase during infection, hormonal stimulation and cirrhosis, especially when obstructive jaundice is present (35). In contrast, the extremely low serum levels of α1AT under homozygous deficiency conditions do not respond to the above stimuli (36).

Many polymorphic variants of α1AT have been uncovered by applying serum samples to an acid starch medium followed by utilization of an antigen antibody crossed electrophoresis technique (15). At least 24 different alleles for this gene have been identified (14). This protease inhibitor (Pi) pheno-typing system classifies the variants by letters in the alphabet. The slowest moving glycoprotein is labeled PiZ while faster moving protein complexes are identified by earlier letters in the alphabet. PiM is the predominant phenotype. Inheritance is co-dominant with each gene contributing its own active protein (13). For example the serum levels of protein and activity for PiZZ are between 10-15% of normal whereas a PiMZ is roughly 60%. The PiP and PiS alleles contribute 12.5 and 30% activity respectively (16). A variant with little or no protein (Pi—) has been found in family studies by Talamo (39) and confirmed by others (27). An increased incidence of both cirrhosis and emphysema has been found in individuals with the PiZZ, PiPZ (7) PiSZ (2) or the Pi— phenotype, i.e., those with low activity.

LIVER DISEASE IN THE PEDIATRIC PIZZ PATIENT

We have adequate studies and follow-up on the liver disease in 24 PiZZ patients from 19 families (tables 1, 2, 3). Past family histories have been positive for previous children dying of liver disease, and emphysema and carcinoma of the liver in adults. The average birth weight was one pound below normal (table 1). Premature delivery was not a factor and patients

Table 1.

PiZZ patients with liver disease	24
T.I.C. = 0.32/mg/ml (0.18-0.45)	
Average birth weight	6½ lbs.
Presented with infantile jaundice	18
Elevation of bilirubin prior to cellular enzymes	4
Coombs negative hemolytic anemia during infancy	8
Persistent hepatosplenomegaly and enzyme elevation	20

not ill during infancy had higher weights at birth. Seventy-five percent of the patients were evaluated for infantile jaundice, usually of the obstructive variety. When studied in the first weeks of life, the bilirubin elevation may occur prior to hepatocellular enzyme alteration. Although perhaps suggestive of early preferential bile duct injury, hepatocyte changes were present at the time of liver biopsy. Only four infants underwent abdominal exploration to rule out extrahepatic biliary atresia prior to the advent of more sophisticated diagnostic tests. Of these 4, two died of liver failure as young children, the other two are still alive; one was a sibling of one who died. She has normal liver function and no hepatosplenomegaly. Therefore, this series is indicative of the natural course of the liver disease uncomplicated by needless surgical procedures and emphasizes the discrepancy in a clinical outcome between siblings. Similar to other intrinsic liver disease during infancy, a mild hemolytic anemia was present and disappeared along with the cholestasis. Nevertheless, hepatosplenomegaly and enzyme elevation persisted in most patients. Besides the above mentioned patient, two others with normal liver function have biopsy evidence of mild residual hepatic fibrosis and one with resolution of his hepatosplenomegaly still has significant enzyme elevation. Mortality resulted from complications of their cirrhosis with two exceptions (table 2). One girl also had cystic fibrosis and died from overwhelming pseudomonas infection.

Except for the child with a non-cholestatic cystic fibrosis, no other infec-

Table 2.

Total mortality to date	*11*
1. Liver failure	4
2. Variceal hemorrhage	2
3. Complications of liver transplantation	2
4. Subdural hemorrhage from Vitamin K deficiency	1
5. Respiratory failure from cystic fibrosis	1
6. Drowning	1

Table 3. Negative studies in α1AT deficiency.

1. Other known causes of infantile cholestasis
2. Immunoglobulins
3. Australian antigen
4. Alpha fetoprotein
5. Serum and urine copper
6. Cholesterol
7. Bile acids
8. Blood type

Table 4. Blood types on 20 PiZZ individuals.

	C	E	hr	Du
A+	—	+	+	
A+	+	—	+	
O+		+	+	+
A+	+	—	+	
O+	+	—	+	
A+	+	—	+	
O+	+	+	+	
A+	+	—	+	
O+			—	
A+	+	—	+	
	M + N	+ Fya +	Kell —	
A+	—	+	+	
A+	—	+	+	
AB+				
AB—	—	—	+	—
AB—	—	—		—
A+	+	—	+	
B+	+	—	+	
O+	—	+	+	
O+				
O+	+	—	+	

tions or metabolic cause for their liver disease could be found (table 3). Extrahepatic atresia was never found nor developed in any of the patients or former family members. Although intrahepatic bile ducts are harder to find as the child gets older, none has developed pruritus or hyperlipidemia; clinical features that are associated with the syndrome with this anatomic abnormality. No consistent abnormality in immunoglobulins was found, and particularly no early increase in IGM was present to indicate intra-uterine infection except for an IGM of 39mg% at two weeks of age in one patient. Australian antigen was always negative and alpha fetoprotein was only slightly elevated one time during recovery from cholestasis. Serum and urine coppers even after penicillamine were unremarkable. The blood types had a normal distribution (table 4).

PATHOLOGIC FINDINGS IN PIZZ CHILDREN

The early and late pathologic findings in the liver of PiZZ patients are summarized in tables 5 and 6. Other than the previously described PAS positive cytoplasmic globules, no specific pathologic findings characterize

Table 5. Pathology of the injured α1AT livers.

Infancy

Hepatocytes - variation in size, some tendency for acinar formation, giant cell transformation usually absent to mild, rarely moderate. No inclusion bodies, specific PAS bodies present but may be difficult to discern, necrosis mild if present, mild fat and hemosiderin.

Bile stasis - hepatocytes, canalicular and within bile ducts.

Extramedullary hematopoiesis - mild

Portal areas - bile duct proliferation, mild to moderate inflammatory cells (poly and eos) plus prominent macrophages and Kuppfer cells. Increased connective tissue.

Table 6. Pathology of the injured α1AT livers.

After infancy

Hepatocytes - prominent PAS positive globules in periportal hepatocytes, necrosis mild if present. Mild fat, bile stasis is a late finding.

Portal areas - usually cirrhotic, rarely portal fibrosis. Mild to moderate chronic inflammation. Bile ducts less easy to find as the age of the patient increases.

the liver disease in α1AT deficiency (34). α1AT deficient patients have been
misdiagnosed as extrahepatic biliary atresia in the first few months of life or
later on as either intrahepatic biliary atresia or chronic active hepatitis on
the basis of liver biopsy findings.

Similar to the pathology under the light microscope, the only distinguishing ultrastructural characteristic of the liver in α1AT deficiency from
PiZ individuals is the amorphous material within the endoplasmic reticulum
(fig. 1). Because of the ribosomes along the outer membranes (→) we have
localized this accumulating glycoprotein to the rough endoplasmic reticulum.
As can be seen in this figure and those to follow, these membranes are not

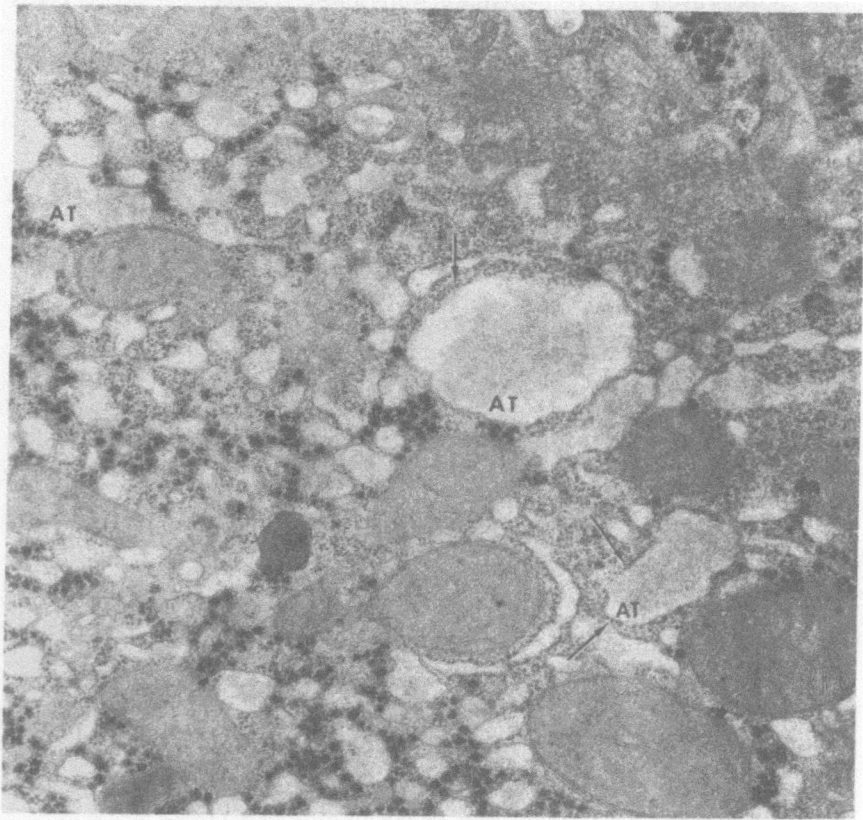

Fig. 1. Electron micrograph of a portion of hepatic cell cytoplasm from a PiMZ patient
demonstrating α1AT (AT) within the lumen of dilated rough endoplasmic reticulum.
Ribosomes are denoted by→. Also note α1AT in endoplasmic reticulum not studded by
ribosomes. (× 19,812)

always completely studded with ribosomes. In fact, in the majority of instances it may be difficult to find ribosomes on the membranes. Thus,the accumulation of this material having antigenic characteristics of α1AT is more prudently localized to just the endoplasmic reticulum. We have never felt that material seen in the golgi apparatus or in any other organelle or in the cytoplasm has ultrastructure characteristics of α1AT (fig. 2).

During the infantile disease period we have seen the amorphous material within the endoplasmic reticulum of some epithelial cells composing the small perilobular bile ducts (fig. 3). Marked accumulations of bile are seen

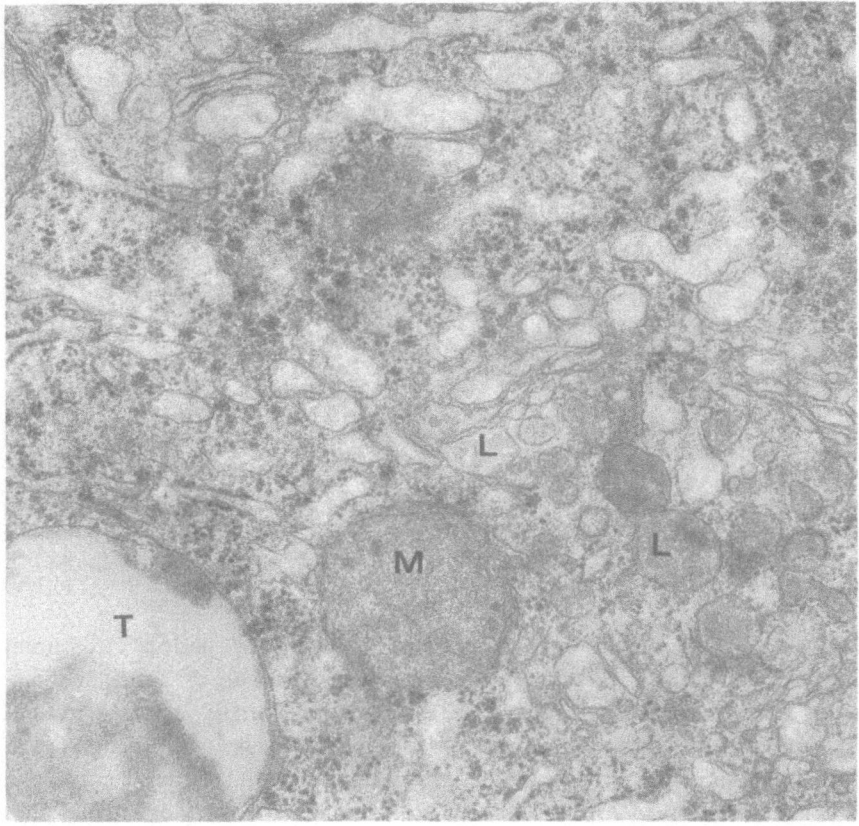

Fig. 2. Electron micrograph of the golgi apparatus in the hepatic cell cytoplasm of a PiZZ infant. The usual lipid particles (L) are present in the vesicles but no definite α1AT material is seen although some vesicles contain an ill-defined material (M) mitochondria, (T) triglyceride. (× 36,250)

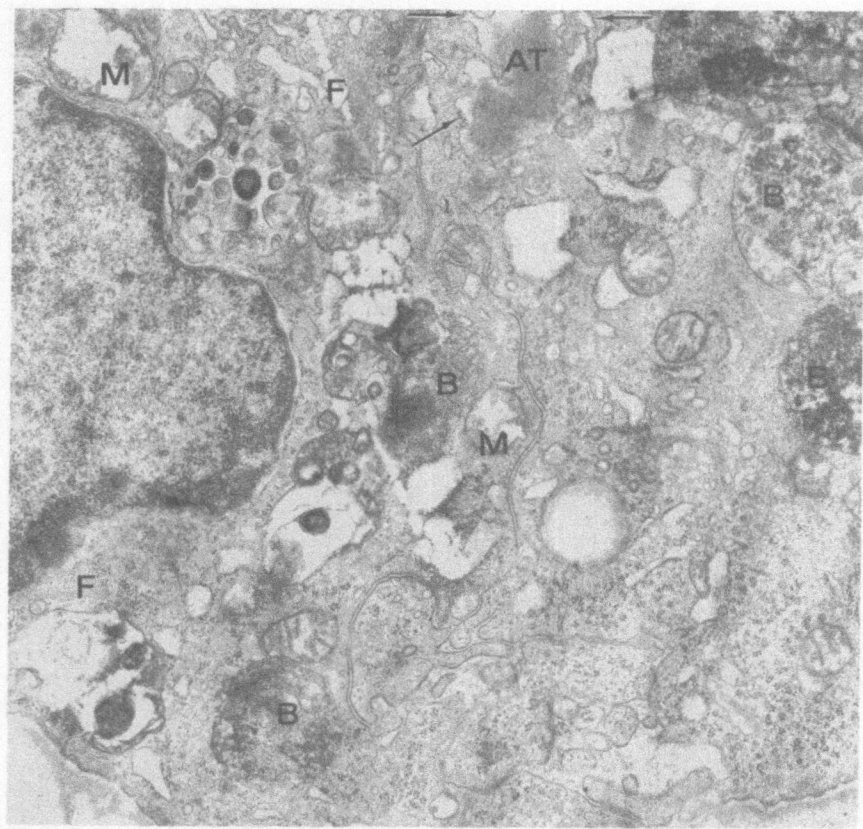

Fig. 3. Electron micrograph of a portion of a small bile duct just beneath the lumen and villous surface. α1AT (AT) at the top within endoplasmic reticulum. Arrows (→) denote occasional ribosomes. Also note numerous lysosomes containing bile constituents (B), altered mitochondria (M) and numerous fibrils (F) in the bile duct epithelium. (× 13,750)

in the lysosomes of bile duct epithelial cells during this period. Occasional mitochondria appear to be undergoing degenerative changes. Fibrillar structures are quite prominent in these bile ducts. Occasionally, crystal-like lipid material is seen in the bile duct epithelium as well as in the hepatocytes. Polymorphonuclear cells are frequently seen immediately adjacent to the bile duct structures, although actual invasion of the integrity of the bile duct epithelium was not seen (fig. 4).

Figure 5 is representative of the various membranous forms seen in the hepatic cell cytoplasm that is termed bile stasis at the light microscopic level from a patient with normal hepatocellular enzymes. Dense membranous bile

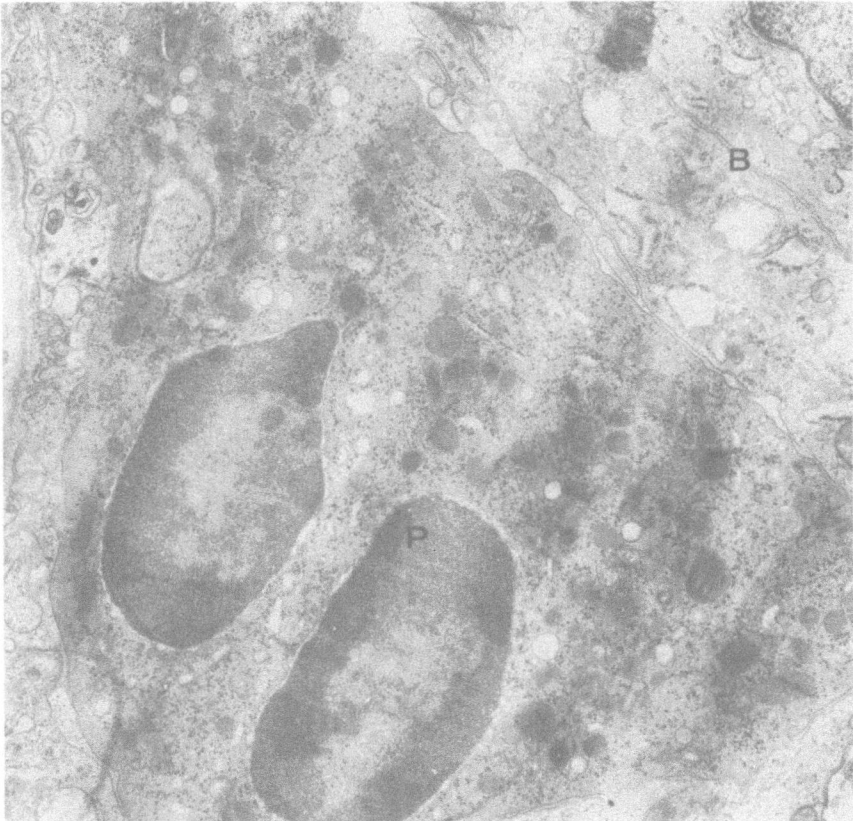

Fig. 4. Electron micrograph of a polymorphonuclear leukocyte (P) at the base of bile duct epithelium (B). (× 13,750)

may also be seen in distended bile canaliculi (fig. 6). Figure 7 shows the composite pathologic findings in the hepatocyte consisting of small amounts of α1AT material, bile stasis and triglyceride. No viral particles have ever been seen in these patients but occasionally ill-defined configurations with the nucleus are present in mononuclear cells in the portal regions.

Perhaps the most important findings in these livers are the cells with small and large lysosomes seen close to periportal hepatocytes (fig. 8, 9, 10). Some of these cells have multiple small lysosome-like structures containing a dense matrix material plus a dilated endoplasmic reticulum. Other cells have extremely large lysosomes with perhaps occasionally some bile pigment. Presently we can not identify the source of these cells but histochemical stains

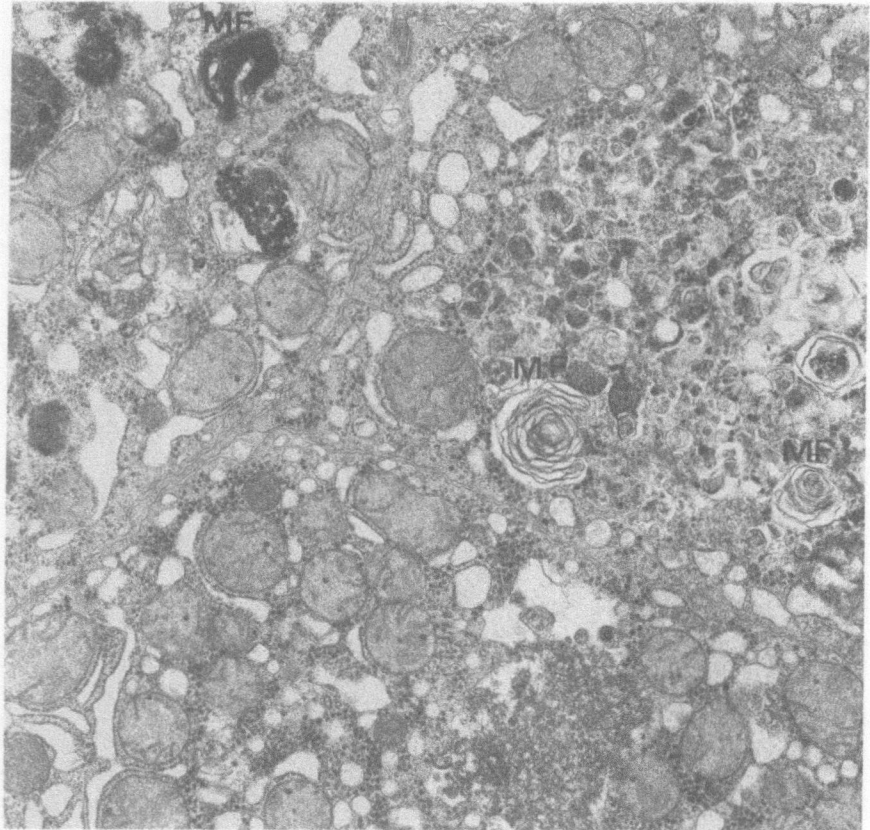

Fig. 5. Electron micrograph of portions of 3 hepatocytes whose cytoplasm contains various membranous forms (MF) in a 2 week old PiZZ with cholestasis and a normal serum OCT. (× 13,750)

in future studies may help clarify the cell type. Nevertheless, it is conceivable that they are a source of proteolytic enzymes capable of injurying the liver if uninhibited.

In PiZZ children with cirrhosis, we have routinely noted a diffuse glomerular lesion characterized by minimal thickening and splitting of the glomerular basement membranes and mild hypertrophy and hyperplasia of the mesangium confirmed by PAS and Jones stains. No fibrosis was noted within the glomeruli or interstial areas, and the vessels appeared histologically normal. Although our patients had no evidence of kidney damage, membranoproliferative glomerulonephritis may be symptomatic in young

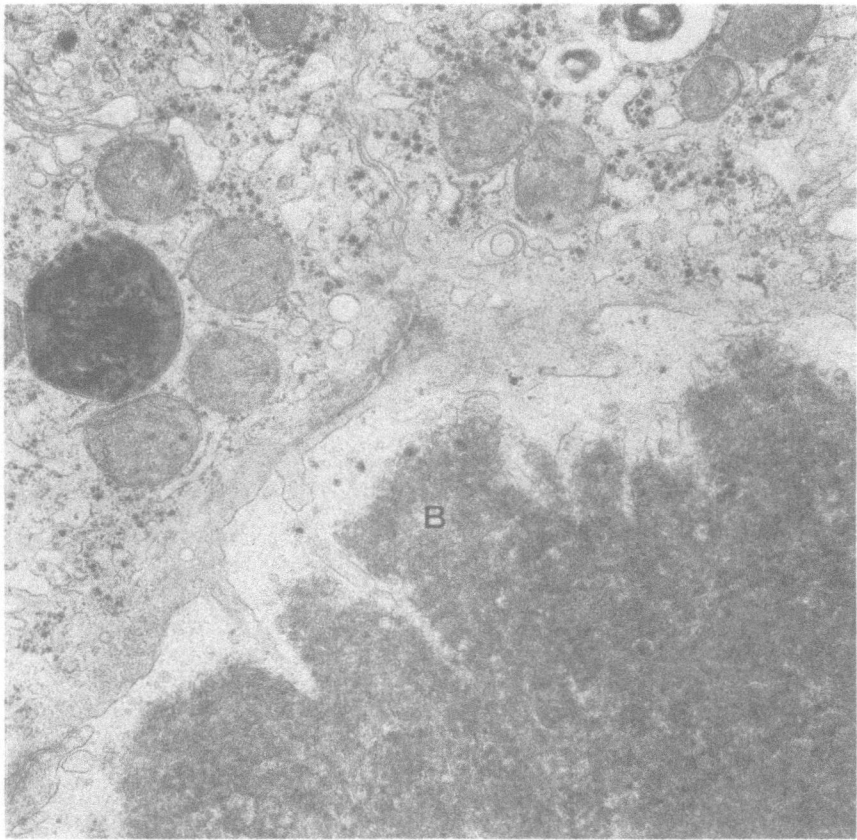

Fig. 6. Electron micrograph of a portion of a distended bile canaliculus containing dense membranous bile (B). (× 19,812)

adults. Cutz and associates in Toronto have elegantly studied this glomerulo-nephritis in three patients (8). Kidney ultrastructure in one case demonstrated subendothelial electron-dense deposits which may be represented by the small PAS particles (→) seen in figure 11. This same patient revealed confluent basement membrane deposits of IgG, IgM, IgA, C_3 and α1AT. Complement levels generally have been normal in most patients with α1AT deficiency but LePrevast et al. noted low levels of C_4 for unexplained reasons in PiZZ patients with liver disease (26). Although speculative, the glomerular lesion may be caused by an immune complex disease precipitated by the release of foreign α1AT into the circulation following hepatic cell death or by an undefined virus which also causes the liver disease.

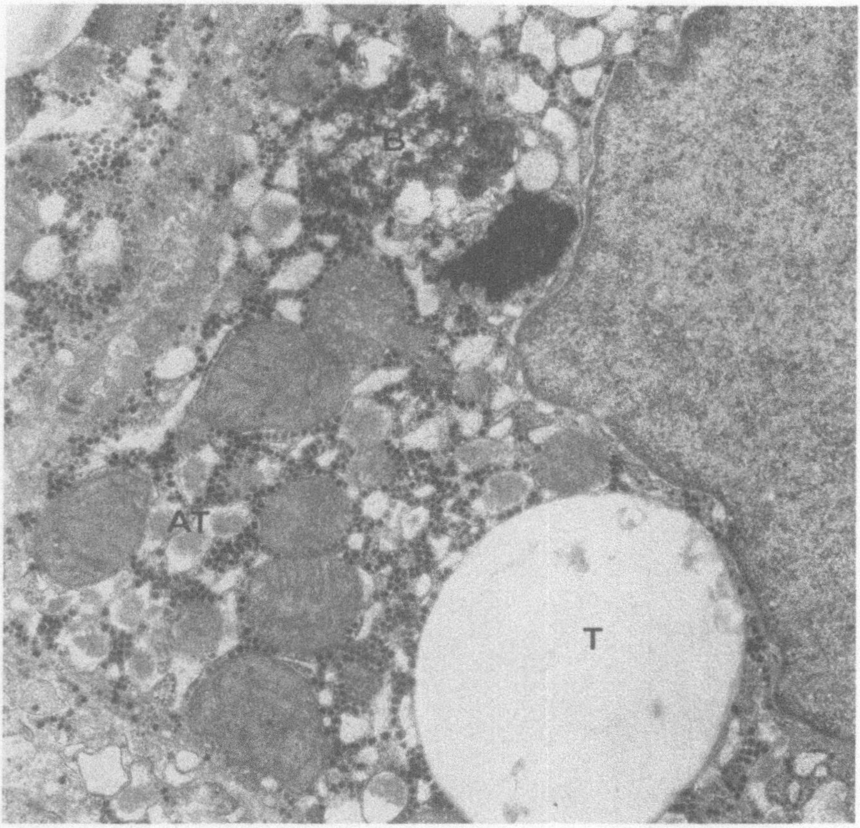

Fig. 7. Electron micrograph of hepatic cell cytoplasm in a PiZZ infant showing bile stasis (B)α1AT (AT) and triglyceride (T) (× 13,750)

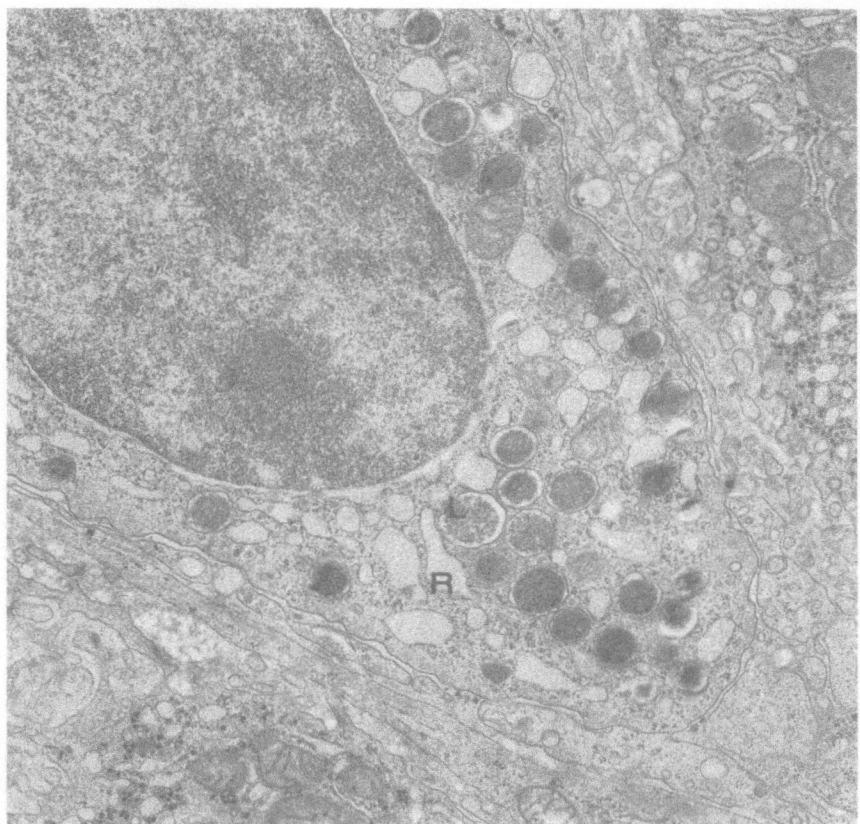

Fig. 8. Electron micrograph of a unidentified cell with numerous small lysosomes (L) and dilated endoplasmic reticulum (R). (× 13,750)

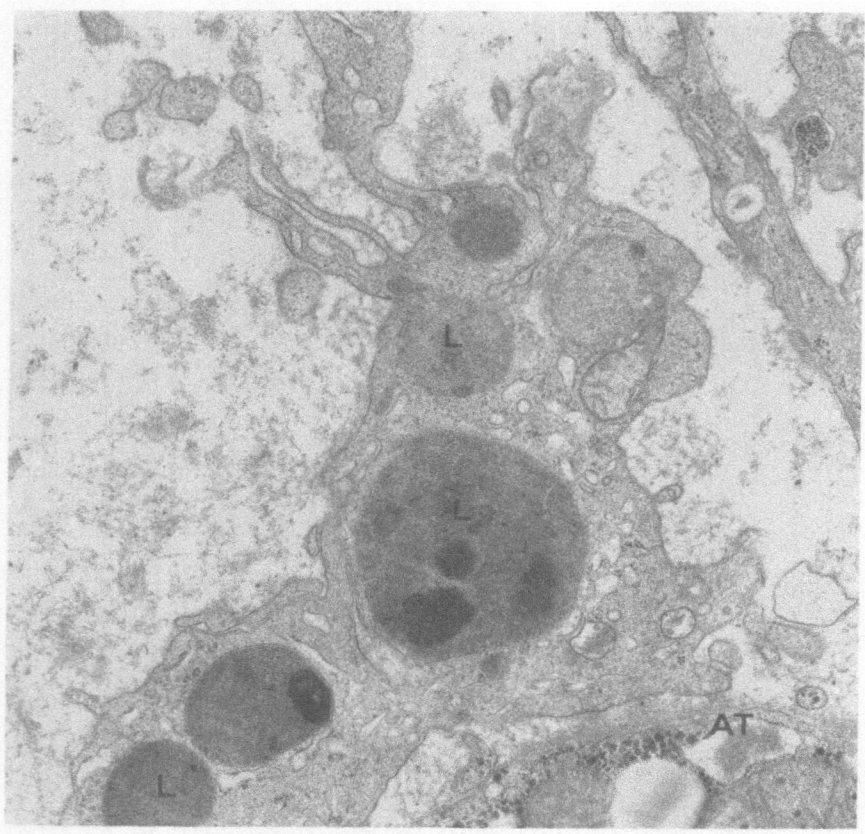

Fig. 9. Electron micrograph of unidentified cells with numerous larger lysosomes (L) bordering a periportal hepatocyte with α1AT (AT). (× 13,750)

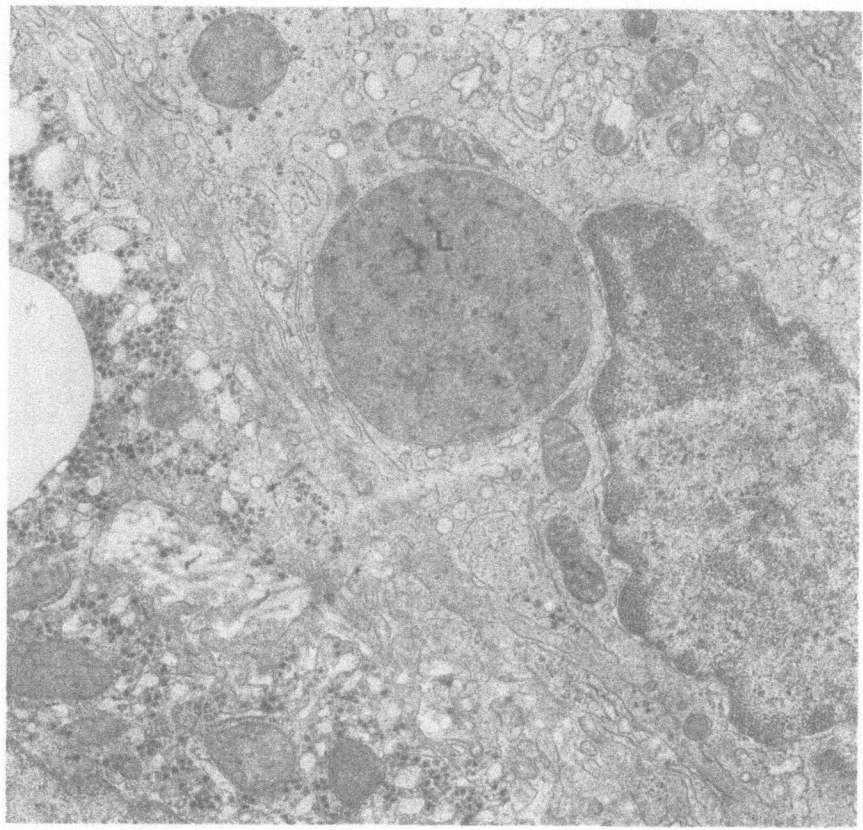

Fig. 10. Electron micrograph of unidentified cell with a very large lysosome (L). (× 13,750)

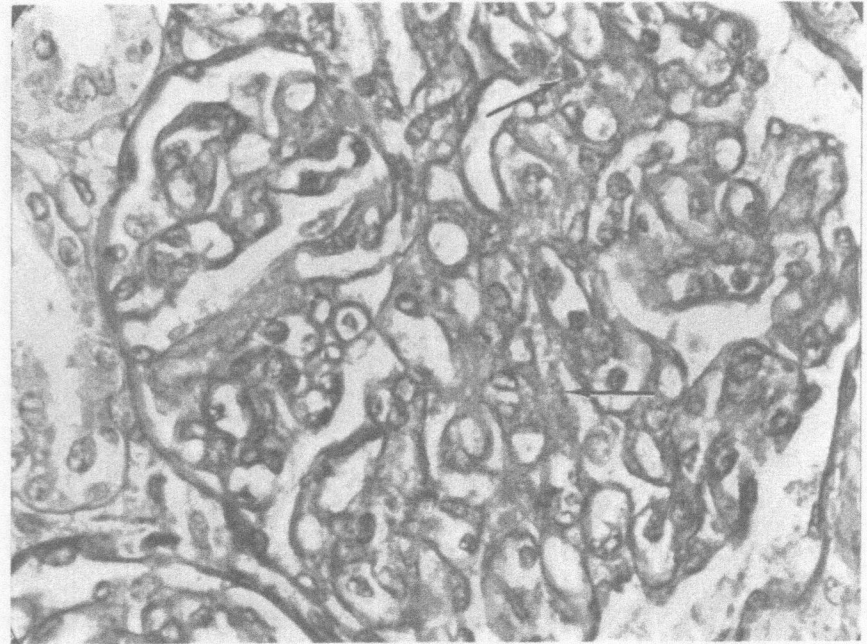

Fig. 11. Photomicrograph of a glomerulus of a PiZZ who died following a variceal bleed. Urinalyses were essentially normal up to demise. Note small PAS positive particle (× 556).

CANCER AND LIVER DISEASE IN ADULTS

An intriguing new observation is the finding of 6 hepatomas in 9 cirrhotics from Ericksson's registered adult ZZ population of which 5% have cirrhosis (10). Four were hepatocellular carcinomas and two were cholangiocellular. Alpha fetoprotein and Australian antigen were not present nor were antinuclear, smooth muscle, or anti-mitochondrial antibodies. For unexplained reasons, the hepatoma cells do not contain $\alpha 1AT$ globules. It has been suggested that heterozygotes may be predisposed to cirrhosis (2). Larger series with liver disease do not substantiate this observation. Morin et al. found the incidence of the heterozygous PiZ to be the same in alcoholic and cryptogenic cirrhosis as in their blood donor population (28).

α1AT ISOLATION STUDIES

Numerous investigations indicate that α1AT is a glycoprotein with a molecular weight in the 50,000 range, that it is probably a single polypeptide with the site of action present within the disulfide bond of cysteine, and that the ratio of amino acids are generally similar. One the other hand, the roughly twelve percent carbohydrate content of galactose, mannose, N-acetyl-glucosamine, and particularly sialic acid seems to be in dispute (19).

Recently, Chan and Rees compared the composition of α1AT from MM and ZZ plasma (3). The percentages of various amino acids shows minimal deviation except for the presence of more arginine and glycine in ZZ glycoprotein. In addition, the total carbohydrate content of the ZZ protein was 75% of the MM proteins; a finding attributed to not only lower sialic acid ratios but more importantly to three-quarters as much mannose signifying alteration of the main carbohydrate chain rather than one of its branches. Thus, they propose the presence of only 3 carbohydrate chains in the ZZ protein rather than the 4 carbohydrate chains in the MM glycoprotein.

Kuhlenschmidt (25) working with a team of investigators at Pittsburgh under the direction of Dr. Glew, studied an 8 year old PiZZ girl with advanced cirrhosis. The PAS positive globules in her hepatocytes did not stain with alcian blue, aldehyde fuchsin, or colloidal iron indicating the absence of detectable mucopolysaccharide and sialic acid. Her serum was markedly deficient in cytidine 5-mono phosphate-N-acetylneuraminic asialoglycoprotein sialic acid transferase when assayed using asialo derivatives of α1AT, fetuin, and ceruloplasmin. To rule out a diffuse liver enzyme depletion in the same serum, a rather high concentration of uridine diphosphate galactose; glycoprotein galactosyltransferase and normal levels of several hydrolytic enzymes of lysosomal origin were present. Since the parents also exhibited decreased sialyltransferase levels suggesting heterozygosity, we joined forces with Dr. Glew's group to test if a sialyltransferase deficiency could account for the defective secretion or transport of α1AT (24). The serum sialyltransferase activity in 6 patients with PiZZ and marked hepatic cirrhosis was low. However, serum from other PiZZ family members with or without hepatic cirrhosis failed to exhibit marked sialyltransferase deficiency. Similar assays were carried out on liver homogenates from one of the patients with very low serum sialyltransferase levels who died following a complication of her marked cirrhosis. Normal sialyltransferase activity was present in 10 different samples of her liver. Kinetic studies failed to detect differences in substrate affinities that might account for the decreased functional sialyltransferase capacity in PiZZ patients with marked hepatic cirrhosis. There fore, sialyltransferase deficiency appears to be secondary to the development of chronic and extensive liver disease in PiZZ patients, perhaps combined with the α1AT accumulation in their hepatocytes, rather than being a primary enzyme deficiency.

Eriksson and Larson (11) have recently isolated and analyzed the PAS positive globules from cirrhotic portions of the livers of PiZZ patients who died of hepatic carcinoma. The main component protein traveled in poly-acrylamide gels at a rate comparable to serum α1AT implying a similar molecular weight compound. Neuraminidase failed to alter the mobility of this isolated immunologically proven α1AT. Chemical analysis substantiated the complete absence of sialic acid. Since sialyltransferase levels (24, 12) are normal according to one methodology, these Swedish investigators postulate a steric hindrance to the incorporation of sialic acid into the deforme d ZZ type antitrypsin molecule. Alternatively, other glysyltransferases might explain this finding or gentler extraction methodology is necessary for isolating hepatic α1AT.

WHY LIVER DISEASE?

Alpha-1-antitrypsin is an enzyme inhibitor, more specifically a binder of various proteolytic enzymes whose function in the deficient individual is either absent (Pi—) or markedly decreased. Since its molecular weight is slightly lower than albumin, it easily leaves the circulation to enter other tissue fluids during normal circumstances. During inflammation, an increased synthesis of α1AT occurs along with the increased transport of this inhibitor to the damaged area to counteract the release of proteolytic enzymes by cells responding to this injury (38). In the lung these cells can actually incorporate α1AT, as demonstrated by fluorescent antibody techniques against α1AT, in pulmonary alveolar macrophages (5) presumably to inhibit proteolytic enzymes.

The PiZZ fetus is uniquely unprotected from injurious agents. Besides other normal immunologic deficiencies, he has no α1AT either of his own or from his mother since there is virtually no transfer of α1AT across the maternal fetal barrier (22). He may even have difficulty handling the enzymes released during normal extramedullary hematopoiesis in utero. If a noxious agent reaches the liver, how do his Kuppfer cells, macrophages and other normally protective cells react to this insult? It would seem reasonable that he is unduly exposed to the proteolytic enzymes released during inflammation whether viral initiated or otherwise. The early jaundice and low birth weight are clinical signs of prenatal injury. Whether other inhibitors such as α2 macroglobulin are protective has not been carefully examined.

In addition other immunologic protective mechanisms uniquely altered in alpha-1-antitrypsin deficiency patients must be considered to understand why these susceptible individuals are unable to counteract liver and/or lung destruction as opposed to those escaping any permanent injury. Alpha-1-antitrypsin deficient patients with emphysema have been found to lack adequate chemotactic factor inactivator (40). Hence, the situation exists in the deficient patient for an inordinate delivery of neutrophils and their uninhibited enzymes to the site of injury. Galdston et al. have made an interesting observation concerning the leukocyte proteases in two kindred with α1AT deficiency (17). Those individuals with emphysema had normal leukocyte lysosomal elastase and leukoprotease activity whereas deficient individuals without diseases had lower intermediate levels for these enzymes. Does a correlation exist between clinical disease and the degree of leukocyte and Kuppfer cells lysosomal protease antiprotease imbalance?

The high incidence of hepatoma may implicate either carcinogenic agents and/or lack of regulatory defense mechanisms. Patients with malignant neoplasms have high serum levels of antiproteolytic activity (4). It has been suggested that proteases including collagenase excreted into the interstitial fluid may destroy the tissue surrounding the tumors, thus promoting invasive growth (37). The role of α1AT in controlling 'malignant' proteases remains to be explored.

SUMMARY

Extremely deficient levels of α1AT predispose such individuals, especially at birth, to the development of liver disease. Hepatic injury appears unrelated to the glycoprotein present in the hepatocyte cytoplasm but rather to the low circulatory levels of α1AT.

ACKNOWLEDGEMENTS

I wish to thank Julie Judge for her help with the illustrations and Linda Hammen for her secretarial help. This work was supported in part by the

National Foundation, a grant (RR-400) from the General Clinical Research Centers Branch, Division of Research Resources, National Institutes of Health, and grants from the Graduate School of the University of Minnesota and the Minnesota Medical Foundation and the Beckman Liver Research Fund.

REFERENCES

1. Blan, A. K., R. J. Grand, H. R. Coltan, et al., Liver in alpha-1- antitrypsin deficiency. Morphological observation and in vitro synthesis of alpha-1-antitrypsin. *Pediat. Res.* *10*: 35-40 (1976).
2. Campra, J. L., J. P. Craig, R. L. Peters et al., Cirrhosis associated with partial deficiency of alpha-1-antitrypsin in adults. *Ann. intern. Med. 78*: 227-232 (1973).
3. Chan, S. K. and D. C. Rees, Molecular basis for the alpha-1-protease inhibitor deficiency. *Nature 255*: 240-241 (1975).
4. Clark, D. G. C., E. E. Clifton and B. L. Newton, Antiproteolytic activity of human serum with particular reference to its change in the presence and consideration of its use for detection of malignant neoplasia. *Proc. Soc. exp. Biol. Med. 69*: 276-279 (1948).
5. Cohen, A. B., Interrelationships between the human alveolar macrophage and alpha-1-antitrypsin. *J. clin. Invest. 52*: 2793-2799 (1973).
6. Crawford, G. M. P. and D. Ogston, The influence of alpha-1-antitrypsin on plasmin, urokinase and hageman factor cofactor. *Biochim. biophys. Acta 354*: 107-113 (1974).
7. Crawford, I. P., A. Dawson and D. D. Stevenson, Alpha-1-antitrypsin deficiency associated with PZ and MP phenotypes. *Amer. J. Med. 57*: 210-216 (1974).
8. Cutz, E., S. P. Moroz, J. W. Balfe, et al., Glomerulonephritis in patients with cirrhosis of liver associated with alpha-1-antitrypsin deficiency. *Amer. J. Path. 74*: 12a (1974).
9. Eisen, A. Z., K. J. Block and T. Sakai, Inhibition of human skin collagenase by human serum. *J. Lab. clin. Med. 75*: 258-263 (1970).
10. Eriksson, S. and J. Hagerstrand, Cirrhosis and malignant hepatoma in alpha-1-antitrypsin deficiency. *Acta med. scand. 195*: 451-458 (1974).
11. Eriksson, S. and C. Larsson, Purification and partial characterization of PAS- Positive inclusion bodies from the liver in alpha-1-antitrypsin deficiency. *New Engl. J. Med. 292*: 176-180 (1975).
12. Eriksson, S. and C. Larsson, Role of sialyltransferases in alpha-1-antitrypsin deficiency. *New Engl. J. Med. 292*: 925-926 (1975).
13. Fagerhol, M. K., Genetics of the Pi system. In: *Pulmonary emphysema and proteolysis.* C. Mittman (ed.). (Academic Press, New York 1972) pp. 123-131.
14. Fagerhol, M. K., Pi typing techniques. In: *22th Ann. Colloq. Protides of the Biological Fluids*, H. Peters (ed.). (Elsevier, Amsterdam 1974). pp. 493-495.
15. Fagerhol, M. K., Quantitative studies on the inherited variants of serum alpha-1-antitrypsin. *Scand. J. clin. Lab. Invest. 23*: 97-103 (1969).
16. Fagerhol, M. K. and H. E. Hauge, Serum Pi types in patients with pulmonary diseases. *Acta Allergol. 24*: 107-114 (1969).
17. Galdston, M., A. Janoff and A. L. David, Familial variation of leukocyte lysosomal protease and serum alpha-1-antitrypsin as determined in chronic obstructive pulmonary disease. *Amer. Rev. resp. Dis. 107*: 718-727 (1973).
18. Gans, H., K. Mori and B. H. Tan, In vitro turnover of bovine alpha-1-antitrypsin. In: *Pulmonary emphysema and proteolysis.* C. Mittman (ed.). (Academic Press, New York 1972) pp. 379-386.

19. Heimberger, N., H. Haupt and H. G. Schwick, Proteinase inhibitors of human plasma·
    In: *Proc. Int. Res. Conf. on Protease Inhibitors.* H. Fritz and H. Tschescher (eds.).
    (Walter de Gruyter, Berlin 1971) pp. 1-22.
20. Jacobson, K., Studies on the trypsin and plasmin inhibitor in human serum. *Scand. J.
    clin. Lab. Invest. Suppl. 14*: 55-102 (1955).
21. Janoff, A., Inhibition of human granulocyte elastase by serum alpha-1-antitrypsin.
    Amer. Rev. resp. Dis. 105: 121-122 (1972).
22. Kaiser, D., O. M. Rennert, H. W. Goedde, et al., Studies of amniotic fluid and cord.
    blood in an infant with alpha-1-antitrypsin deficiency. *Humangenetik 25*: 241-245 (1974)
23. Kueppers, F. and A. G. Bearn, A possible experimental approach to the association
    of hereditary alpha-1-antitrypsin deficiency and pulmonary emphysema. *Proc. Soc.
    exp. Biol. Med. 121*: 1207-1209 (1966).
24. Kuhlenschmidt, M. S., C. J. Coffee, S. P. Peters et al., Serum sialyltransferase activity
    in alpha-1-antitrypsin deficiency and hepatic cirrhosis. Protease and biological con-
    trols; In E. Welch, D. B. Rifkin and E. Shaw (eds.), *Coldspring Harbor Conference on
    Cell Proliferation*, vol. 2: 415-428 (1975).
25. Kuhlenschmidt, M. S., E. J. Yunis, R. M. Iammarino, et al., Demonstration of sialyl-
    transferase deficiency in the serum of patients with alpha-1-antitrypsin deficiency and
    hepatic cirrhosis. *Lab. Invest. 31*: 413-419 (1974).
26. LePrevast, C., D. Frommel and J. Dupay, Complement studies in alpha-1-antitrypsin
    deficiency in children. *Fed. Proc. 33*: 647 (1974).
27. Martin, J. B. D. Vandeville and C. Robartz, Alpha-1-antitrypsin deficiency: PiO.
    Lancet 2: 845 (1973).
28. Morin, T., G. Feldman, J. P. Benhamou, et al., Heterozygous alpha-1-antitrypsin
    deficiency and cirrhosis in adults, a fortuitous association. *Lancet 1*: 250-251 (1975).
29. Ohlsson, K., Neutral leukocyte proteases and elastase inhibited by plasma alpha-1-
    antitrypsin. *Scand. J. clin. Lab. Invest. 28*: 251-253 (1971).
30. Ohlsson, K. and I. Olsson, The neutral proteases of human granulocytes isolation and
    partial characterization of two granulocyte collagenases. *Europ. J. Biochem. 36*: 473-
    481 (1973).
31. Rawley, P. T. and L. L. Miller, Serum antitrypsin synthesis by the isolated perfused
    rat liver. *Proc. Soc. exp. Biol. Med. 148*: 145-150 (1975).
32. Schultz, H. E. and J. F. Heremans, *Synthesis of the plasma proteins, molecular biology
    of human proteins*. Vol. 1, pp. 321-449 (Elsevier, Amsterdam 1966).
33. Schwick, V., N. Heimburger and H. Haupt, Anti proteinase des human serums. *Z. Ges.
    inn. Med. 21*: 193-198 (1966).
34. Sharp, H. L., Alpha-1-antitrypsin deficiency. *Hospital Practice 6*: 83-96 (1971).
35. Sharp, H. L., R. A. Bridges, W. Krivit, et al., Cirrhosis associated with alpha-1-anti-
    trypsin deficiency: a previously unrecognized inherited disorder. *J. Lab. clin. Med. 73*:
    934-939 (1969).
36. Statement on methods for detecting alpha-1-antitrypsin abnormalities. In: *Pulmonary
    emphysema and proteolysis*. C. Mittman (ed.). (Academic Press, New York 1972) pp.
    141-143.
37. Sylven, B. and L. Bois-Svensson, On the chemical pathology of interstitial fluid I prot-
    eolytic activities in the transplantated mouse tumors. *Cancer Res. 25*: 458-468 (1965).
38. Talamo, R. C., C. E. Langley, J. C. Barker, et al., Distribution and quantitation of
    alpha-1-antitrypsin in dilute biological fluids – its localizing increase in tears of patients
    with corneal ulcerations. *Pediat. Res. 6*: 119 (1972).
39. Talamo, R. C., C. E. Langley and S. Makino, Alpha-1-antitrypsin deficiency: a variant
    with no detectable alpha-1-antitrypsin. *Science 181*: 70-71 (1973).
40. Ward, P. A. and R. C. Talamo, Deficiency of the chemotactic factor inactivator in
    human sera with alpha-1-antitrypsin deficiency. *J. clin. Invest. 52*: 516-519 (1973).

REYE'S SYNDROME:
CAUSE-AND-EFFECT RELATIONSHIPS

M. MICHAEL THALER, M.D.

This paper examines a series of postulates concerning the pathogenesis of Reye's syndrome (16). These hypotheses are derived from available clinical, pathologic and biochemical observations and are selected on the basis of their verifiability by clinical or experimental means. No claim is made for their ultimate correctness. Rather, the aim is to organize data in a manner which may serve to orient further inquiry into underlying mechanisms, and may reveal unsuspected relationships among metabolic processes involved in the clinico-pathological changes described by Reye et al.

GENERAL OBSERVATIONS

The incidence of Reye's syndrome appears to be on the increase throughout the world. The disease is distributed in 2 distinct patterns: the epidemic form, generally encountered in cities, and associated with outbreaks of influenza B or other common viral infections; the endemic form, associated with chicken pox, ingestion of drugs or poisons, or exposure to hepatotoxic insecticides. The endemic form has been increasing strikingly in rural areas of most 'developed' countries.

Extensive experience with Reye's syndrome over the past decade has had two contradictory effects: while the clinical manifestations, evolution and histopathology of the disorder have been clarified, considerable confusion has resulted from the multiplicity of potential 'causes' which are being reported. Drugs such as aspirin, and poisons such as warfarin, natural toxins such as aflatoxin and hypoglycin, and most disease-producing viral agents have been associated with Reye's.

Direct links between these widely distributed agents and pathogens and Reye's syndrome are difficult to visualize, since relatively few among the vast numbers of treated or infected children develop the disorder. For example, the association between influenza B epidemics and Reye's syndrome is well documented, and it can be shown that most infected children are treated with aspirin. Nevertheless, Reye's syndrome occurs in a very small subpopulation of these patients, usually less than 0.1% (17, 6). A similar point can be made about endemic cases associated with chicken pox. Crocker et al (7) have shown that newborn mice infected with encephalomyocarditis virus and treated with an organophosphate-DDT combination developed a lethal disease resembling Reye's; either chemical agent was relatively harmless in infected mice. It may be significant, also, that newborn or very young mice were selected, rather than adult animals. A parallel is thereby suggested to the unique susceptibility of infants and children to Reye's. These epidemiologic and experimental observations are consistent with the possibility that Reye's syndrome may require concurrence of several synergistic factors acting on a susceptible subpopulation of individuals.

Despite their apparent complexity, the mysterious antecedents of Reye's syndrome may be clarified or at least identified by exploring the nature of a hypothetical defect which renders certain children more vulnerable than others to the disease process. It may be postulated that in such susceptible individuals, viral infection and exposure to potential hepatotoxins, singly or in combination, may inhibit or overwhelm marginal metabolic capacities for utilization of essential precursors or elimination of toxic metabolites.

CLINICAL OBSERVATIONS

Several varieties of 'Reye's syndrome' due to isolated or combined deficiencies in interdependent metabolic pathways may be eventually distinguished by analysis of clinical, histological and biochemical aspects of the disorder. An underlying inherited or acquired metabolic deficiency may be reflected in the temporal sequence of events as the disease process develops. The bland 'flu-like' prodrome is nearly always superceded by severe vomiting, which may be the first manifestation of central nervous system involvement. Elevated blood ammonia levels are generally recorded during this early phase (14). It is of interest that initial blood ammonia concentrations correlate relatively well with depth of subsequent coma and eventual outcome, whereas ammonia levels obtained later in the course do not differ significantly in survivors and non-survivors (14). SGOT and prothrombin values are usually elevated by the time patients are brought to the hospital. However, signs of neurotoxicity may be occasionally observed before abnormalities in liver function can be detected (1). Hypoglycemia is an inconstant finding in patients above 2 years of age.

The typical course of Reye's syndrome is one of progressive deterioration in brain functions. A noteworthy feature of this phase of the disease is the observation that patients who persist in stage II or III coma for about 24 hrs after onset generally recover, whereas progression to stage IV coma is usually rapid when it occurs, and carries an extremely grave prognosis.

Several tentative conclusions which may point toward underlying pathogenetic mechanisms are suggested by these clinical observations. The course and outcome of the disease process may be entirely dependent on the extent of CNS injury sustained at the onset. Ammonia appears to be involved during this early phase. The possibility that hyperammonemia may also be responsible for liver damage (rather than reverse) should be considered, as hepatic dysfunction can precede, develop concurrently with, or follow the appearance of neurological abnormalities.

HISTOPATHOLOGIC OBSERVATIONS

These considerations suggest that the role of the liver in the pathogenesis of Reye's syndrome deserves closer scrutiny. The relatively benign histological appearance of liver in Reye's contrasts sharply with hepatic changes observed in other types of 'hepatic encephalopathy'. The normal hepatic lobular architecture, inconspicuous inflammatory reactions, and absence of extensive cell damage are as characteristic of Reye's as the panlobular lipid microdeposits which are the accepted hallmark of the syndrome (fig. 1). Ultra structural changes in hepatocytes are remarkably non-specific and transient: crops of peroxisomes engaged in degradation of lipid, and variable mitochondrial swelling which may reflect primary or secondary changes in these organelles (fig. 2). In keeping with this unremarkable pathologic picture, biochemical evidence of disturbed hepatocellular function disappears within days after termination of the acute phase. In contrast with such common causes of hepatic coma. as fulminant hepatitis, terminal cirrhosis and severe toxic hepatitis, residual liver damage is not found in survivors of Reye's syndrome. These observations support the impression that a specific lesion or defect, rather than massive injury to liver cells, may be responsible for encephalopathy in this disorder.

The appearance of the brain at autopsy suggests a toxic or metabolic encephalopathy. Gross swelling and neuronal degeneration are the main findings, and evidence of infection or inflammation is lacking.

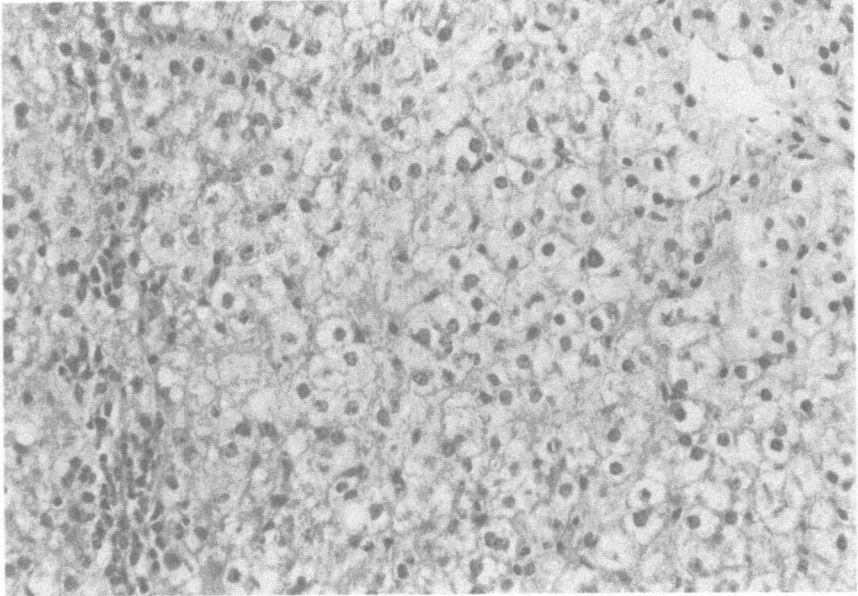

Fig. 1. Typical appearance of liver in Reye's syndrome. Extensive panlobular cytoplasmic vacuolization of hepatocytes (portal zone at lower left, central vein at upper right). Hematoxylin and eosin. (× 338)

CONDITIONS RESEMBLING REYE'S SYNDROME

The possibility that a susceptible subpopulation may develop Reye's syndrome during outbreaks of viral infection has previously been mentioned. Similarly, Reye's syndrome appears to be triggered in a small proportion of children ingesting aflatoxin, a fungal poison prevalent in Northern Thailand (2). However, the mechanism whereby aflatoxin produces these manifestations is unknown. A somewhat analogous illness is caused by hypoglycin, a toxic 7-carbon carboxylic acid component of an edible plant indigenous to the Caribbean (3). The resemblance between 'Jamaica vomiting sickness' and Reye's syndrome was originally noted by Reye et al. (16). Isovaleric acid, a short-chain fatty acid of proven neurotoxicity, accumulates in hypoglycin-treated animals (21) and in infants with isovaleric acidemia, an inherited disorder associated with vomiting, coma, and fatty liver (9).

Other inherited metabolic defects which manifest themselves early in life by vomiting, fatty liver, toxic encephalopathy and hyperammonemia include

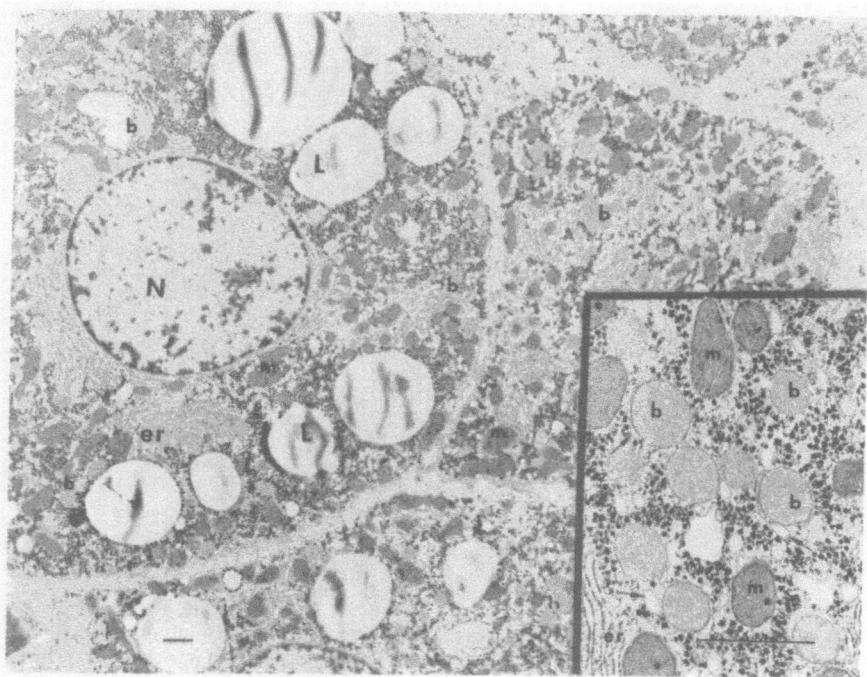

Fig. 2. Ultrastructural appearance of liver in Reye's syndrome. Cytoplasmic lipid micro-droplets (L) which do not displace the nucleus (N). Marker represents 1μ ($\times$ 4,167). Higher magnification (*inset*) reveals peroxisomes (b) associated with smooth endoplasmic reticulum (arrows), pleomorphic mitochondria (m) and normal rough endoplasmic reticulum (er). Marker represents 1μ. ($\times$ 13,889)

abnormalities of branch-chain amino acids (hypervalinemia, branched-chain ketonuria), disorders of propionate and methylmalonate metabolism, and lactic aciduria. The clinical features of these acquired and inherited 'organic acidurias' suggest that fatty acids of short and intermediate chain length and closely related compounds such as hypoglycin, may induce an illness which closely resembles Reye's syndrome in clinical expression. Indeed, coma and characteristic fatty changes in liver cells can be rapidly induced in experimental animals with infusion of fatty acids (10).

Another group of genetically transmitted metabolic disorders with features which occur in Reye's syndrome are inherited errors in conversion of ammonia to urea. Several enzymatic deficiencies are known, the most common being ornithine transcarbamylase (OTC) deficiency (19). Male infants with classical X-linked OTC deficiency die soon after birth of an acute illness clinically indistinguishable from Reye's syndrome. The females generally survive but may become critically ill after a mild viral infection. Severe vomiting precedes the appearance of coma during such crises, blood ammonia and SGOT values are markedly increased, and cerebral edema and hepatomegaly may develop and regress rapidly.

Evidence of a novel protein-tolerant form of OTC deficiency was obtained in a boy with 'recurrent' Reye's, whose younger brother had died from a similar disease. An unrelated girl who survived a single episode of Reye's exhibited a similar defect in OTC activity and kinetic properties (22) (fig. 3).

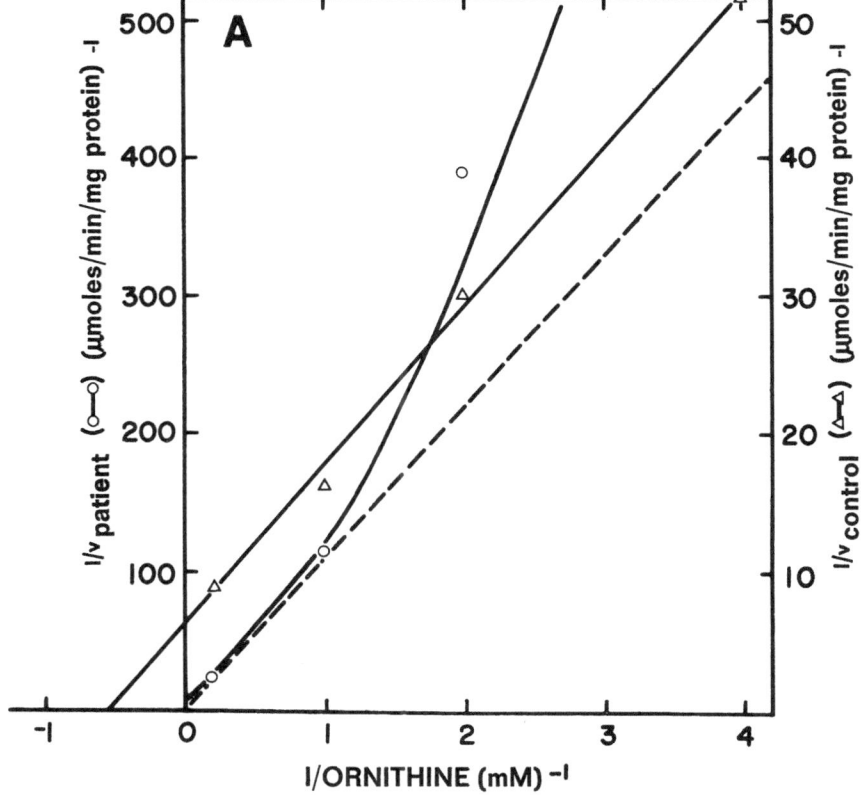

Fig. 3. Kinetics of ornithine transcarbamylase (OTC) in a patient with Reye's syndrome in whom hepatic OTC activity was 20.7% of the control value. Solid lines represent actual best-fit lines from which inhibition constants (K_i) were determined; broken lines represent best-fit lines calculated as if there were no substrate inhibition from which apparent affinity

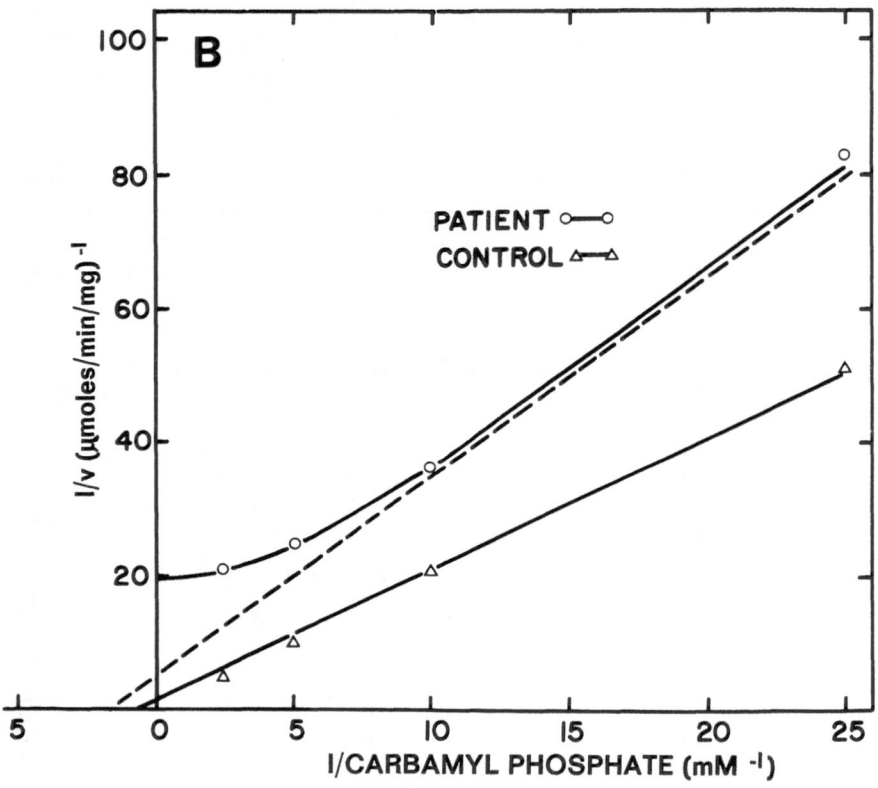

constants (K_m) were derived. (A) Carbamyl phosphate concentration was constant (0.4 mM) and ornithine was varied. (B) Ornithine concentration was constant (10 mM) and carbamyl phosphate was varied. (For detail of assay, see ref. 22.)

More recently, combined deficiencies in OTC and carbamyl phosphate synthetase (CPS), the 2 enzymes of the urea cycle located in mitochondria, were found in 4 patients with Reye's reported by Brown et al. (5) and in 6 reported by Sinatra et al. (20). These findings suggest that a majority of patients with Reye's may suffer from induced or precipitated defects in ammonia metabolism, whereas a minority with recurrent Reye's may represent true errors in ammonia metabolism.

HYPOTHETICAL CONSIDERATIONS

The clinical observations outlined above suggest that Reye's may occur in children made susceptible by inherited errors of metabolism, or in those with similar deficiencies created by a rare concurrence of several pathologic factors (e.g. virus + toxin + drug). It may be predicted that the acquired forms of the disease may be more frequently encountered, whereas the occasional patient with recurrent episodes may suffer from the inherited form of the disease. Thus, at least 2 possible mechanisms suggest themselves as potentially responsible for the fatty liver and neurologic abnormalities in patients with Reye's (fig. 4).

1. A block at the OTC step in the urea cycle due to deficient or defective enzyme, or interference with intramitochondrial transport of ornithine, the amino acid substrate of OTC, may be responsible for the inherited type of Reye's syndrome. Under these circumstances, the other OTC substrate, carbamyl phosphate (a condensation product of ammonia and CO_2) leaks out of the mitochondria and is converted to orotic acid by a cytoplasmic pathway (15). Orotic acid inhibits pre-beta and beta lipoprotein synthesis in man (12). Since these lipoproteins are active in export of fat from the liver, the cytoplasmic deposits of neutral fat in Reye's may reflect interference with release of hepatic lipids, as demonstrated in young rats by Windmueller et al. (23). Hypolipoproteinemia has been observed in Reye's syndrome during the acute phase of the disease (4) and orotic aciduria was provoked with a protein load in a patient with 'recurrent' Reye's syndrome after complete clinical recovery (11).

2. Selective damage to mitochondrial membranes and their constituent enzymes active in ammonia metabolism (CPS and OTC) may underlie Reye's syndrome of the acquired type. Exogenous compounds, and endogenous metabolites with detergent properties such as fatty acids, may interfere with intramitochondrial transport and enzyme activity in a variety of ways. Short chain fatty acids may trap carnitine, a factor essential for fatty acid transport into mitochondria, in a manner analogous to the action of hypoglycin (3). Depressed ATP production due to interference with fatty acid oxidation and gluconeogenesis may inhibit the urea cycle, causing hyperammonemia, while unoxidized fatty acids may be incorporated into lipids within hepatocytes.

Considerable evidence is also beginning to accumulate suggesting that fatty acids of various chain lengths inhibit the conversion of ammonia to urea. Thus, the metabolic and physiologic consequences of treatment with 4-pentenoic acid, a short chain fatty acid, are entirely consistent with the

LIVER CELL

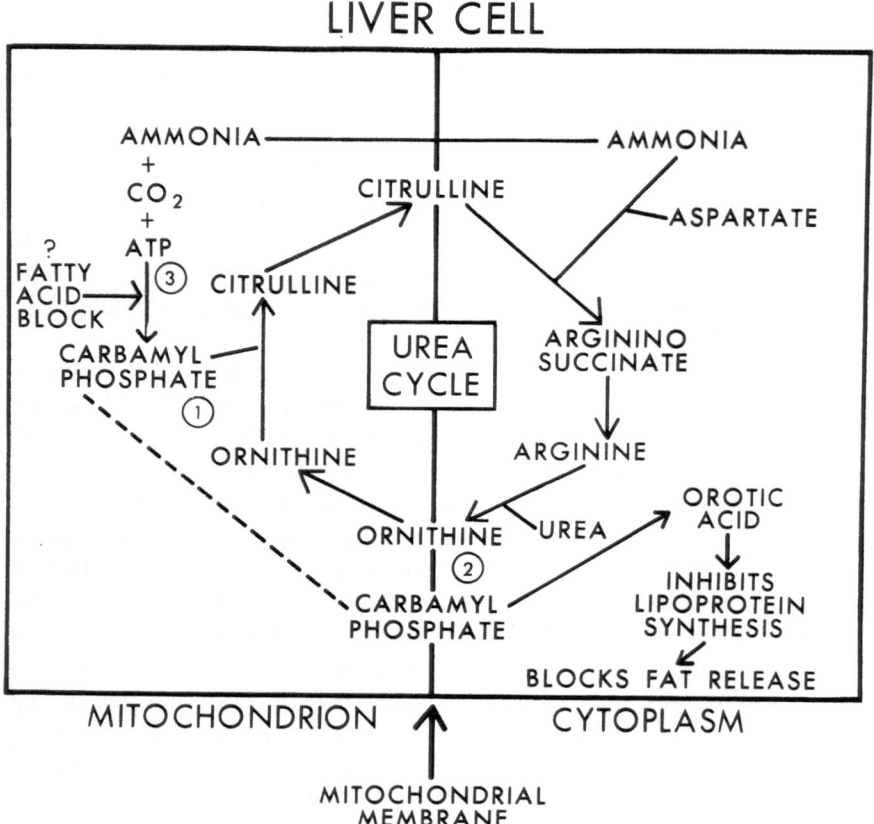

Fig. 4. Postulated abnormalities in ammonia metabolism in Reye's syndrome. Block at the ornithine transcarbamylase step (1) or inhibition of intramitochondrial transport of ornithine (2) would cause accumulation of ammonia and carbamyl phosphate which may leak out of mitochondria (broken line) to be converted to orotic acid in the cytoplasm. Block at the carbamyl phosphate synthetase step (3) would cause accumulation of ammonia. Blocks at 1, 2, 3 may be induced by organic acids. Administration of arginine or ornithine may overcome blocks 1 and 2; administration of citrulline may assist in removal of ammonia by an alternate cytoplasmic pathway.

hypothesis that Reye's syndrome may be due to inherited or acquired defects in interrelated pathways which affect ammonia and fatty acid metabolism. Experiments in rats have shown that 4-pentenoic acid induces coma, convulsions, fatty liver, hyperammonemia and transaminase elevation (10) and combined deficiency in hepatic CPS and OTC (20). Conversely, a 30-fold elevation in plasma propionic acid (3-carbons) has been recently detected in a child with hyperammonemia due to classical X-linked OTC deficiency (13). The postulated connection between hereditary acidurias and hyperammonemic states may be demonstrated experimentally in the near future.

Intermediate and long chain fatty acids are known to be neurotoxic (18). Zieve et al. (25) have shown that fatty acids 8 to 18 carbons in length act synergistically with ammonia in inducing coma in rats and cats when sub-coma doses of each are administered simultaneously. More recently, these investigators have reported inhibition of several steps in the urea cycle by hepatic concentrations of octanoate that exist in pathological stages associated with coma (24). An intimate relationship between ammonia and fatty acid metabolism is suggested by these findings.

The proposed hypothesis has 2 advantages: 1. it can be tested with systematic kinetic analysis of urea cycle enzymes in liver biopsy tissue from patients with organic acidurias, and from those with Reye's syndrome; concentrations of short, intermediate and long chain fatty acids can be determined in plasma and urine of children with hereditary hyperammonemia and with Reye's syndrome, and correlated with blood ammonia levels, urinary orotic acid, and clinical course; 2. postulated involvement of urea cycle activities in the pathogenesis of Reye's syndrome suggests a specific therapeutic approach which may be evaluated in controlled clinical trials.

THERAPEUTIC IMPLICATIONS

A block at the OTC step may be ameliorated or corrected with oral administration of amino acid substrates such as ornithine or its precursor arginine. Administration of citrulline, the amino acid product of OTC activity, may enhance removal of ammonia by an alternate pathway when both OTC and CPS are deficient (8).

The clinical data summarized at the beginning of this paper suggest that treatment of Reye's syndrome should be initiated as soon as the diagnosis is suspected, preferably at a time when vomiting and the first manifestations of neurological involvement become apparent. Recognition at an early stage may be especially important in this disorder, since the outcome may be largely dependent on the severity of the initial insult. The effectiveness of aminotherapy should be correlated with such variables as the interval between the beginning of the vomiting phase and initiation of treatment, or prior duration of stage II or III coma at initiation of therapy. These clinical signposts may also assist in clarifying the efficacy of other treatments, such as exchange blood transfusion, peritoneal dialysis, hemodialysis and procedures aimed at cerebral decompression.

REFERENCES

1. Applebaum, M. N. and M. M. Thaler, Reye's syndrome without initial hepatic involvement. *Amer. J. Dis. Child.* Submitted.
2. Bourgeois, G., L. Olson, D. Comer, et al., Encephalopathy and fatty degeneration of the viscera: A clinicopathologic analysis of 40 cases. *Amer. J. clin. Path. 56*: 558-571 (1971).
3. Bressler, R., L. Corredor and K. Brendel, Hypoglycin and hypoglycin-like compounds. *Pharmacol. Rev. 21*: 105-130 (1969).
4. Brown, R. E., G. E. Madge and D. A. Trauner, Lipid and lipoprotein studies in Reye's syndrome. *Virginia med. Mth. 99*: 622 (1972).
5. Brown, T., G. Hug, K. Bove, et al., (letter) Reye's syndrome. *Lancet 2*: 716 (1974).
6. Corey, L. and R. J. Rubin, Reye's syndrome 1974: An epidemiologic assessment. In: *Reye's Syndrome.* J. D. Pollock (ed.). (Grune & Stratton, New York 1974) pp. 179-187.
7. Crocker, F. S., K. R. Rozee, R. L. Ozere, et al., Insecticide and viral interaction as a cause of fatty visceral changes and encephalopathy in the mouse. *Lancet 2*: 22-24 (1974).
8. DeLong, G. R., T. H. Glick and D. C. Shannon, Citrulline for Reye's syndrome. *N. Engl. J. Med. 290*: 1488 (1974).
9. Efron, M. L., Isovaleric acidemia. *Amer. J. Dis. Child. 113*: 74-76 (1967).
10. Glasgow, A. M. and H. P. Chase, Production of the features of Reye's syndrome in rats with 4-pentenoic acid. *Pediat. Res. 9*: 133-138 (1975).
11. Hoogenraad, N. J. and M. M. Thaler. Unpublished observations.
12. Kelley, W. N., M. L. Green, I. H. Fox, et al., Effects of orotic acid on purine and lipoprotein metabolism in man. *Metabolism 19*: 1025-1035 (1970).
13. Krieger, I., W. Gronemeyer and J. Cejka, Further evidence of a link between urea cycle and short chain fatty acid metabolism (abstract). *Pediat. Res. 9*: 352 (1975).
14. Lovejoy, F. H., Jr., A. L. Smith, J. J. Bresman, et al., Clinical staging in Reye's syndrome. *Amer. J. Dis. Child. 128*: 36-41 (1974).
15. MacLeod, P., S. Mackenzie and C. R. Scriver, Partial ornithine carbamyl transferase deficiency: an inborn error of the urea cycle presenting as orotic aciduria in a male infant. *Canad. med. Assoc. J. 107*: 408 (1972).
16. Reye, R. D., G. Morgan and J. Baral, Encephalopathy and fatty degeneration of viscera. A disease entity in childhood. *Lancet 2*: 749-752 (1963).
17. Reynolds, D. W., H. D. Riley, Jr., D. S. LaFont, et al., An outbreak of Reye's syndrome associated with influenza B. *J. Pediat. 80*: 429-432 (1972).
18. Samson, F. E., Jr. and D. R. Dahl, A study of the narcotic action of the short chain fatty acids. *J. clin. Invest. 35*: 1291-1298 (1956).
19. Shih, V. E. and M. L. Efron, Urea cycle disorders. In: *The Metabolic Basis of Inherited Disease.* J. B. Stanbury, J. F. Wyngaarden and D. S. Fredrickson (eds.). (McGraw-Hill, New York 1972) pp. 370-392.
20. Sinatra, F., T. Yoshida, M. N. Applebaum, et al., Abnormalities of carbamyl phosphate synthetase and ornithinetranscarbamylase in liver of patients with Reye's syndrome. *Pediat. Res. 9*: 829 (1975).

21. Tanaka, K., K. J. Isselbacher and V. Shih, Isovaleric and α-methylbutyric acidemias induced by hypoglycin A: Mechanism of Jamaica vomiting sickness. *Science 175*: 69-71 (1972).
22. Thaler, M. M., N. J. Hoogenraad and M. Boswell, Reye's syndrome due to a novel protein-tolerant variant of ornithinetranscarbamylase deficiency. *Lancet 2*: 438-440 (1974).
23. Windmueller, H. G., R. I. Levy and A. E. Spaeth, Selective inhibition of hepatic but not intestinal *b*-lipoprotein production and triglyceride transport in rats. *Adv. exp. Med. Biol. 4*: 365 (1969).
24. Zieve, L. and R. Derr, Effect of fatty acids on the disposition of ammonia. *Clin. Res. 23*: 521A (1975).
25. Zieve, F. J., L. Zieve, W. M. Doizaki and R. B. Gilsdorf, Synergism between ammonia and fatty acid in the production of coma: implications for hepatic coma. *J. Pharmacol. exp. Ther. 191*: 10-16 (1974).

HEPATIC PORTO-ENTEROSTOMY.
SURGICAL PROBLEMS AND RESULTS

J. VALAYER, M.D.

Surgery of biliary atresia has been radically modified since the introduction by Kasai in 1954 and the first publications in the English literature in 1968 of the so-called hepatic porto-enterostomy (1).

The principal aim of this operation is to open up, by a transverse section at the level of the porta hepatis, the biliary ducts at the point where they are supposed to emerge from the hepatic parenchyma. Microscopic examination of fibrous tissue removed from this site at operation may show a number of small ductules, some of which may still be in communication with functional intrahepatic ductules.

All reports on biliary atresia give an account of two different groups. 1. Correctable cases – 20% – with a very low cure rate; and 2. Uncorrectable cases in which surgical attempts invariably failed to cure the disease.

Definite improvement in results has been obtained in these latter cases by hepatic porto-enterostomy, with good bile excretion in a reasonable number of cases, and even cure with more than ten year follow-up in some cases recently published by Kasai.

However new problems have arisen in the clinical courses of these children in spite of bile flow recovery.

One complication is the long term risk of infection, which is supposed to be due to angiocholitis, and is observed in practically all cases with a functional jejunal loop anastomosis.

The other complication is portal hypertension.

In this report, we will first give our experience with 95 explorations of children with biliary atresia, operated upon between 1968 and the end of 1974. Results will be given for a total of only 49 cases, for reasons to be discussed later.

Before coming to the surgical part, it seems important to underline certain points.

Diagnosis of atresia is practically always made before the operation. Of more than 100 children referred to us for surgical exploration in the last 7 years, only 15% were shown to have a normal biliary tree at operation. This better selection of patients by the pediatricians seems to be due to greater clinical experience rather than better interpretation of biologic or histologic tests.

Contraindication to operation is essentially related to low coagulation factors in long term jaundiced infants. At the usual age of the operation, one or two months, this should not be a problem after correction by vitamin K. Young age is not a contraindication; in fact, at one month, liver changes may already be quite marked.

A further point to emphasize is the importance of giving full information on the subject to the families of these children. Even though bile stained stools may be observed soon after the operation, we think that parents should be warned that the general outlook remains guarded even after apparently successful surgery.

The last important point is the improvement in anesthesia techniques resulting in lower operative risks and more accurate surgical techniques.

SURGICAL TECHNIQUE

I. Laparotomy
Abdominal approach is by transverse laparotomy sectioning of both rectus muscles, quite a distance above the umbilicus, at a site which is best determined by examination once the child is asleep: one should then try to visualize the level of the porta hepatis so that the cutaneous incision is made at the same horizontal level.

We have had no complications related to this kind of laparotomy.

II. Exploration
1. First, one should evaluate the state of the liver. It may be quite variable from one patient to another, but we should like to emphasize the following points:

The liver never looks quite normal, even in very young patients, so that one can almost diagnose atresia by the macroscopic appearance of the liver alone.

Fibrous changes may be noted, even at one or two months of age, by palpation of the liver.

Hypertrophy of the entire liver is usually found but it may predominate in one lobe or in one segment; it may be necessary then to remove a small fragment of parenchyma in front of the porta hepatis to have good access to that region.

2. Ascites may be noted on opening the abdomen; but never much more than a few milliliters. Extensive ascites is a contraindication to operation.

3. Measurement of portal pressure has been performed at each explora-

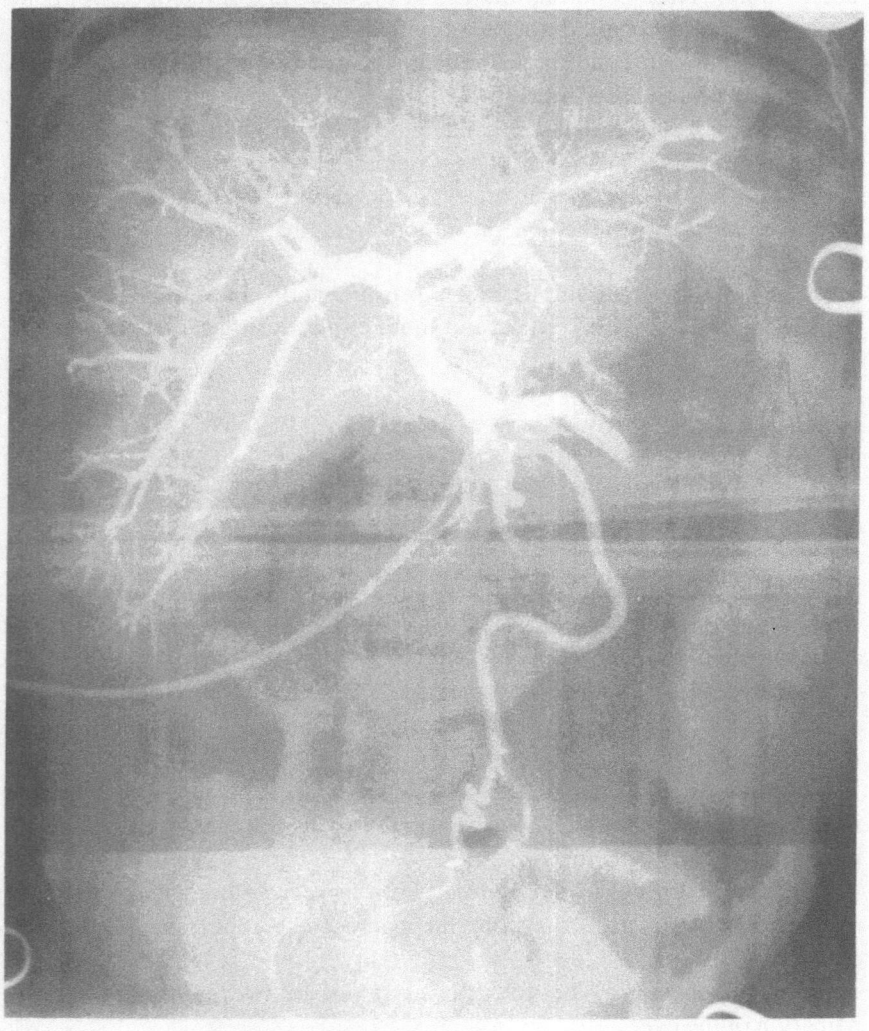

Fig. 1. Opacification of the portal system via the umbilical vein. Reverse flow into portal vein, splenic vein and mesenteric veins. Portal pressure: 27 cm H_2O.

tion during the past year, by umbilical vein catheterization. It was always found possible to push the catheter up to the level of the left portal vein inside the liver and to measure the pressure simply by holding the catheter upwards and measuring the distance between the level of serum used to rinse the catheter and the level of the umbilical vein.

This was done in 26 patients, 3 of whom had normal bile tracts and were operated upon for other reasons, one with hepatitis and two with pyloric stenosis. In these 3 patients, the pressures were 7, 8 and 12 cm of water. In the 23 patients with atresia, 14 had between 13 and 20 cm pressure, 7 had between 22 and 27, and 2 had 34 cm.

These numbers seem to correlate well with the age of the patients at operation since in the first group, the mean age was 6 weeks, in the second group, 15 weeks and, in the last group, each child was 5 months old.

4. Using the same catheter, portography is done with an injection of a radiopaque medium. As this examination has not proved to be valuable in biliary atresia, in our series, we have given up this exploration. In 23 portographies, only twice did we notice any reverse flow from the liver (fig. 1).

5. Alterations in the gall-bladder are the next notable findings during exploration.

Usually, the gall-bladder is hard to visualize due to hypertrophy of surrounding parenchyma and to its small size. This hypoplasia of the gall-bladder was noticed in 72 of 95 cases. In this condition, no injection of radiopaque medium trhough the gall-bladder is possible.

In one case out of 4 (23 in our series), one may find a firmer gall-bladder, rather small, and containing a $\frac{1}{2}$ ml of colourless, syrupy liquid. It may then be possible to radiograph the extra-hepatic biliary tree to the exclusion of the common hepatic duct, where later dissection will show the fibrous changes of atresia. It is striking to see how massive injection of dye into the duodenum may be obtained through this route in spite of the apparent minute diameter of the common duct (fig. 2).

If the gall-bladder contents should appear the least bile stained, there should be no doubt that it is not an atresia of the biliary tract.

6. Next, dissection is undertaken towards the porta hepatis.

It is essential to have a good view under the liver. For this, electro-coagulation of the smallest bleeding points is necessary.

The best land mark is the right branch of the hepatic artery, in front of which the biliary tract of the fibrous remnants should be isolated. In some cases with a deep operating field and a very large liver, it may be useful to detach the gall-bladder and use it as a guide for dissection.

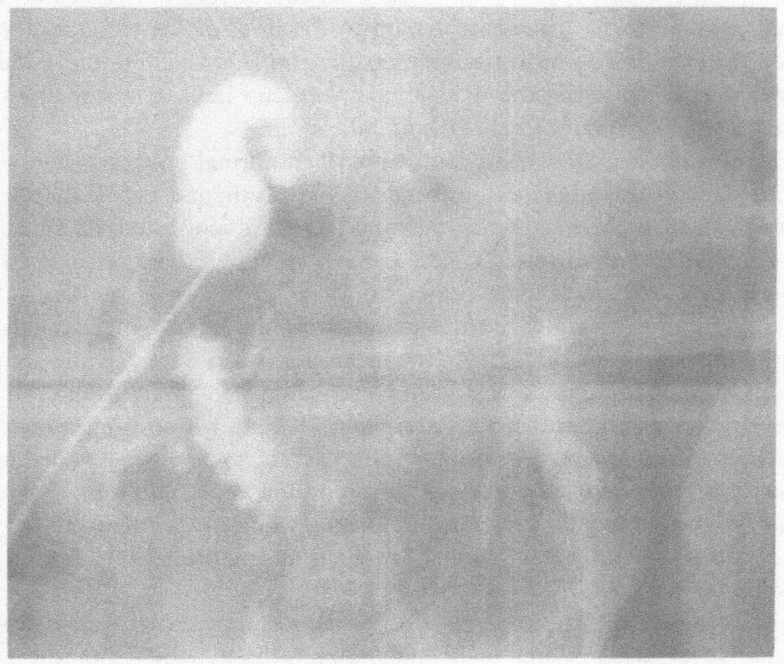

Fig. 2. Extra hepatic atresia limited to the common hepatic duct. Good flow is obtained from injection of dye into the Gall bladder in spite of the small size of the main duct.

As regards classification of different types of biliary atresia, we do not completely agree with Kasai (2). He considers correctable cases as obstruction of the common bile duct with a dilatation of the proximal portion similar to that of a congenital choledochal cyst. We have only once observed such a case, with a rather peculiar dilatation of the intra-hepatic bile ducts. Atresia of the hepatic duct with dilatation of the proximal portion or small cyst-like structures at the porta hepatis, are both described by him to communicate in some cases with intrahepatic radicles, and are therefore considered to be correctable cases also. We have found such lesions, pea-sized nodules, emerging from the liver at the porta hepatis, in 17 of 95 cases. Kasai himself now agrees that these cysts may well be simply 'bile lakes', from extravasation of bile into interstitial tissue, and this seems to be the case, as histologic analysis may not show a continuous epithelial border in these cysts, and also as attempts to inject a contrast medium have always failed, in our experience, to show correspondence with intra-hepatic biliary ducts. That is probably why very few cures are recorded in the literature from among the 20% so-called curable cases.

As to the non-correctable cases, where no bile is discovered during dissection, the state of the biliary tract in these cases is variable. It may be totally absent between the porta hepatis and the gall-bladder, the right hepatic artery being immediately apparent without any fibrous tissue in front of it; or more commonly, it will be represented as a fibrous band or cord whose edges are not well defined, but is quite easy to separate from the posterior vascular plane.

Trans-section of this fibrous tissue is done at the converging point with the cystic duct or below that point if the gall-bladder is used to direct the dissection, as proposed by Kasai. Some kind of a fibrous cone will thus be isolated, containing possible biliary ductules, and still fixed at its base at the point of the porta hepatis. This is where the second section should take place in the hope of opening some ductules in communication with the intra-hepatic biliary tract. In the early cases of our series, this section was done a few millimeters below the level of the porta hepatis; in more recent cases, section is done just at the level of the porta hepatis and without any attempt to cut inside liver parenchyma. We think there is a greater risk in that case of causing permanent hemorrhage which would certainly create difficulties for the construction of the anastomosis. Even in those cases where dissection of fibrous tissue is interrupted just at the level of the porta hepatis, a small hemorrhage is quite frequent at the posterior aspect of the section plane. This accounts for the difficulties we find as a rule in assuming at operation that bile has been seen or ducts individualized during trans-section of the porta hepatis. Another point is that lymphatic drainage may also be quite abundant and to such an amount sometimes, that we wonder if it could not be at least partly responsible for staining of intestinal contents or even more of the secondary so-called angiocholitis, which then should better be called lymphangitis.

Tissue from the region of the porta hepatis has thus been available in 23 cases. Histologic examination was done by Dr. M. Gauthier using Kasai's method for preparation. Studies are done at different levels. Bile ducts of different sizes were found in 18 cases: 2 were 1 mm in diameter, 5 about 300 or 400 microns, and 7 showed numerous ductules less than 50 microns. All these findings are at the porta hepatis level; in 5 cases, no duct could be traced in the fibrous tissue, and yet in 2 of these, there was some bile flow recovery. In more than half of the cases, numerous inflammatory cells were seen in the fibrous tissue, and often may be found clustered around the bile ducts. At a lower level, histologic analysis of the fibrous remnants has never shown any duct at all. This is consistent with the diagnosis of complete atresia and not just hypoplasia of the biliary tract. Also, an analysis of the fibrous tissue shows some large lymphatic lumina in a number of preparations.

7. We believe one of the most important problems in extra-hepatic biliary atresia is the anatomical state of the main intra-hepatic biliary canals. If obstruction should be limited to the extra-hepatic part of the biliary tree, one should expect some dilatation of the intra-hepatic part. To our knowledge, this has not been demonstrated in any case. Our experience with trans-hepatic tapping during exploration has not been rewarding and we have given up these attempts. Post-mortem studies are not often available with biliary atresia, as death often occurs outside the hospital; besides, liver changes from fibrosis certainly alter the general architecture of the biliary tract inside the liver. Nevertheless, we did manage to get pictures of the intra-hepatic structures in 4 cases: 2 during exploration, one through a small cyst and the other by injection of the gall-bladder which seemed directly connected to the hepatic duct via the cystic duct; also 2 cases where a trans-cutaneous injection of the liver was done and showed the complete intra-hepatic biliary system and flow into the jejunal loop (fig. 3).

The anatomical disposition of the principal biliary canals inside the liver seems to be quite different in these cases from that in the normal child of the same age. We believe that the disease is not located only at the extra-hepatic site but may also affect the ducts to some extent inside the liver. Yet specimens from liver biopsies taken from a subcapsular site during surgical exploration do not always show the exact state of the interlobular ductules. Agenesis of intra-hepatic ducts, such as described in MacMahon's syndrome, has not been seen in association with extra-hepatic biliary atresia in our series.

8. Associated congenital anomalies were not frequently encountered in our experience: 3 cases of situs inversus, one of which was associated with poly-splenia; one case of duodenal stenosis operated soon after birth, elsewhere, and only 2 cases where an abnormal right hepatic artery was found coming from the superior mesenteric artery. No other major malformation was noted in this series.

Our conclusions as regards surgical exploration in biliary atresia are:
1. Extension of the disease to the main collecting ducts inside the liver,
2. Early co-existing portal hypertension, in relation to fibrosis,

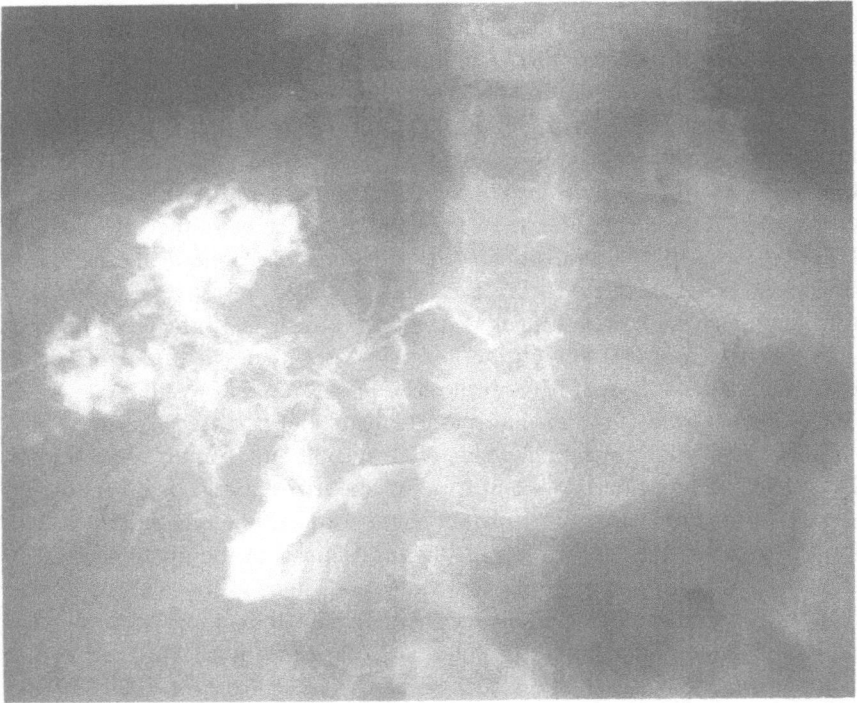

Fig. 3. Opacification of the jejunal loop by transhepatic cholangiography 2½ years after hepatoportoenterostomy.

3. Great varieties of extra-hepatic duct anomalies, which can not be fitted into a rigid classification,
4. Infrequent associated congenital anomalies, which added to the preceding remark, would lead to the assumption of acquired lesions of previously normal biliary tract, rather than a congenital lack of development.

III. Repair

1. In our entire series of 95 cases, only 25 children were submitted to simple exploration without any attempt to correct the anomaly. Although 10 of these were early cases at a period when HPS was not yet performed, there are still 15 cases operated on more recently, where any attempt at repair was given up because of different conditions, including very large fibrous livers in children four of five months of age, and also local difficulties due to bleeding or too small a surface at the site of the porta hepatis for anastomosis. The

aim should remain to construct an anastomosis at any price since there is no other chance to offer to these children.

2. Repair modalities depend on local conditions.

a. Considering the hepatic end of the anastomosis, a small nodule with bile contents was used in 16 cases for a cysto-jejunal anastomosis. As we have said above, we now feel that these cysts are not to be qualified as correctable lesions, because they may not connect with the intra-hepatic biliary system. In 54 cases, a hepatic portostomy was done using the stump of fibrous tissue in the 19 first cases, and in the 35 more recent ones, performing the anastomosis at the liver and just at the level of the porta hepatis.

b. For the intestinal part of the anastomosis, either a jejunal Roux-en-Y loop was used, or the gall-bladder in recent cases, if it was available.

The jejunal loop is the second one; its distal end is closed by interrupted sutures and a small opening is made close to that end, for the anastomosis. Repair of the intestine is done at a point about twenty cm from the closed end. This may appear a short distance, but we have the feeling that a long loop carries a risk of separation of the anastomosis at the porta hepatis, in relation to post-operative atony and stagnation, since we have observed this complication in one case. Whatever the length of the jejunal loop, prevention of a later angiocholitis is not assured by means of this procedure. Temporary external derivation, such as described by Kasai in 1974 (2), and other Japanese authors (3), seems to be a good way of dealing with this problem. Our experience was rather disappointing, so we abandoned this rather lengthy procedure. We must admit that it was not a very serious trial since we did it only once as a primary operation and also once with an external T tube, and in another case as a secondary procedure in a child with unremitting angiocholitis. Having recently heard from Kasai that external derivation is now systematically performed in Japan, our intention is to do the same in future cases. Hepato-porto-enterostomy using a jejunal loop has been done 44 times.

The gall-bladder may be used instead of a jejunal loop, providing the ducts have remained patent right through to the duodenum. The gall-bladder is completely detached from the liver, with care to preserve its irrigation by the cystic artery, then opened up its entire length and anastomosed to the fibrous tissue at the porta hepatis. This type of procedure, which we call hepato-portocholecystostomy has been used in 10 cases. If it does prevent ascending cholangitis, it seems to carry the risk of secondary rupture, probably because of the very minute caliber of the main duct in regard to the flow of possible bile, lymph and blood.

Anastomosis between porta hepatis and jejunum or gall-bladder is constructed with very fine nylon sutures No. 6/0: on the hepatic side, sutures are passed through the posterior aspect of the fibrous tissue, rather than on the very thin adventitium of the portal vein. The anterior sutures are passed directly into the liver capsule. On the other end, jejunal loop or gall-bladder, the sutures are passed through the whole thickness of the wall so that mucosa should not be too redundant inside the lumen of the anastomosis.

OPERATIVE COMPLICATIONS

Before discussing the results, we should like to say that complications from this surgery are, on the whole, not frequent, since we had only 10 post-operative intestinal obstructions, and those in the early cases of this series when anesthesia was more difficult and many manipulations of the intestine necessary.

RESULTS

Our results will be analyzed in a limited number of cases, for the following two reasons:
– Justification of HPS in non-correctable cases, such an operation being either questionable as regards principles of surgery,
– A homogeneous group could only be one followed by the same team of pediatricians.
So we have excluded from the study of results all cases with cysto-jejunal anastomosis (3 survivors out of 16, one the oldest child in this study) and 5 HPS for children followed by other pediatricians (1 survivor, four years old, without jaundice but with portal hypertension).
This leaves 49 cases of HPS for non-correctable cases for study.

I. Mortality
26 out of the 49 patients died during the five year period.
– 5 children died in the early post-operative period, 4 from sepsis and 1 from severe gastro-intestinal bleeding.
– 11 children died with unchanged cholestasis.
– 10 children died in spite of restoration of bile flow, 3 from acute attacks of cholangitis, 2 from progressive hepatic insufficiency, and 5 from what

has been thought to be bile leakage into the peritoneum from the site of the anastomosis, especially in cases where the gall-bladder was used for repair.

Overall mortality seems to be greater in children operated upon after 3 months of age than in the younger ones, but the difference has no statistical significance.

II. Survivors

23 patients have survived until the present.

The follow-up time is over 3 years for 8 patients and less than 3 years for 15 patients.

2 of the survivors have unchanged cholestasis, and unfortunately, there is no hope for improvement.

Restoration of bile flow was observed in the 21 other patients, but 6 of them still had recurrent episodes of angiocholitis at the time of the study.

Another of these has also developed ascites from bile leakage.

At present, this is the condition of the survivors:

Among the 15 patients less than 3 years old, only one child is in good condition, eleven months after surgery. The others still suffer from repeated attacks of cholangitis (7 cases), and 5 have definite portal hypertension.

Among the 8 patients over 3 years old, 6 have no cholestasis. 2 still suffer from cholangitis. All but one have portal hypertension

III. Conclusions

1. First, about correction of cholestasis by HPS in supposedly uncorrectable cases, we can say that 31 patients, of 49, did recover bile flow after the operation.

Staining of stools may start in the immediate post-operative period, but sometimes, especially when the gall-bladder is used for the anastomosis, the first bile-stained stool may not be apparent before 2 or 3 weeks.

Later, normal colored stools may coexist with a slight degree of clinical jaundice. We should like to emphasize that our cases said to have no cholestasis have normal bilirubinemia.

Correlation between recovery of bile flow and the size of the bile ducts in the fibrous tissue collected from the operations has not yet been established in our series as Kasai did for his cases.

2. Angiocholitis was a definite problem in 20 of the 31 patients with post-operative bile excretion.

Infection may start as soon as the first month after the operation (15 patients), or later, even after the second month for 2 patients. Recurrence of episodes of infection is rather unpredictable, since some patients had angiocholitis up to 3 years after surgery. However, some improvement is usually noted after the first post-operative year is over.

Symptoms are always the same: high temperature, severe jaundice, white stools, and often some degree of enlargement of the liver, which may be quite tender. Coliform bacilli, proteus, and other Gram negative organisms were occasionally cultured from blood samples of liver tissue obtained by liver biopsy.

A fatal outcome seemed directly related to angiocholitis in 3 cases.

Trials for prevention of angiocholitis by medical treatment, such as long term cure by sulfonamides, have not been conclusive. As for surgical prevention, the safest method is to use the gall-bladder for anastomosis if possible. Nevertheless, there is a risk of either rupture or non function of this type of anastomosis: of our 10 patients with HPC, only 4 survive, one of whom has unchanged cholestasis.

3. Portal hypertension is now the main concern in long term survivors; it has been demonstrated in 13 patients one year or more after surgery.

All these patients have esophageal varices, and hemorrhage has occurred in 2 cases; both were submitted to a porto-caval shunt.

Among the factors causing portal hypertension, it seems that neither late correction of biliary retention, nor recurrent angiocholitis, have much influence on its degree; all survivors with HPC have portal hypertension.

Patients with portal hypertension all have large and hard livers. Evaluation of periportal fibrosis is not possible by needle biopsy, because of fragmentation of the specimen.

The future of this serious problem is still uncertain. However, there may be some hope for improvement during the growth of the child, since the Kasai's recent publications about his long-term survivors hardly mention the problem of portal hypertension.

SUMMARY

Definite progress in the treatment of biliary atresia has been achieved since the technical procedure described by Kasai has become the prevalent operation by pediatric surgeons for correction of the so-called uncorrectable type.

This report deals with our HPS experience during the period 1968-1974.

Surgical problems are analysed on the basis of 95 explorations of children with confirmed biliary atresia. Subdivision of anatomical types into correctable and non-correctable cases may not be a proper classification, since the small cystic lesions found in the correctable types may not communicate with the intrahepatic biliary system.

No attempt at correction was made in 25 cases. 70 children were submitted to some repair procedure.

16 cases had a cysto-jejunal anastomosis; most of these cases concern children operated in the first two years of this series.

54 cases had HPS, using the stump of fibrous tissue in the first 19 cases, and in the 35 more recent ones, performing the anastomosis just at the level of the porta hepatis. Repair was done by means of a Roux-en-Y jejunal loop in 44 cases, and by use of the gall-bladder in 10 cases. Our experience with external derivation for prevention of angiocholitis is small and not conclusive.

Only 49 cases have been analysed: all were followed by the same team of pediatricians, and were all of the so-called uncorrectable type.

26 children have died, 10 in spite of restoration of bile flow.

23 children survive at the present date, with a follow-up time of over 3 years for 8 of them. In 6 there was complete suppression of cholestasis.

Correction of cholestasis has thus been obtained in 31 of 49 cases.

Angiocholitis was a problem for 20 children among these 31. Prevention of infection by medical means was not effective. The safest method was the use of the gall-bladder for anastomosis if possible.

The main concern in long-term survivors is portal hypertension. High levels of portal pressure can be demonstrated at the time of operation as early as one or two months of age. 13 patients have esophageal varices one year or more after surgery; 2 have presented with hemorrhage and were submitted to a porto-caval shunt procedure.

REFERENCES

1. Kasai, M., S. Kimura, Y. Azakura, H. Suzuki, Y. Taira and E. Ohashi, Surgical treatment of biliary atresia. *J. pediat. Surg. 3*: 665-675 (1968).
2. Kasai, M., Treatment of biliary atresia with special reference to hepatic porto-enterostomy and its modifications. *Progr. pediat. Surg. 6*: 5-50 (1974). (Masson/Urban & Schwarzenberg, Paris/München).
3. Sawaguchi, S., Y. Akiyama, M. Saeki and Y. Ohta, The treatment of congenital biliary atresia, with special reference to hepatic porto-entero-anastomosis. In: *Annu. Meeting of the Pacific Ass. Pediat. Surgeons.* Tokyo, Japan 1972 (Personal communication).

LIVER REPLACEMENT IN CHILDREN*

T. E. STARZL, PH.D., M.D.,** K. A. PORTER, M.D.,
C. W. PUTNAM, M.D., R. W. BEART, M.D.,
C. G. HALGRIMSON, M.D., AND A. F. A. GADIR, M.R.C. PATH.

In the $10\frac{1}{2}$ years between the spring of 1963 and the fall of 1974, liver transplantation was attempted in 93 patients by removing the diseased native liver and replacing it with a cadaveric homograft in the natural (orthotopic) location. Fifty-six of the liver recipients were 18 years old or younger; the other 37 were adults.

The following report will be concerned with the 56 pediatric patients, of whom 40 carried the diagnosis of biliary atresia. Attention will be directed to the need in the treatment of biliary atresia to develop a unified philosophy in which the porticoenterostomy of Kasai and liver transplantation are perceived to be complementary rather than competitive components of the continuum of care.

CASE MATERIAL

The indication for operation was something other than biliary atresia in only 16 of the 56 pediatric recipients. The mean age of these 16 patients at the time of transplantation was 12.9 ± 4.6 (S.D.) years (range 1 to 18 years). Nine of the 16 patients had some variant of chronic aggressive hepatitis without HB_sAg antigenemia (table 1). Three more had hepatomas for which conventional partial hepatectomy was not feasible. Two had Wilson's disease. There was one example each of congenital biliary cirrhosis and cirrhosis associated with homozygous alpha-1-antitrypsin deficiency of the PiZZ phenotype.

The 40 patients who had biliary atresia were 42.0 ± 37.7 (S.D.) months old (range 3 to 191 months) at the time of transplantation. The four oldest

* The work was supported by research grants MRIS8118-01, 7227-01 from the Veterans' Administration; by Grants AI-AM-08898 and AM-07772 from the National Institutes of Health; by Grants RR-00051 and RR-00069 from the General Clinical Research Centers Program of the Division of Research Resources, the National Institutes of Health; and by a grant from the Medical Research Council of Great Britain.
** Faculty Scholar of the Josiah Macy jr. Foundation.

Table 1. Pediatric patients with diagnosis other than biliary atresia.

	Number	Survival > 8 months	Alive now**
Chronic aggressive hepatitis	9*	3 (33 %)	2 (2/3, 1½ years)
Hepatoma	3	2 (67 %)	0
Wilson's disease	2	2 (100 %)	2 (4¼, 6 years)
Congenital biliary cirrhosis	1	1 (100 %)	1 (3 years)
Alpha-1-antitrypsin deficiency	1	1 (100 %)	1 (1½ years)

* None of these 9 patients was HBsAg positive.

** The three late deaths were after 13, 14 and 26 months (see text and table 4 for causes).

children, who were 7, 11, 11 and 15 years old (OT 80, 26, 67 and 43*), were diagnosed as having intrahepatic atresia largely because of their long survival. Histopathologically, these 4 livers showed a micronodular biliary cirrhosis compatible with congenital intrahepatic biliary atresia. Two of the 4 livers also contained liver cell carcinomas (hepatomas); only one such malignancy was found in the other 36 patients suffering from extrahepatic biliary atresia.

Excluding the four oldest children, the collective age of the other 36 patients with biliary atresia was 31.3 ± 15.7 (S.D.) months (range 3 to 67 months).

Although they will not be considered in this report, it is worth mentioning that the 37 adult patients treated during this same time were 39.0 ± 11.1 (S.D.) years old (range 21 to 68 years). Their most frequent diagnoses were primary hepatic malignancy, chronic aggressive hepatitis and alcoholic cirrhosis.

MANAGEMENT PRINCIPLES

Most aspects of the care of these patients have been described (7). Here, a few details will be mentioned.

In recent years, only stable brain dead donors have been accepted. Preliminary arteriography has been routinely performed. Complicated preservation devices are no longer used for the grafts. With almost all infant and

---

* These orthotopic transplant (OT) numbers are frequently given so the reader may follow given patients through different publications from our center. This method of identification has been used since 1969 (7).

child donors, the only preservation used has been perfusion with a chilled electrolyte solution through the portal vein just before and after liver removal. To protect the larger livers of adolescents and adults, these donors are often placed on cardiopulmonary bypass and cooled by means of a heat exchanger preparatory to a final infusion with cold electrolyte solution (7).

HL-A typing was obtained on all donors and recipients since 1964, but the match was not used as an instrument of donor-recipient matching. In 51 of the 54 pediatric cases in which typing data were obtained (table 2), major

Table 2. HL-A typing of primary grafts in 56 pediatric cases.

Match*	No.	Survival > 8 months	Alive now
A	1**	1 (100%)	0
B	2	1 (50%)	0
C	8	3 (38%)	2 (25%)
D	16	3 (19%)	2 (13%)
E	25	11 (44%)	9 (36%)
F	2	0	0
Not done	2	1 (50%)	0
Total	56	20 (36%)	13 (23%)

* A-Match: HL-A identity between recipient and donor.
  B-Match: Compatibility between donor and recipient, but fewer antigens determined in the donor.
  C-Match: One antigen incompatible.
  D-Match: Two antigens incompatible.
  E-Match: Three or four antigens incompatible.
  F-Match: ABO violation or positive cytotoxic crossmatch.
** Retransplanted after 68 days with C-match graft. Thus the extended survival reflects the result with the second or less well matched graft.

incompatibilities were present. The presence and severity of incompatibilities did not seem to influence the outcome, although the force of such a conclusion was weakened by the fact that good matches were a rarity.

Preformed anti-red cell isoagglutinins and leukocyte cytotoxins are apparently less injurious for liver grafts as compared to kidneys. These antibodies, which immediately destroy many renal homografts that are transplanted in violation of a 'positive crossmatch' (4, 7) do not usually cause a comparable hyperacute rejection of the liver (5). In two patients of the pediatric series, liver transplantation was carried out in confrontation of such preformed antibodies (table 2).

One significant change has been made in the technique of transplantation.

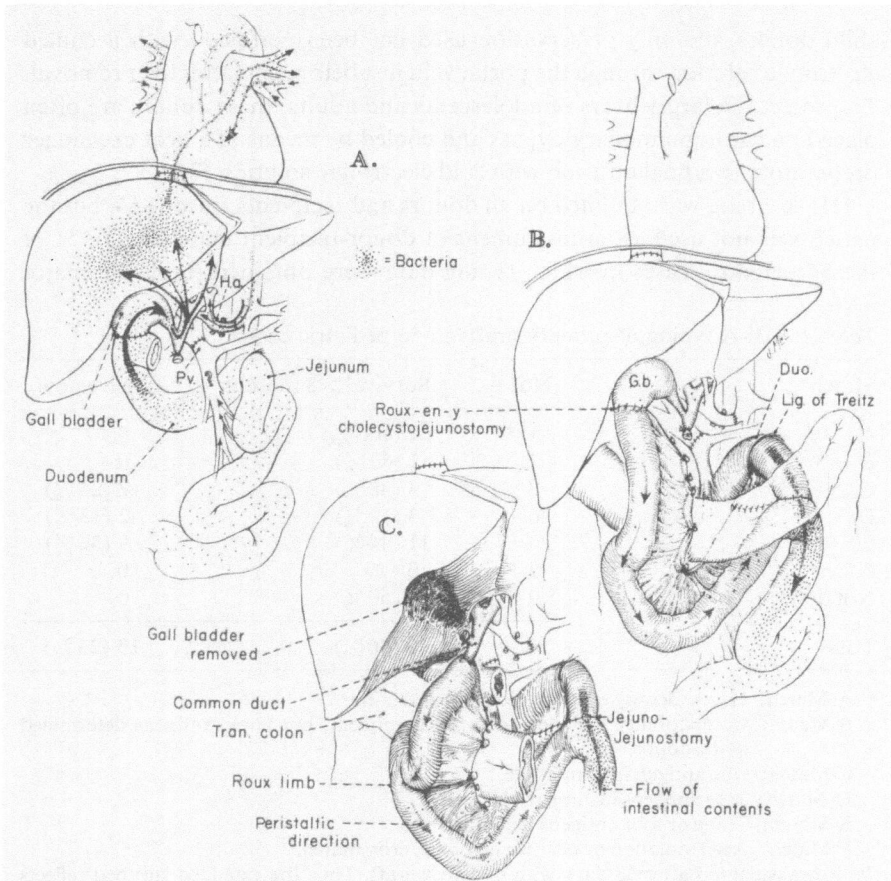

Fig. 1. Commonly used methods of biliary reconstruction. (A) Cholecystoduodenostomy. This extremely simple operation probably carries the greatest risk of graft infection. (B) Roux-en-Y cholecystojejunostomy. This operation protects from hepatic sepsis by placing the new liver outside the main gastrointestinal stream. The isoperistaltic limb is made at least 18 inches long. (C) Roux-en-Y choledochojejunostomy. The end-to-end duct-to-bowel anastomosis is simple if the duct is dilated, as would be the case if a conversion became necessary from B to C because of biliary obstruction. If the common duct is not dilated, the end of the Roux limb is closed and the common duct is anastomosed to the side of the jejunum an inch or so from the tip. (By permission of *Transplant. Proc. 6*: 129, 1974.)

Provision for graft biliary drainage in most of our early experience was with cholecystoduodenostomy after ligation of the common duct (fig. 1A). Since November 1973, the gall bladder usually has been anastomosed to the jejunum by the Roux-en-Y technique (fig. 1B), thus placing the transplant outside the main continuity of the gastrointestinal tract. In a few cases, choledochojejunostomy (fig. 1C) or choledochocholedochostomy with T-tube splinting has been used instead after removal of the gall bladder.

Splenectomy was carried out at the time of transplantation or had been performed previously (3 cases) in 42 of the first 51 pediatric patients, being omitted only if it seemed excessively dangerous. In the last five cases of this report, splenectomy was omitted.

Triple agent immunosuppression with azathioprine, prednisone and horse antilymphocyte globulin (ALG) has been standard treatment for most cases since 1966 (7). If hepatotoxicity with azathioprine is suspected, cyclophosphamide may be substituted with the expectation of a comparable therapeutic effect (8).

RESULTS IN PEDIATRIC CASES

Other than Biliary Atresia
Mortality in the first half year. Seven of the 16 patients died from one to 188 days after operation (table 3). The longest survivor amongst the early deaths was a 15 year old girl (OT 65). She developed inexorable rejection of her first graft. After 157 days, retransplantation was carried out. She died one month later with a multiplicity of complications including intra-abdominal infection, pneumonitis and pulmonary insufficiency. Total survival was 188 days. Histopathologic analysis of the successive grafts showed that the first transplant was severely damaged by rejection while the only damage to the second graft was chronic venous congestion. By 37 days the first graft was undergoing cellular rejection and the portal tracts were densely infiltrated by lymphoid cells, about 20 per cent of which had pyroninophilic cytoplasm. By 147 days there was loss of bile ductules and obstruction of hepatic arterioles and small arteries by fibrous intimal thickening. When the graft was removed at 157 days there was marked centrilobular cholestasis and frequent scattered areas of old ischemic damage and recent infarction. At autopsy, the second graft had no evidence of rejection.

The second longest survivor amongst those who died early was a 15 year old boy whose homograft was eventually invaded and destroyed in 143 days by metastases from the hepatoma which had been the original disease in the excised native liver (OT 23).

Omitting the foregoing recipients with survivals of 188 and 143 days, the

Table 3. Transplantation for indications other than biliary atresia. Causes of death in the first half year after transplantation.

OT No.	Age at operation (years)	Survival (days)	Last bilirubin (mg%)	Clinician's opinion** of cause of death	Pathologist's opinion
65	15	188	1.5	First homograft rejected and replaced after 157 days; died of abdominal sepsis and pulmonary insufficiency 31 days later.	First graft: Loss of bile ductules and obliterative intimal thickening in small arteries following rejection. Second graft: Chronic venous congestion. No evidence of rejection.
23	15	143	40	Carcinomatosis	Multiple metastases of liver cell carcinoma. Severe centrilobular cholestasis. Rejection not definite.*
7	16	64	3.0	Intra-abdominal sepsis following perforation of right colon diverticulum.	Few tiny focal necroses associated with sepsis. No evidence of rejection.
41	16	61	13	Systemic sepsis and hepatic abscesses after delayed correction of partial biliary obstruction (cholecystoduodenostomy to choledochoduodenostomy).	Slight bile retention and evidence of partial bile duct obstruction. No evidence of rejection. No obvious liver abscesses seen.
44	11	34	14	Partial biliary obstruction and dilated intrahepatic duct communicating with ruptured hepatic abscess (diagnosed at autopsy).	Partial biliary duct obstruction. Ruptured hepatic abscess and cholangitis. Widespread fatty infiltration. No evidence of rejection.
31	15	9	30	Massive hepatic necrosis; possible arterial insufficiency of graft.	Acute cellular rejection.

Table 3. (continued).

OT No.	Age at operation (years)	Survival (days)	Last bilirubin (mg%)	Clinician's opinion** of cause of death	Pathologist's opinion
20	8	1	too soon	Massive hepatic necrosis; probable arterial insufficiency of graft.	Extensive hepatic necrosis. No rejection.

* In all the tables, the phrase 'rejection not definite' was used in an equivocating sense. The classical findings of cell-mediated rejection were not present, but abnormalities such as intrahepatic cholestasis cannot yet be excluded as manifestations of the rejection process, either early or late after transplantation (see reference 7 for full description of histopathology of rejection).
** The clinician's opinions in this and the other tables were reached after the gross autopsy findings were known, but without knowledge of the histopathology of the grafts.

five other patients shown in table 3 died 33.8±28.9 (S.D.) days postoperatively (OT 20 1 day; OT 31 9 days; OT 41 61 days; OT 44 34 days; and OT 57
64 days). Graft rejection accounted for only one of these failures. Technical
complications accounted for three more fatalities. The fifth death after 64
days resulted from perforation of a posterior diverticulum in the ascending
colon.

The two earliest deaths were of patients who had massive necrosis of the
liver at autopsy, one (OT 20) and nine days (OT 31) postoperatively.
Although the hepatic artery of one of these patients (OT 20) was patent at
autopsy, it was thought that it had been distorted or kinked with consequent
poor flow. Alternatively, the transplant may have sustained unrecognized
damage from ischemia before, during or just after its removal from the donor
and during implantation. The graft of the other patient (OT 31) was found
at autopsy to be undergoing uncontrolled cellular rejection (fig. 2).

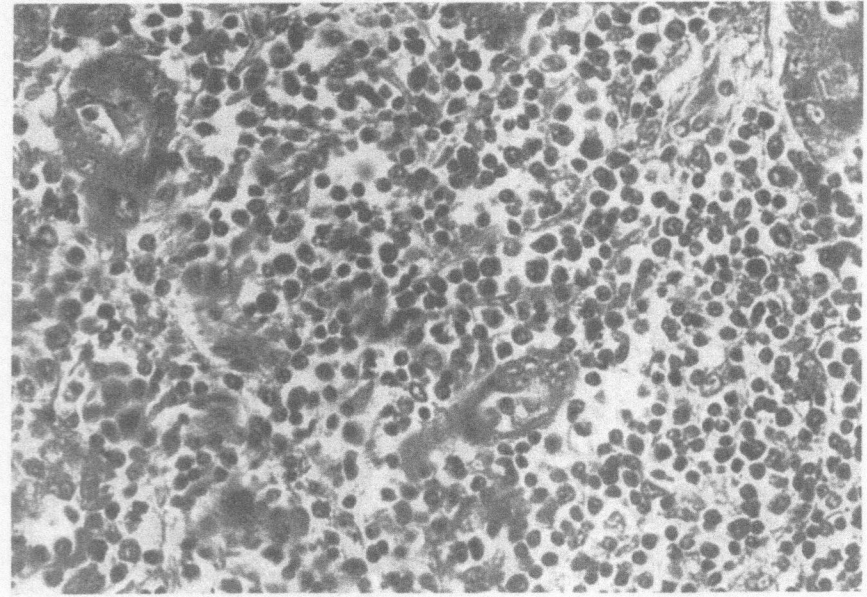

Fig. 2. Acute cell-mediated rejection (OT 31). The portal tract is diffusely infiltrated with
lymphoid cells. Hematoxylin and eosin. ($\times$ 300)

Two of the patients died 61 and 34 days after transplantation (table 3) as
a consequence of partial obstruction of the homograft cystic duct following
cholecystoduodenostomy. The results were dilatation of the intrahepatic

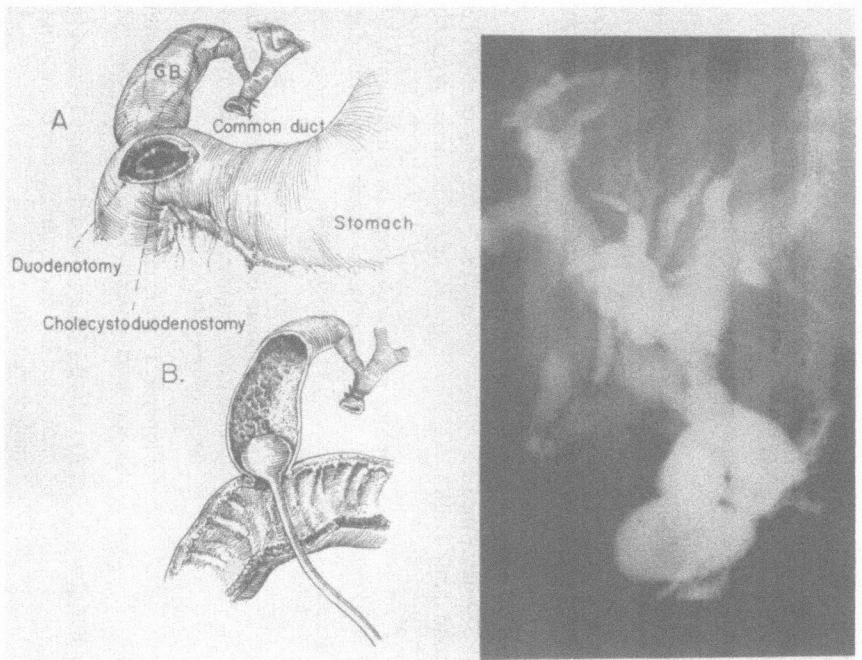

Fig. 3. Cholangiography of hepatic homograft. (A) and (B). Technique of dye injection through a duodenotomy and through the anastomosis. Right ... the obstructed duct system in patient OT 43. Operative and radiographic findings were almost identical in patient OT 41. In both cases cytomegalovirus of the cystic duct was present and may have been partially responsible for the complication. (By permission of *Surgery 72*: 604, 1972.)

biliary tree similar to that shown in figure 3, and bacteremia that presumably originated from the liver. The complication was diagnosed at autopsy in one case after a right hepatic duct had ruptured first into an abscess and then into the subphrenic space (OT 44). The diagnosis in the other recipient (OT 41) was made at reoperation. Secondary conversion to choledochoduodeno-stomy was carried out, but too late. The grafts of these patients at autopsy had no evidence of rejection.

Late mortality. Nine of the 16 recipients had long survival (tables 1 and 4). Eight lived for at least a year and since a ninth child has reached the eight month mark with normal liver function, the one year survival is almost certain to be 56 per cent. Of the nine children who lived for a long time, six are still alive (table 4).

Two late deaths at 13 and 14 months were caused, at least in part, by

Table 4. Liver transplantation for indications other than biliary atresia. Ultimate fate of the nine patients who had prolonged survival.

OT No.	Age at operation (years)	Survival (months)	Last bilirubin (mg%)	Clinician's opinion of cause of death	Pathologist's opinion
8	1½	13	15	Carcinomatosis from original hepatoma	Recurrence of liver cell carcinoma. Chronic cholangitis and obstruction of biliary tree by inspissated bile. Thrombosis of both branches of hepatic artery. Arterial collateral from right phrenic artery.
14	16	14	5	Carcinomatosis; first graft rejected and removed after 379 days; died 57 days after second graft (with disrupted cholecystoduodeno-stomy)	First graft: Micronodular cirrhosis and cholangitis. Narrowing of small hepatic artery branches probably as a result of chronic rejection. No evidence of rejection or bile duct obstruction. Second graft: Widespread fatty infiltration. No evidence of rejection or bile duct obstruction.
27	11	72	20	Alive	Biopsy at 4 years 10 months shows slight increase in amount of connective tissue in portal tracts. Liver copper levels normal. No evidence of rejection.
42	16	51	0.5	Alive	Biopsy at 3½ years showed normal liver. Liver copper levels normal. No evidence of rejection.
55	6	26	30	Undiagnosed main bile duct obstruction	At necropsy biliary tree dilated and blocked by inspissated bile due to stricture at choledocho-choledochostomy.

Table 4. (continued).

OT No.	Age at operation (years)	Survival (months)	Last bilirubin (mg%)	Clinician's opinion of cause of death	Pathologist's opinion
56	18	37	2.5	Alive	Biopsy at 5 months showed early evidence of bile duct obstruction. Two months later choledocho-cystoduodenostomy converted to choledocho-duodenostomy.
74	16	19	10.0	Alive	Biopsy at 133 days showed some centrilobular cholestasis with bile thrombi following a rejection episode.* No evidence of bile duct obstruction or recurrence of alpha-1-antitrypsin enzyme deficiency hepatic changes.
77	16	17	0.5	Alive	Never biopsied.
92	11	8	1.0	Alive	Biopsy at 90 days showed changes consistent with acute viral hepatitis. No evidence of rejection or large bile duct obstruction.

* By 1 year 5 months rebiopsy showed no cholestasis, but slight cellular infiltration of portal tracts and swelling of hepatocytes suggestive of some drug toxicity.

metastases from the hepatomas for which the transplantation had been originally performed (OT 8 and OT 14).

A third child whose original disease was chronic aggressive hepatitis died 2 years and 2 months after transplantation (OT 55). At autopsy, which was performed by Dr. Fred Germuth of St. Louis, Missouri, the total intra- and extrahepatic duct systems were crammed with chalk-like sludge. The complication was apparently caused by an underlying stricture at the choledocho-choledochostomy that had been constructed more than two years earlier without T-tube drainage. The diagnosis was not made premortem in spite of two attempts to perform transhepatic cholangiography. Failure to enter the intrahepatic ducts was incorrectly taken as assurance against duct obstruction.

The liver in this tragic case had little evidence of rejection. The predominant findings were those of bile stasis. All the bile ductules were dilated and many lacked lining epithelium and were blocked by inspissated bile (fig. 4).

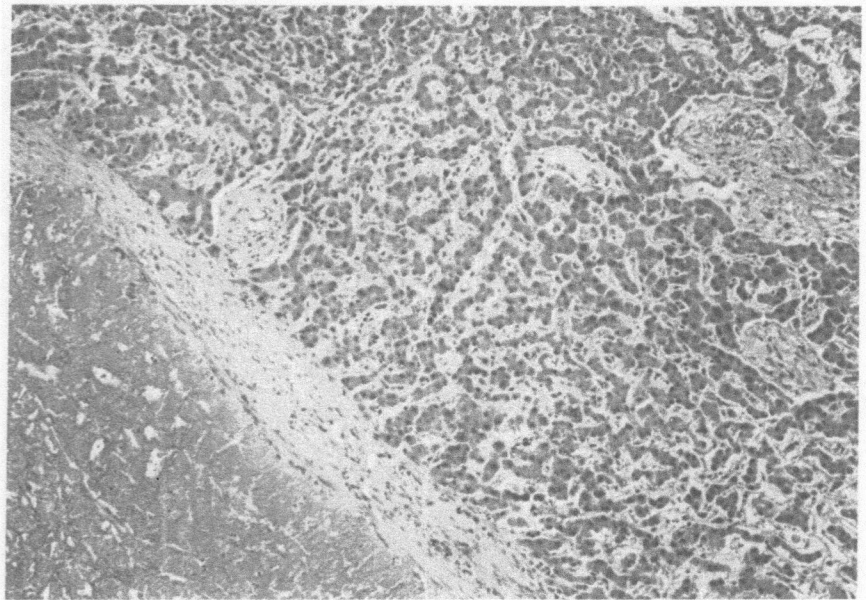

Fig. 4. Biliary obstruction caused by a stricture at the common duct anastomosis (OT 55). In the lower left of the picture, a greatly dilated bile ductule is filled with inspissated bile. Hematoxylin and eosin. (× 120)

Some ductules had ruptured with extravasation of bile and subsequent focal fibrosis and calcification. There was also great narrowing of many of the hepatic artery branches by intimal thickening composed of smooth muscle cells and connective tissue. In several of the arteries the internal elastic lamina was ruptured. This arterial narrowing seemed to be mainly endarteritis caused by proximity to bile extravasation and cholangitis but chronic rejection may have contributed in part to the vascular obliterative changes.

Cases of biliary atresia
Mortality in the first half year. Twenty-nine of the 40 patients died early after transplantation (intraoperatively to 188 days). The mortality occurred in progressive waves to which specific etiologic factors selectively contributed at successive times.

Ten patients died 4.9 ± 6.3 (S.D.) days postoperatively (range intraoperatively to 20 days) because of failure to obtain a satisfactory technical result, or in one case because of a mistake in management (table 5). The most common accident was inability to arterialize the new liver, either because of hepatic artery thrombosis (three cases) or because of nonthrombotic occlusion of this vessel by compression or twisting (two cases). Operative and postoperative hemorrhage killed two more recipients and contributed to the death of a third. Portal vein thrombosis, obstruction of the venous outflow from the liver (caused by excessive cuff lengths of the vena caval anastomosis at the diaphragm) and blood volume mismanagement accounted for the other three failures.

hepatic artery thrombosis and wound hemorrhage, respectively) were of patients who were undergoing retransplantation after the first grafts had failed after 85 and 33 days for reasons that may not have involved rejection (see table 5). The primary graft of one patient (OT 70) appeared to have been irreversibly damaged by viral infection. The other primary graft (OT 52) was obtained from an anencephalic monster. It provided excellent function except for the persistence of jaundice. When the graft was removed after 85 days, intrahepatic ducts could not be found. It was considered possible that the donor had unrecognized intrahepatic biliary atresia.

A second group of five early deaths occurred 21.8 ± 11.9 (S.D.) days (range 7 to 36 days) after transplantation because of what the clinicians diagnosed as an inability to control rejection. Jaundice (table 6) and other perturbations of liver function tests showed hepatic failure but infections elsewhere were almost invariably present as a contributory cause of mortality. In one of the cases, a chimpanzee heterograft was used to replace a failed homograft after

Table 5. Biliary atresia. Early deaths from faulty technique or management (excluding duct problems).

OT No.	Age (years)	Time to death or graft loss (days)	Main complication	Pathologist's opinion
1	3	0	Bleeding	Massive necrosis of hepatocytes of allograft due to ischemic damage before transplantation.
18	1	4	Hepatic artery clot	Homograft completely necrotic except for single layer of surviving liver cells beneath capsule.
21	2	1	Portal vein clot	Necrosis of hepatocytes in central and middle zones of lobules and fat accumulation in liver cells in peripheral lobular zones of homograft.
24*	3	11	Liver necrosis from arterial insufficiency	Necrosis of hepatocytes in central and middle zones of homograft. No evidence of rejection.
34*	2	7	Outflow obstruction	Homograft completely necrotic.
38	3	20	Hepatic artery clot	Necrosis of hepatocytes in central zones of lobules of homograft. No evidence of rejection.
48	2	2	Liver necrosis from arterial insufficiency; bleeding	Massive necrosis of hepatocytes of allograft.
52	¼	85 (first graft)	Rejection	First graft: Marked cholestasis due to congenital intrahepatic biliary atresia. Little evidence of rejection.
		1 (second graft)	Hepatic artery clot	Second graft: Massive necrosis of hepatocytes.

Table 5. (continued).

OT No.	Age (years)	Time to death or graft loss (days)	Main complication	Pathologist's opinion
76	2	33 (first graft)	Rejection	First graft: Massive necrosis of hepatocytes in central and middle zones of lobules of homograft due to extensive viral infection of unknown kind. No evidence of rejection.
		2 (second graft)	Bleeding	Second graft: Normal-looking liver homograft.
80	7	1	Hypovolemia from inadequate fluid replacement	Normal-looking liver homograft.

* A complex of anomalies was present consisting of an absent retrohepatic inferior vena cava, hepatic artery originating from superior mesenteric artery, preduodenal portal vein and intestinal rotation (3, 7).

Table 6. Biliary atresia. Early deaths from rejection.

OT No.	Age (years)	Time to death or graft loss (days)	Complication	Last bilirubin (mg%)	Pathologist's opinion
7	11/12	7	Rejection; liver failure	15	Acute cellular rejection
35	2	36	Rejection; liver failure; infection	17.5	No rejection. Liver failure possibly secondary to infection.
50	1	31	Rejection; liver failure	12.6	Acute cellular rejection
71	2	10 (first graft)	Rejection; liver failure		First graft: Acute rejection of mixed cellular and humoral type.
		14 (second graft; chimp)	Rejection; liver failure	14.7	Second graft: (xenograft): No evidence of rejection.? liver failure secondary to pulmonary insufficiency.
86	3	21	Rejection; liver failure; partial duct obstruction repaired after 10 days.	29	Acute cellular rejection

Table 7. Biliary atresia. Delayed deaths after technical complications.

OT No.	Age (years)	Time to death (days)	Complication	Last bilirubin (mg%)	Pathologist's opinion
26	11	76	Late intra-abdominal bleed; pancreatitis; gastrointestinal bleed; infections	10	Necrosis of centrilobular hepatocytes due probably to hypotension. No evidence of rejection, obstruction or cholangitis. No fungal invasion of liver.
30	11/12	37	Partial duct obstruction; infections	22	Virus infection of unknown kind (not cytomegalovirus) causing bile ductule obstruction and focal liver necrosis (see fig. 5). No evidence of rejection.
43	15	47	Partial duct obstruction*; liver abscesses	7.4	Marked evidence of partial large duct obstruction and cholangitis. No evidence of rejection.
47	3	81	Bile fistula; intra-abdominal abscesses	5.0	Evidence of infection of graft with cytomegalovirus. No evidence of rejection or cholangitis.
49	2	73	Partial duct obstruction and fistula*; gastrointestinal haemorrhage	2.9	Evidence of infection of graft with cytomegalovirus. No evidence of rejection or cholangitis.
68	5	28	Disrupted cholecystoduodenostomy*; multiple abdominal abscesses; bowel perforation	10.4	Necrosis of most of centrilobular and midzonal hepatocytes due probably to hypotension. No evidence of rejection or cholangitis.
84	2½	84	Partial duct obstruction; infection	11.0	Partial duct obstruction of large bile ducts. No evidence of rejection.

* Attempted secondary duct reconstruction. In the cases in which obstruction was relieved, the final histopathologic picture at autopsy did not always clearly reflect the earlier complication.

rejection of the first organ in 10 days. The chimpanzee liver was much less severely damaged than the homograft (table 6).

The histopathology of the transplants in these five cases is summarized in table 6. The diagnosis of cell mediated rejection was usually confirmed but in case OT 35, the histopathologic findings were not compatible with rejection by customary criteria of diagnosis. In the other cases which had typical rejections there were large numbers of lymphoid cells infiltrating the portal tracts, and the areas around the central veins. The findings were like those shown in figure 2. Lymphocytes were present in smaller numbers in and around the sinusoids. Many of the lymphoid cells were large with pyroninophilic cytoplasm and mitoses were common. The portal tracts were oedematous and there was necrosis of hepatocytes in the central and middle zones of the lobules. The reticulin framework of the liver retained a lobular pattern but there was collapse of reticulin around the central veins. Cholestasis with bile 'thrombi' in the canaliculi was not a dominant feature.

Seven additional patients passed through the first few postoperative weeks in spite of very serious and eventually lethal technical complications (table 7). Six of the seven had defective biliary reconstructions, four with the kind of cystic duct obstruction shown in figure 3 after cholecystoenterostomy. Two other patients had bile fistulas, and in one of these cases there was also a delayed bowel perforation at the site where the intestine had been mobilized from its adhesion to the portal structures of the native liver. Only one of the seven patients, an 11 year old girl (OT 26), had a complication not related to the biliary tract of the homograft. In this case, an injury of the pancreatic tail apparently occurred during splenectomy. Later, this general area became the site of intra-abdominal hemorrhage and an invasive retroperitoneal fungal infection. Shortly after, gastrointestinal hemorrhage also occurred.

The histopathology of the homografts after 60.9 ± 22.9 (S.D.) days (range 28 to 84 days) in these mechanically flawed seven cases is summarized in table 7. Histopathologic evidence of partial obstruction of the large biliary ducts was the main feature in three of the seven liver allografts. In one of these cases (OT 30) the cause was a massive viral infection of the epithelial cells lining the biliary tree causing swelling, necrosis and shedding of the infected cells to form obstructing casts (fig. 5). Obstruction in the other two livers (OT 43 and OT 84) was due to the same cystic duct lesion shown in figure 3. Two of the livers were severely infected with cytomegalovirus. Hypotension, associated with the patient's terminal illness, appeared to be the cause of the predominantly centrilobular necrosis in two other grafts. There was no evidence of rejection in any of these hepatic transplants.

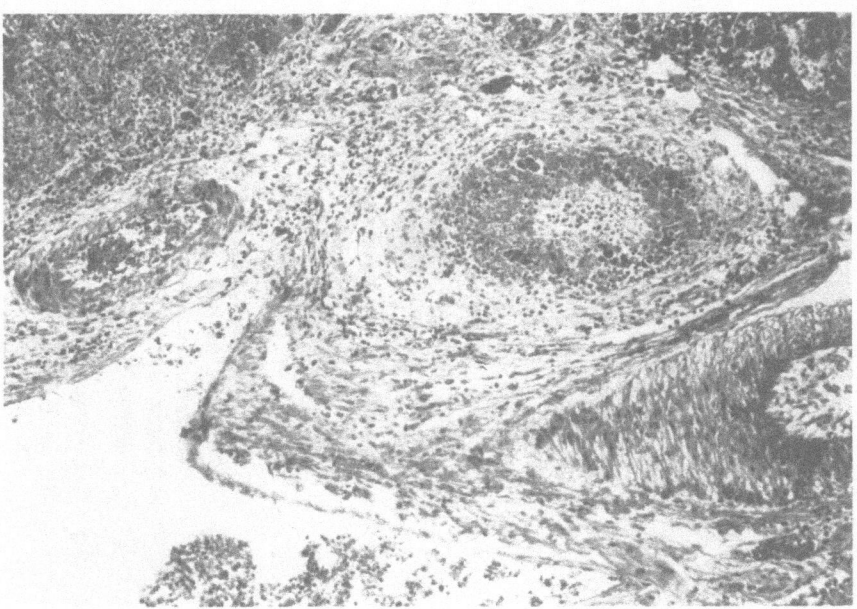

Fig. 5. Biliary obstruction caused by virus infection of the lining epithelium of the biliary ductules (OT 30). A portal tract containing a greatly narrowed bile ductule is in the upper right of the picture. Some of the lining epithelial cells are necrotic and others contain viral inclusions. Hematoxylin and eosin. (× 120)

The final wave of seven deaths came after 110 ± 56.3 (S.D.) days (range 51 to 186). All but one of these patients had abnormal liver function but the final event in each of their lives was uncontrolled infection with bacteria, fungi or viruses (table 8). Four of these seven delayed deaths were of patients who had a complication that has been called 'septic hepatic infarction' (7). Portions of the liver became necrotic and were invaded with bacteria from the intestinal tract. The four patients were tided over the immediate effects of the partial liver infarction, but they all eventually died with local plus systemic sepsis. Septic hepatic infarction is now thought to be due at least in part to under-immunosuppression and thus to be a manifestation of rejection. Mechanical factors such as twisting of the fragile hepatic arterial branches of these tiny recipients could contribute (7).

The livers from patients OT 37, 59 and 67 did not have regional infarctions; these patients had overwhelming systemic infections (table 8).

Table 8. Biliary atresia. Complex delayed deaths.

OT No.	Age (years)	Time to death (days)	Complication	Last bilirubin (mg%)	Pathologist's opinion
9	1	133	Septic hepatic infarctions	5	Micronodular cirrhosis, cholestasis, and obliterative intimal thickening in small arteries due to chronic rejection. Also multiple small septic infarcts due to thrombosis of hepatic artery branches. Bile duct obstruction not definite***.
10	1	186	Septic hepatic infarctions; general sepsis	23	Hepatic fibrosis, cholestasis, and obliterative intimal thickening in small arteries due to chronic rejection. Also multiple small septic infarcts due to thrombosis of hepatic artery branches. Bile duct obstruction not definite.***
11	1	61	Septic hepatic infarctions; general sepsis	12	Micronodular cirrhosis and cholestasis due to chronic rejection. Also multiple small septic infarcts due to thrombosis of right hepatic artery. Bile duct obstruction not definite.***
12*	1	105	Septic hepatic infarctions; general sepsis	3	Biliary tree dilated and blocked by inspissated bile due to kink at junction of cystic and common duct. Also multiple small septic infarcts due to thrombosis of right hepatic artery. No evidence of rejection.
37	3	51	Nocardia and Candida sepsis	4.9	Marked non-specific fatty infiltration of hepatocytes in homograft. No evidence of rejection or bile duct obstruction.

Table 8. (continued).

OT No.	Age (years)	Time to death (days)	Complication	Last bilirubin (mg%)	Pathologist's opinion
59**	11/12	175	? septicemia	normal	Arterial and arteriolar narrowing as a result of past rejection. No evidence of bile duct obstruction at autopsy. No infection found to account for sudden death following brief fever.
67	11	59	Pneumonia (? herpes)	4.2	Marked fatty infiltration of hepatocytes in homograft. No evidence of rejection or bile duct obstruction.

* Also probably had partial biliary obstruction.
** Had apparently successful reconstruction of partially obstructed duct four months previously. Death occurred suddenly after an illness of a few hours.
*** The term 'bile duct obstruction not definite' means that an opinion was not possible about the cause of the cholestasis. Obstruction was considered unlikely but it could not be ruled out. The same term is used in table 9.

Table 9. Biliary atresia. The ultimate fate of the 11 patients who had extended survival.

OT No.	Age at operation (months)	Survival (months)	Last bilirubin (mg%)	Clinician's opinion of cause of death	Histopathology of graft
13	25	30	52	First homograft chronically rejected and removed after 881 days; died 20 days later with rejection.	First graft: Narrowing of small arterial branches and infiltration of large lymphoid cells due to chronic rejection. Severe cholestasis. Bile duct obstruction not definite.**
					Second graft: Massive necrosis of hepatocytes in central and middle zones of lobules. The necrotic areas contain aspergillus. This liver was only given an arterial supply. No evidence of rejection.
16	23	13½	9.7	First homograft subacutely rejected and removed after 65 days; died 339 days later with chronic rejection	First graft: Severe narrowing of small arterial branches and infiltration by large lymphoid cells due to chronic rejection. Some cholestasis. Multiple old and new infarcts.
					Second graft: Chronic rejection with severe arterial narrowing and lymphoid cell infiltration. Focal areas of old ischemic atrophy and recent infarction. No cholestasis.

Table 9. (continued).

OT No.	Age at operation (months)	Survival (months)	Last bilirubin (mg%)	Clinician's opinion of cause of death	Histopathology of graft
19	52	41	23	Liver injury following hemophilus septicemia; ? chronic rejection	Severe narrowing of small arterial branches due to chronic rejection. Marked cholestasis. Bile duct obstruction ruled out by cholangiography. CMV in gall bladder mucosa at autopsy. Lungs contained CMV, aspergillus and pneumocystis.
29	67	12½	15	? hepatitis; ? chronic rejection	Viral hepatitis. No evidence of rejection or bile duct obstruction.
33	46	65	normal	Alive	Never biopsied.
46	46	47	normal	Alive	Biopsy at 9 months showed cellular infiltration of portal tracts probably representing mild homograft rejection. No evidence of persistence or progression of viral hepatitis. No evidence of bile duct obstruction.
53	20	40	normal	Alive	Never biopsied.
64	36	28	normal	Alive	Never biopsied.
73	58	20	normal	Alive	Never biopsied.
89	45	10	normal	Alive	Never biopsied.
91	38	8	normal	Alive	Biopsy at 42 days at time of acute clinical rejection episode showed dense lymphoid cell infiltration including lymphoblasts and cells in mitosis. No evidence of bile duct obstruction.

* Autopsy report has been published (6).
** See table 8 footnote for definition of statement about obstruction.

The histopathologic appearance of the seven livers recovered from 51 to 186 days postoperative is summarized in table 8. Some evidence of chronic rejection was present in four of the seven livers and in three of these cases it was accompanied by obliterative intimal thickening of the small hepatic arteries (fig. 6). In one homograft kinking at the junction of the cystic and

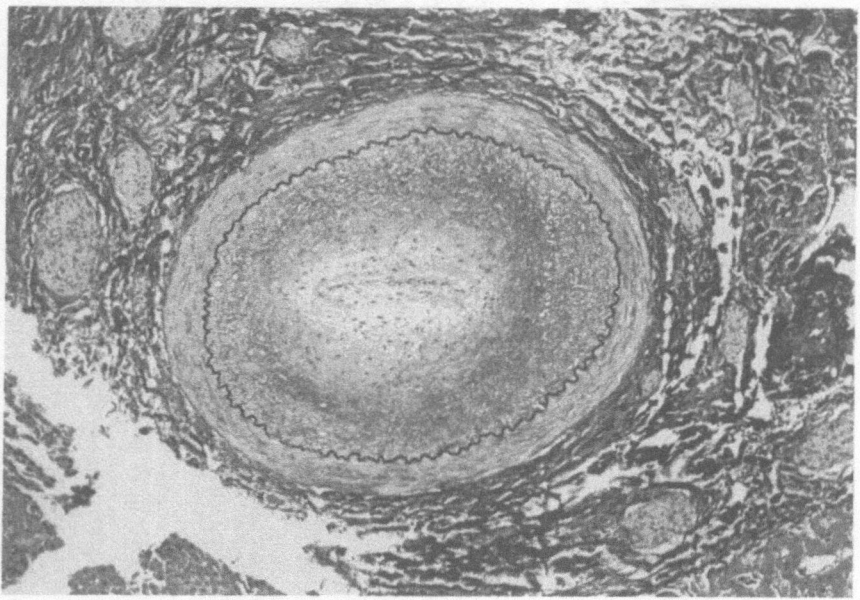

Fig. 6. Chronic rejection of a liver homograft (OT 19) almost 3½ years after transplantation. The small hepatic artery branch in a portal tract is completely occluded by a massively thickened intima. The internal elastic lamina is preserved. Elastic stain. (× 120)

common duct had caused the biliary tree to become dilated and blocked by inspissated bile. The other two livers showed only marked fatty infiltration secondary to infection.

Late mortality. Of the 11 patients who lived for more than a half year, four subsequently died between 12½ and 41 (mean 24.2) months postoperatively for the reasons listed in table 9. All four children became jaundiced, but the reasons for this were probably multiple (table 9).

These four children were given a total of 6 grafts, since 2 of the recipients had retransplantation. The histopathologic findings in the six transplants are shown in table 9. The most important pathologic findings in 4 of the 5 homografts that functioned for the longest time ($2\frac{1}{3}$ to 41 months) were chronic rejection with narrowing of the small arterial branches (fig. 6) and infiltration by lymphoid cells. The fifth chronically functioning liver (OT 29) showed the changes of viral hepatitis with no evidence of rejection or bile duct obstruction after more than a year. The second graft of patient OT 13 was given only an arterial supply. At 20 days after retransplantation it showed massive necrosis of hepatocytes in the central and middle zones of the lobules and infection by aspergillus.

The other seven patients are still alive (table 9) from 8 to 68 months post-operatively (mean 31.1 months). It is of interest that all seven survivors have normal bilirubins and that their liver function tests are normal in other measurable dimensions.

Graft biopsies were obtained early in the course of two of the seven patients who are still living. These showed cellular rejection, mild in one case and marked in the other. Both patients are well, 7 months and $3\frac{1}{4}$ years later (OT 91 and 46) and after total survivals of 8 and 47 months respectively.

EFFECT OF ORIGINAL DISEASE

The only unequivocal effect of the original disease upon the transplant recipient was recurrence of the hepatomas in three cases. The patients with Wilson's disease were relieved of their excessive copper storage in extra-hepatic tissues, and there has been no tendency for the homograft to accumulate copper (table 10). The pediatric victims of chronic agressive hepatitis,

Table 10. Biochemical findings pre- and posttransplantation in a patient with classical Wilson's disease.

	Normal values	Pre-Op	3 months	17 months	24 months
Liver copper	($<20\,\mu g/gm$)	184	—	45	27
Ceruloplasmin	($22\text{-}49\;mg/100\;ml$)	1.0- 1.7	74	48	32
Urine copper	($<30\;\mu g/24\;hours$)	540	119	80	87
SGOT	($3\text{-}27\;Iu./L$)	25	70	25	15
Bilirubin	($<1.0\;mg/100\;ml$)	2.9	.4	.64	.5

HB$_s$Ag negative, have not had an obvious recapitulation of the disease in their grafts although this has probably occurred in one adult who was HB$_s$Ag positive (2).

In an earlier report on immunosuppressed kidney and liver recipients, the appearance of HB$_s$Ag in the serum seemed to be a permanent and consequently sinister finding (9). Therefore the observations on the course of post-transplantation HB$_s$Ag antigenemia which developed postoperatively for the first time in 5 of the chronic survivors were of great interest. Four (OT 29, 42, 55 and 77) of the patients had clinically apparent bouts of HB$_s$Ag-associated hepatitis. A fifth patient (OT 46) had positive sera but had no associated alterations in liver function or clinical symptoms. Three of the 5 patients had subsequent clearing of the virus marker. One of the exceptions (OT 77) is shown in figure 7; although he recovered clinically he is now a carrier.

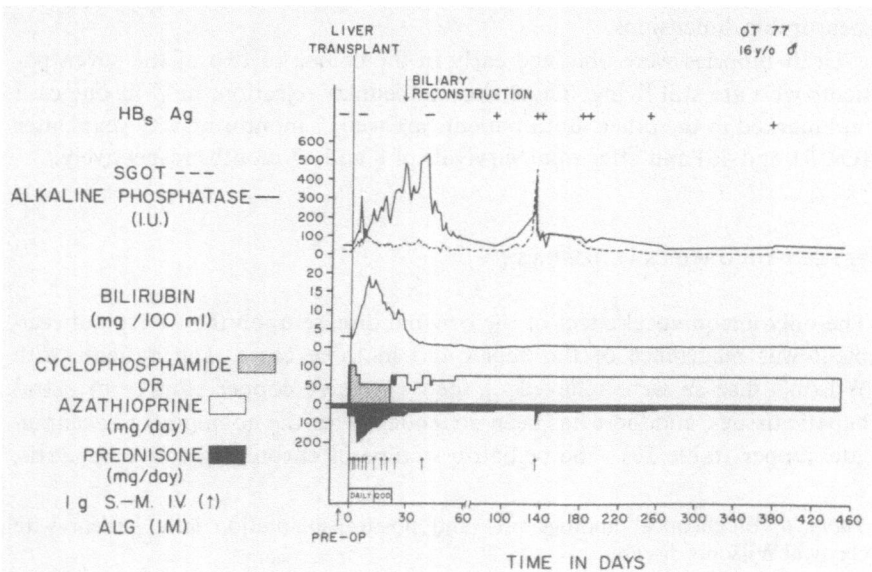

Fig. 7. Recovery after liver replacement for the indication of chronic aggressive hepatitis. The patient (OT 77) is the one whose postoperative transhepatic cholangiogram is shown in 8B. Jaundice persisted until the duct system was relieved of its obstruction by converting the initial Roux-enY cholecystojejunostomy to a choledochojejunostomy at the time indicated by the arrow. Note also that a bout of serum hepatitis complicated the recovery after about 2½ months. The patient recovered but became an HBsAg carrier.

The other patient (OT 29) with persistent HB$_s$Ag died after 12½ months and had findings of hepatitis in his graft (see table 9).

The poor results in 40 patients with biliary atresia, projected at a one year survival of 28%, are in contrast to the 56% figure in pediatric recipients with other preoperative diagnoses. Although atresia patients have other anomalies of which some may jeopardize the transplantation (3, 7) the presence of anomalies is not the main explanation for the difference in outcome between the two groups. Probably, the principal adverse factor has been the small size of the structures to be reconstructed in the younger and smaller population of the atresia subgroup, and a consequent increase in technical errors.

PROSPECTS OF IMPROVEMENT

The statistics given earlier showed that technical and mechanical complications were the main cause of early or late death in 22 cases, or the majority of all patients who have died. In an effort to ameliorate this situation, a number of changes were instituted in the autumn of 1973.

In an effort to minimize vascular accidents, microvascular techniques were used with increasing frequency for the portal venous and hepatic arterial anastomoses. Of even greater importance, techniques were upgraded to diagnose biliary obstruction and manage it effectively by reoperation according to the strategy outlined in an earlier publication (5).

Any patient who becomes jaundiced after transplantation or who develops unexplained bacteremia is now suspected of having biliary obstruction. Transhepatic cholangiography is performed, sometimes on multiple occasions (figs 8 and 9). The yield has been high since this aggressive and consistent policy was instituted. Of the last ten pediatric patients, three have required early conversion of Roux-en-Y cholecystojejunostomy to choledochojejunostomy because of the kind of partial or complete obstruction shown in figures 3 and 8B. All have survived and with prompt relief of jaundice. A fourth patient, who had the same complication plus a bile leak from the ligated common duct (fig. 8C), died before reoperation was possible (table 7, OT 84). Six (60%) of the last ten pediatric recipients are still alive after 8 to 20 months. Without aggressive reintervention this figure would have been 30%.

Even if all the technical problems are solved, it now seems to us that between one and two of every ten liver homografts is going to be rejected early in spite of the best immunosuppression available today. In such cases, early retransplantation will have to be considered after the differential diagnosis of duct obstruction is ruled out, and providing other etiologic factors such as hepatitis or drug hepatotoxicity are not implicated.

The indolent pattern of an inexorably rejecting graft is shown in figure 9,

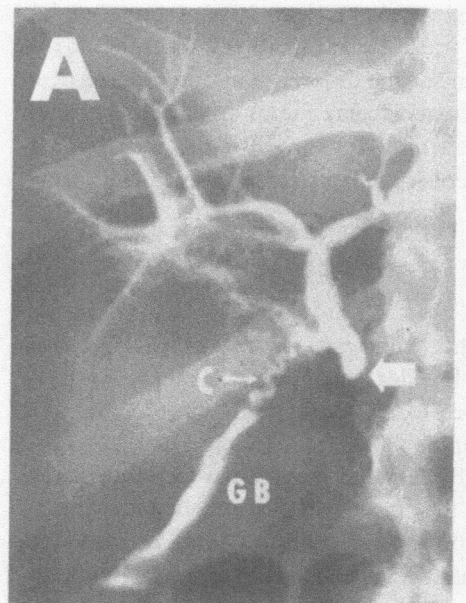
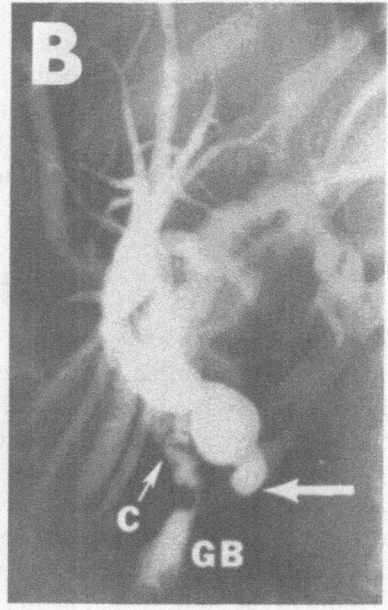
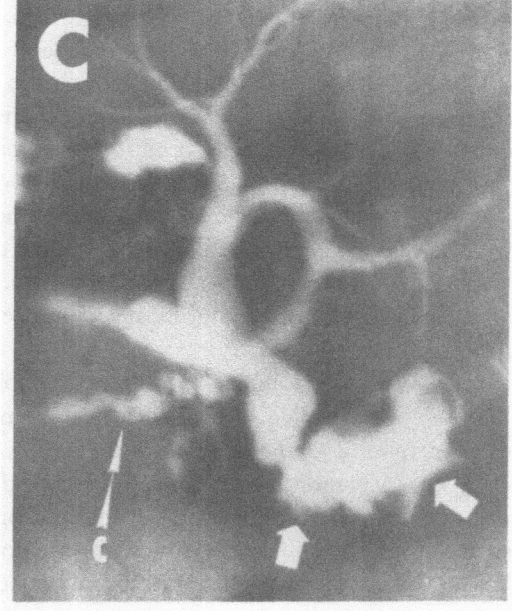

Fig. 8. Transhepatic cholangiography in 3 patients: (A) The demonstration of a nondilated duct system prompted intensification of steroid therapy. Arrow – ligated common bile duct. (B) partially obstructed duct system. The patient was reoperated and the cholecystojejunostomy (see fig. 1B) was converted to the choledochojejunostomy shown in figure 1C. The ultimate result was perfect (see fig. 7). (C) Obstructed cystic duct syndrome plus bile extravasation near distal ligated common bile duct (arrows). This child died of generalized sepsis before reoperation could be carried out. C: cystic duct; GB: gallbladder.

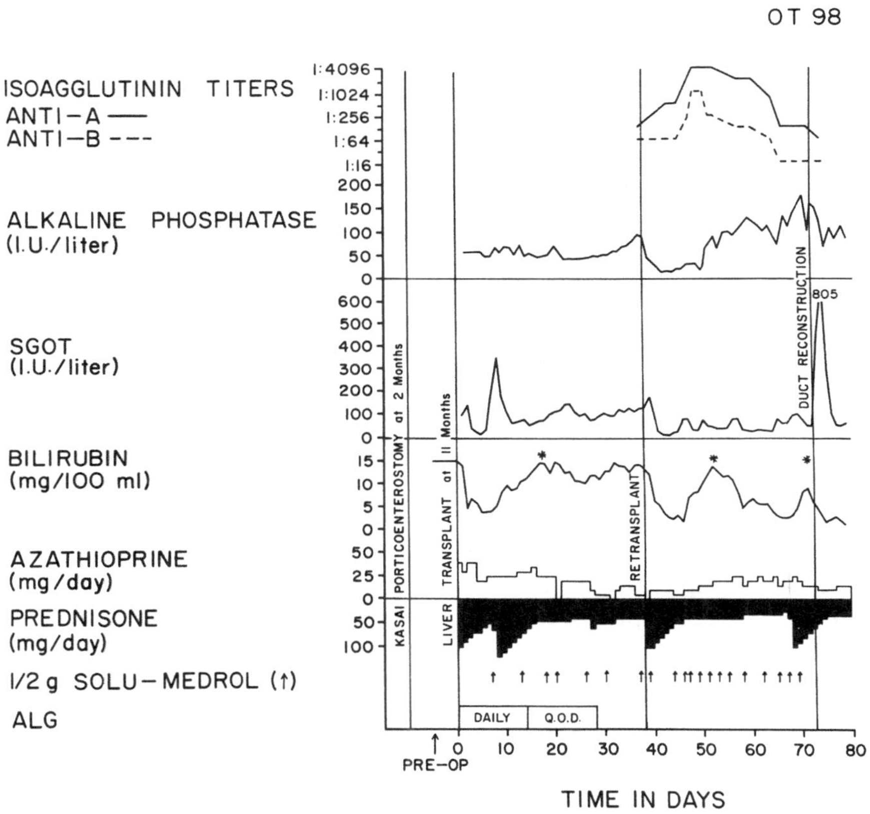
OT 98
ISOAGGLUTININ TITERS
ANTI-A ——
ANTI-B - - -
ALKALINE PHOSPHATASE
(I.U./liter)
SGOT
(I.U./liter)
BILIRUBIN
(mg/100 ml)
AZATHIOPRINE
(mg/day)
PREDNISONE
(mg/day)
1/2 g SOLU-MEDROL (↑)
ALG
KASAI PORTICOENTEROSTOMY at 2 Months
LIVER TRANSPLANT at 11 Months
RETRANSPLANT
DUCT RECONSTRUCTION
805
DAILY
Q.O.D.
PRE-OP
TIME IN DAYS

Fig. 9. Uncontrolled rejection after orthopic liver transplantation (OT 98) in a 9 month old child who had had an unsuccessful porticoenterostomy at the age of 2 months. The rejected primary transplant was removed after 38 days and replaced with another liver. The recipient was O blood type as was the first donor. The second donor was A blood type. Note the prodigious increase in the anti-A isoagglutinins which did not have an obvious adverse effect. The duct system of the second graft became obstructed, and was relieved by converting the cholecystojejunostomy to choledochojejunostomy. The asterisks indicate the performance of transhepatic cholangiograms. The first two were normal but the third revealed obstruction.

with jaundice that is predominantly obstructive and with serum transaminases that are modestly elevated. If the biliary reconstruction is proved sound, there can be little doubt of the diagnosis, and reexploration must be performed as soon as a liver becomes available. In the case depicted (fig. 9) the graft weighed more than 500 grams, an estimated fivefold increase from its weight at its insertion a month earlier. The second graft for this O recipient was from an A donor. In spite of this red blood group mismatch, the organ functioned much better than the red blood group compatible first organ.

Since cadaveric organ donors may not be available at times of desperate need, cautious exploration of chimpanzee liver heterotransplantation is going to be necessary as a possible way out of what otherwise rapidly becomes a hopeless situation. Three liver heterotransplantations have been performed (5, 7) with maximum survival of only two weeks, but with encouragingly minor histopathologic findings in the grafts (for example, see table 6, OT 71).

PORTICO-ENTEROSTOMY AND TRANSPLANTATION IN
BILIARY ATRESIA

Some of the patients with biliary atresia whom we have recently seen have had earlier portico-enterostomy procedures that failed. The prior perform-ance of the Kasai operation has not jeopardized transplantation. In three cases of our experience the previous construction of an isolated Roux-en-Y jejunal segment has proved to be a significant advantage since the Roux limb has been used to accept the graft biliary drainage (figs. 9 and 10).

Although the Kasai procedure apparently alters the natural history of biliary atresia in some cases, the operation will be curative only rarely. Alt-man and Lilly have shown that progressive cirrhosis is almost invariable, even in those patients whose jaundice has been completely relieved by porti-coenterostomy (1). Although some of these children probably will have their lives prolonged, eventually almost all will become candidates for transplan-tation.

Thus, porticoenterostomy and liver transplantation are not competitive procedures. They should be viewed as complementary in the continuum of care that is slowly evolving for children with biliary atresia. If it is to be effective, porticoenterostomy has been urged by its proponents before the age of three months when liver transplantation is not yet a good possibility. Liver replacement is reserved for a later time. Examples of this approach are shown in figures 9 and 10.

In our three patients who had liver transplantation after previous Kasai procedures, one died in less than a month and the other two are still alive after 3 and 20 postoperative months.

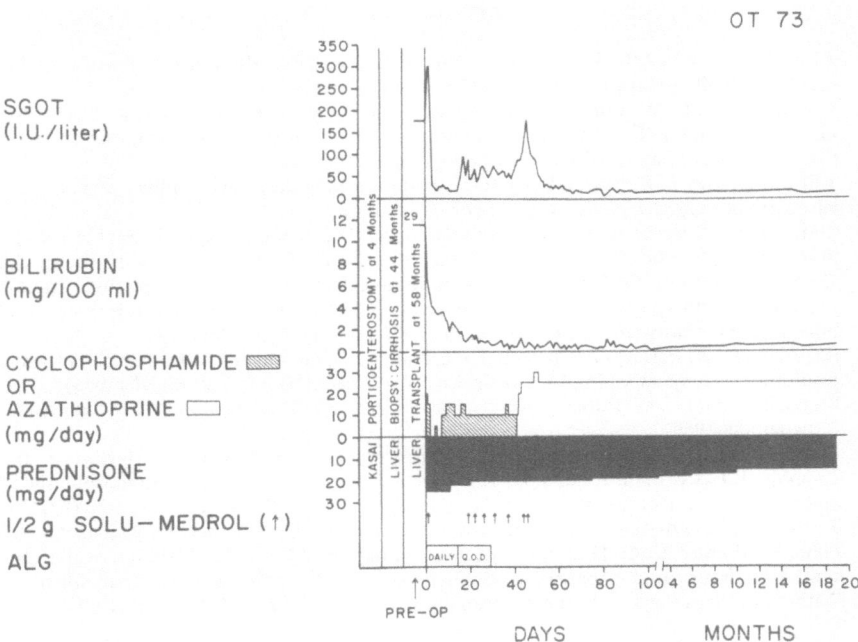

Fig. 10. The course of a child who had a failed Kasai operation but who ultimately was effectively treated with liver replacement. The successive use of the porticoenterostomy and liver transplant is also illustrated in figure 9.

SUMMARY

In the decade ending in the fall of 1974, liver replacement was attempted in 93 patients of whom 56 were 18 years old or younger. Twenty of the 56 pediatric recipients had survival of eight months or more, 17 lived for at least a year and 13 are still alive. The longest survival is now six years.

The results with biliary atresia were poorer than if the original disease was something other than atresia. In both subgroups, the greatest cause for the high failure rate was a variety of technical misadventures of which complications of bile duct reconstruction headed the list. Failure to control rejection was a far less common cause of death. Suggestions to improve the results were made.

REFERENCES

1. Altman, R. P. and J. R. Lilly, Ongoing cirrhosis after successful porticoenterostomy in infants with biliary atresia. *J. pediat. Surg. 10*: 685-691 (1975).
2. Corman, J. L., C. W. Putnam, S. Iwatsuki, A. G. Redeker, K. A. Porter, R. L. Peters, G. Schroter and T. E. Starzl, Liver homotransplantation for chronic aggressive hepatitis, Australia antigen positive. *Gastroenterology.* In press.
3. Lilly, J. R. and T. E. Starzl, Liver transplantation in children with biliary atresia and vascular anomalies. *J. pediat. surg. 9*: 707-714 (1974).
4. Starzl, T. E., *Experience in Renal Transplantation* (W. B. Saunders, Philadelphia 1964).
5. Starzl, T. E., M. Ishikawa, C. W. Putnam, K. A. Porter, R. Picache, B. S. Husberg, C. G. Halgrimson and G. Schroter, Progress in and deterrents to orthotopic liver transplantation; with special reference to survival, resistance to hyperacute rejection, and biliary tract reconstruction. *Transplant. Proc. 6* (suppl. 1): 129-139 (1974).
6. Starzl, T., K. A. Porter, G. Schroter, J. Corman, C. G. Groth and H. L. Sharp, Autopsy findings in a long-surviving liver recipient. *New Engl. J. Med. 289*: 82-84 (1973).
7. Starzl, T. E. and C. W. Putnam, *Experience in Hepatic Transplantation* (W. B. Saunders, Philadelphia 1969).
8. Starzl, T. E., C. W. Putnam, C. G. Halgrimson, G. T. Schroter, G. Martineau, B. Launois, J. L. Corman, I. Penn, A. S. Booth, Jr., and C. G. Groth, Cyclophosphamide and whole organ transplantation in humans. *Surg. Gynec. Obstet. 133*: 981-991 (1971).
9. Torisu, M., T. Yokoyama, H. Amemiya, P. F. Kohler, G. Schroter, G. Martineau, I. Penn, W. Palmer, C. G. Halgrimson, C. W. Putnam and T. E. Starzl, Immunosuppression, liver injury and hepatitis in renal, hepatic, and cardiac homograft recipients: With particular reference to the Australia antigen. *Ann. Surg. 174*: 620-639 (1971).

INTRA-HEPATIC BILIARY ATRESIA
(HEPATIC DUCTULAR HYPOPLASIA)

DANIEL ALAGILLE, M.D.

It is uncommon to discuss intrahepatic biliary atresia without extrahepatic biliary atresia. We have studied 34 children with 'intrahepatic biliary atresia' (5, 6). This condition has been described by many authors under different names (table 1), and there remains great confusion between heterogenous patterns. As the definition of this condition is only anatomical, it is necessary to be very precise about the presence or absence of ductules in portal areas. This is why a laparatomy was performed on each patient in order to confirm the patency of extrahepatic ducts as well as to obtain large surgical biopsies from the left and right lobes of the liver, permitting the study of a sufficient number of portal areas.

SYNONYMS

1. INTRAHEPATIC BILIARY ATRESIA

2. INTRAHEPATIC BILIARY PAUCITY

3. INTRAHEPATIC BILIARY HYPOPLASIA   WITH NORMAL EXTRAHEPATIC DUCTS

4. INTERLOBULAR BILIARY ATRESIA

5. HEPATIC DUCTULAR HYPOPLASIA

Table 1

Two pathologists, working independently, examined each biopsy without prior knowledge of other details or findings. Particular attention was paid to the size and number of portal areas, size and structural features of the interlobular bile ducts, evidence of pseudo ductular proliferation, amount and distribution of fibrous tissue, absence of inflammatory cell infiltrates.

The ratio of interlobular bile ducts to the number of portal areas was compared in livers from 34 patients and from 26 normal children of similar ages, and the differences evaluated statistically according to Student's T test. In 15 the evolution and histologic patterns (fig. 1) were heterogenous, especially the fibrosis. The other 19 showed a distinctly homogenous, readily recognizable clinical syndrome. This report presents the clinical, biochemical and

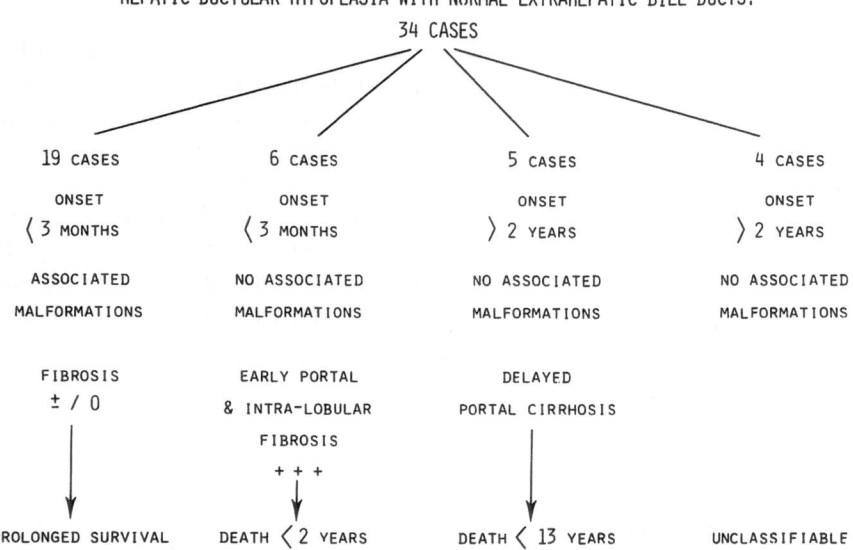

Fig. 1. Hepatic ductular hypoplasia associated with normal extrahepatic ducts: 4 different groups.

histologic features which differentiate this condition from other varieties of biliary disease. Therefore, we shall consider only this homogenous group.

PATIENTS AND METHODS

Eighteen patients were admitted for investigation of chronic cholestatic liver disease and one for growth retardation. Following a thorough evaluation of physical and developmental status, each patient, except two, underwent an exploratory laparotomy and operative cholangiography, which outlined the extrahepatic biliary passages and established their patency in every instance. This patency was verified post-mortem in one patient who did not undergo surgery.

The following laboratory determinations were made: serum bilirubin (total and direct), total lipids, cholesterol, esterified cholesterol, BSP retention, [131]I Rose Bengal fecal excretion (7), serum alkaline phosphatase, glutamic oxaloacetic transaminase, glutamic pyruvic transaminase; total serum protein electrophoresis and immunoelectrophoresis, serum albumin, clotting factors II, V, VII and X (following vitamin K loading). Other tests included routine radiograms of the chest and spinal column, electroencephalograms and electrocardiograms; 9 out of 13 patients with mid-systolic murmurs had an angiocardiography. Serum lipids were analyzed in detail in 8 patients, using previously published methods (18). Basal and post-arginine stimulation levels of growth hormone were measured in 8; testicular volume index (8) and biopsies were performed in 6 boys. Testicular function was studied by Saez and Bertrand's method (16). Serologic tests for cytomegalic inclusion disease, syphilis, rubella and toxoplasmosis were obtained in all patients. During the past 5 years, all patients have been tested for hepatitis-associated antigen. Chromosomal and dermatoglyphic analyses were performed in most.

RESULTS

General aspects
Both sexes were affected approximately equally (10 boys and 9 girls). The outstanding clinical feature of the syndrome is chronic cholestasis. Occasionally, an older patient is brought to the attention of physicians because of intense pruritus, isolated hepatomegaly or for investigation of growth retardation. The other features of the syndrome include (table 2): characteristic facies, a cardiac murmur, vertebral abnormalities, mental retardation and hypogonadism. These are discussed in the order of frequency.

1. Chronic liver disease. The earliest indication of the disease is persistent cholestasis which appears during the first 3 months of life. An unusual aspect of this cholestasis is the combination of intense pruritus with a relatively moderate elevation of serum bilirubin. The urine may be normal in color or dark; the stools may be clay-colored or may reveal the presence of bile. Hepatosplenomegaly is a constant feature; the spleen may be enlarged even in the absence of portal hypertension. Xanthomas are relatively rare, but

HEPATIC DUCTULAR HYPOPLASIA
(19 CASES).

	NO. OF CASES
CHRONIC CHOLESTASIS	19
CHARACTERISTIC FACIAL APPEARANCE	19
CARDIOVASCULAR ABNORMALITIES	13
(DEMONSTRABLE PULMONARY ARTERIAL STENOSIS)	9
VERTEBRAL ARCH DEFECTS	12
GROWTH RETARDATION	12
MENTAL RETARDATION	9
HYPOGONADISM	6

Table 2

suggest the diagnosis when distributed over the palms, extensor surfaces and body creases (fig. 2).

As the disease progresses to the second year of life, the serum bilirubin may be normal or moderately elevated (4 to 8 mg%). In contrast, serum lipid and cholesterol levels rise to extremely high values, frequently exceeding 2,000 mg% for triglycerides and ranging between 500 and 1,000 mg% for cholesterol. Alkaline phosphatase is 3 to 5-fold normal; the transaminases are less strikingly increased. The serum lipoproteins, isolated by ultracentrifugation, sediment with the low density fraction. On immunoelectrophoresis these lipoproteins are predominantly of the alpha type, while they migrate electrophoretically as beta lipoproteins (18). Thus, the serum lipid electrophoretic pattern shows a flattened or absent alpha lipoprotein peak and a sharply increased beta lipoprotein peak. Liver protein synthesis is normal, as reflected in serum 'albumin concentrations and prothrombin time after vitamin K loading. Hepatitis-associated antigen was negative in the 13 living patients.

Histologic findings. When surgical biopsies with 20 or more portal areas were available for examination, it was clear that bile ducts were absent from most portal triads, while other portal areas contained hypoplastic biliary ductules, frequently without a visible lumen (fig. 3). The ratio of interlobular bile ducts to the number of portal areas was between 0 and 0.4 compared

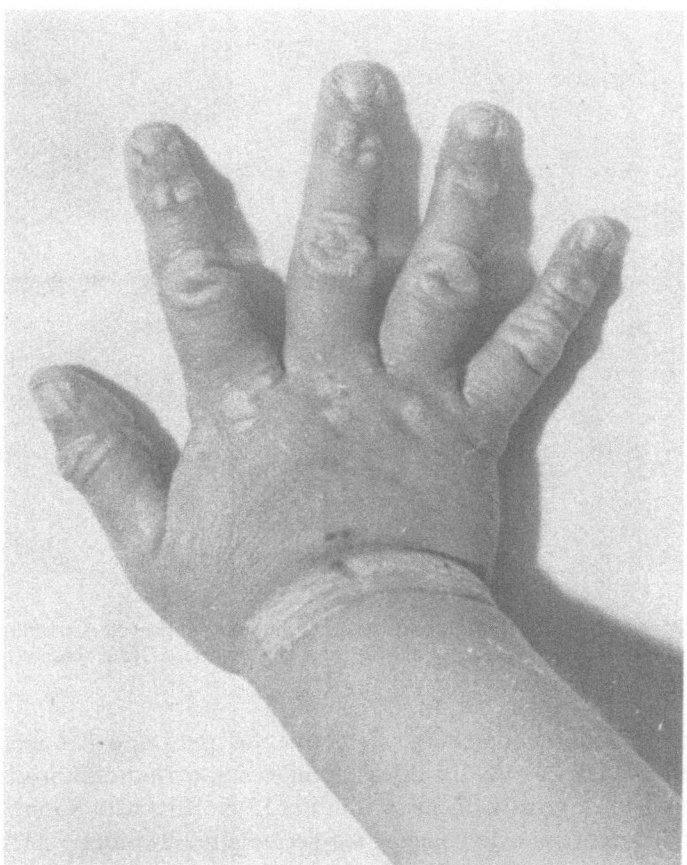

Fig. 2. Xanthomatous formations on hands.

with 0.9 and 1.8 in normal children; the difference was statistically significant (p <0.001). In 3 cases, intrahepatic biliary epithelium in numerous portal areas was altered with occasional picnotic nuclei in the cells. In each patient, the terminal branches of the hepatic artery and portal vein were always normal. However, the portal areas were less numerous than in the normal liver. Periportal fibrosis was absent or mild: intralobular fibrosis was present in but one case and numerous inflammatory cells were seen in portal areas only in another. Hepatocellular damage such as clarification and ballooning was observed particularly during the first months of life when bile stasis was prominent. Giant-cell transformation was occasionally seen unaccompanied

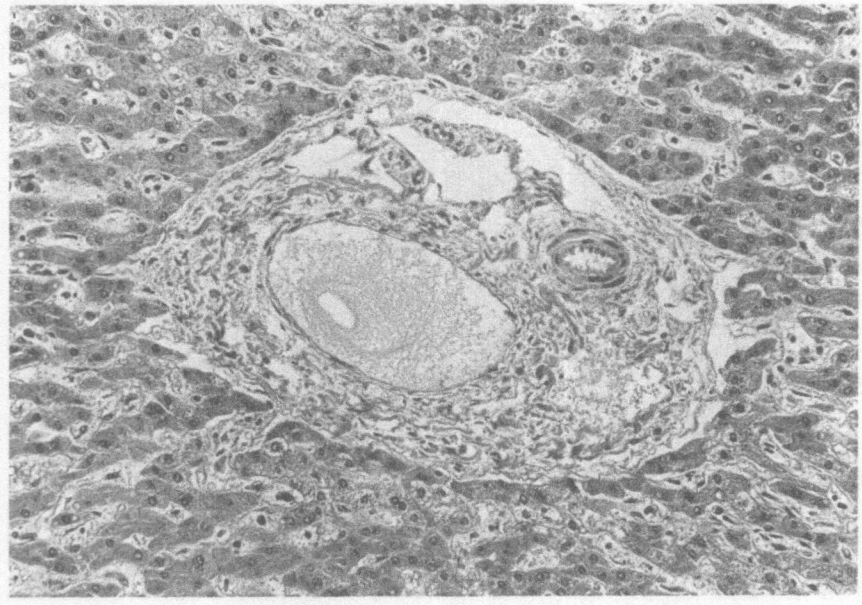

Fig. 3. Biopsy of liver (× 190). Hematoxylin eosin stain. Patient at 3 months of age. Portal area with well developed portal veins and hepatic artery. Note absence of biliary structures.

by mesenchymal reaction. Surgical biopsies of right and left lobes were histologically identical. As the disease progressed, periportal fibrosis, when present, remained grossly unchanged in the 13 patients with a long follow-up, when it was possible to compare surgical and needle biopsies. There was no evidence at any stage of the disease of progressive ductular or ductal destruction.

Two patients presented fatal septicemia at respectively 3 and 6 months of age: examination of the entire liver obtained at autopsy in both instances revealed nearly complete absence of ductules from all lobes.

The remaining 17 patients are alive and relatively well. Most are being treated with large doses of cholestyramine and additional fat-soluble vitamins, are free of pruritus and maintain almost normal concentrations of serum bilirubin, cholesterol and triglycerides. Seven patients, refractory to this form of therapy, were returned to near-normal status after cholecysto-jejunostomy. Despite these encouraging results, currently available follow-up data are still insufficiently complete to make predictions of life expectancy.

2. Characteristic facies are invariably present after the first month of life.

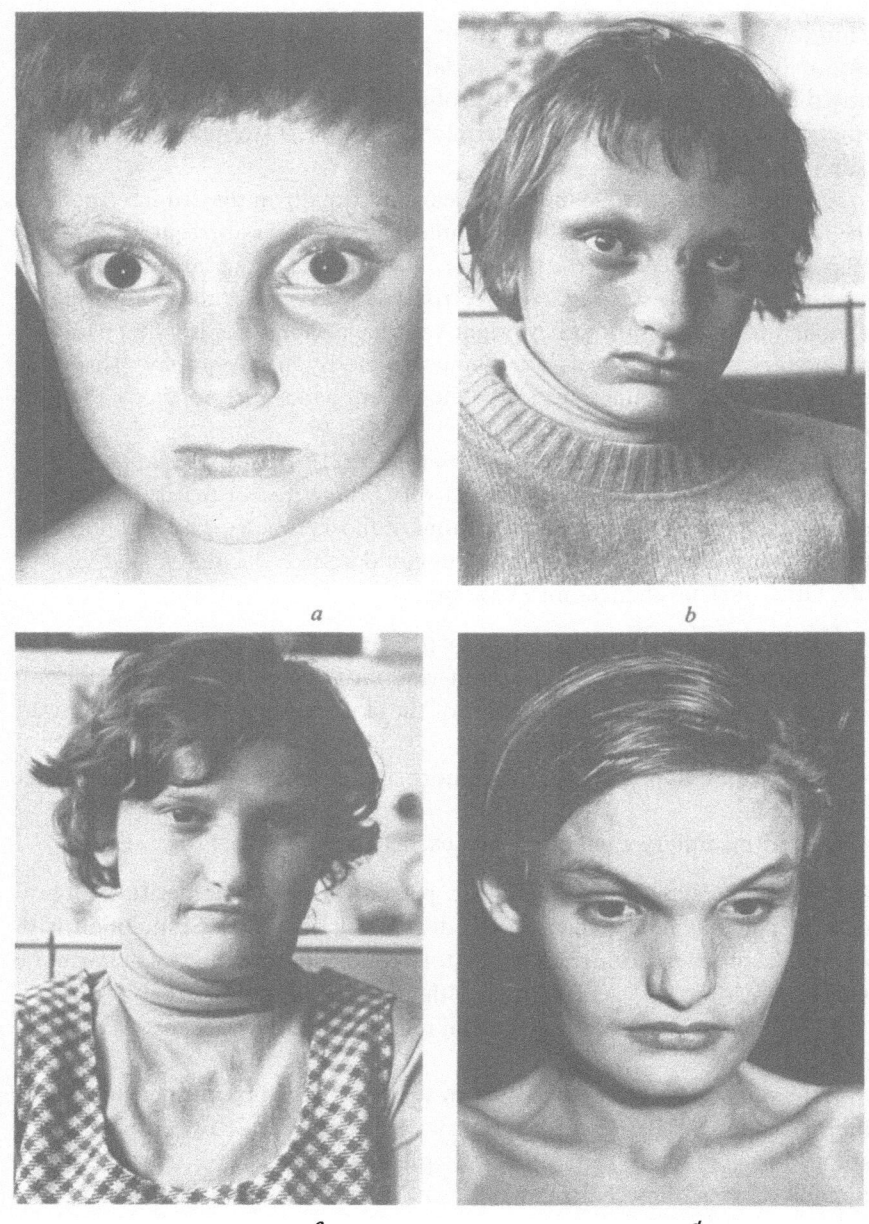

Fig. 4. Characteristic facies in patients at different ages: *a/b.* Boy at 6 years and 12 years; *c.* Girl at 13 years; *d.* Boy at 17 years.

Thus, all patients resemble each other. This characteristic aspect of the disease may reveal the diagnosis at a glance. The typical appearance is illustrated in figure 4. The forehead is prominent, eyes are set deeply and somewhat widely separated, mild hypertelorism above a straight nose, and the chin is small and pointed.

3. A harsh mid-systolic murmur, heard maximally in the 3rd interspace at the left sternal border over the pulmonic valve area, was present in 13 of the 19 patients when seen for the first time. The cardiac silhouette and lung fields were normal on chest x-ray, and electrocardiograms were normal or showed a moderate and non progressive right ventricular hypertrophy. In 9 patients, pulmonary arterial stenosis was demonstrable by arteriography. They had unimpaired cardiac functions (12). One patient had severe aortic coarctation which required surgery at the age of 6.

4. Vertebral arch defects were observed in 12 of the 19 patients. Frequently, the anterior arches of several vertebrae were not fused, resulting in one or more spina bifida defects without scoliosis (fig. 5). These abnormalities were more evident with ageing, but could be seen during the first year of life. Other skeletal changes may be seen:

- Decreased medullary-cortical ratio (6 cases); broad densification of the metaphyseal plates (fig. 6), without vitamin-D overload (7 cases); among these, 4 children had densification of the skull base and 2 of them showed calcification of the falx cerebri.
- Osteoporotic appearance, with abnormally clear and trabeculated aspect (8 cases).
- Dilated medullary cavities of metacarpal and phalanges (fig. 7).

5. Growth retardation was always present in association with vertebral defects, and was independent of the degree of cholestasis. Stimulation with arginine resulted in the highest circulatory concentrations of growth hormone (10) ever recorded by us in children with growth retardation.

6. Mild or moderately severe mental retardation (I.Q. 60 to 80) was present in 9 patients.

7. Hypogonadism was suspected in the 6 boys studied: testicular volume index was low in all; testicular biopsy was normal in 2; in 2 others, interstitial fibrous tissue proliferation was present; in the last 2, spermatogenic hypoplasia was observed (fig. 8). Plasma concentration of testosterone was low in only 1 boy. In 4 others, it was normal and human chorionic gonadotrophin stimulation induced normal response. The oldest boy in this series still shows no evidence of puberty at the age of 17. However, his bone age is

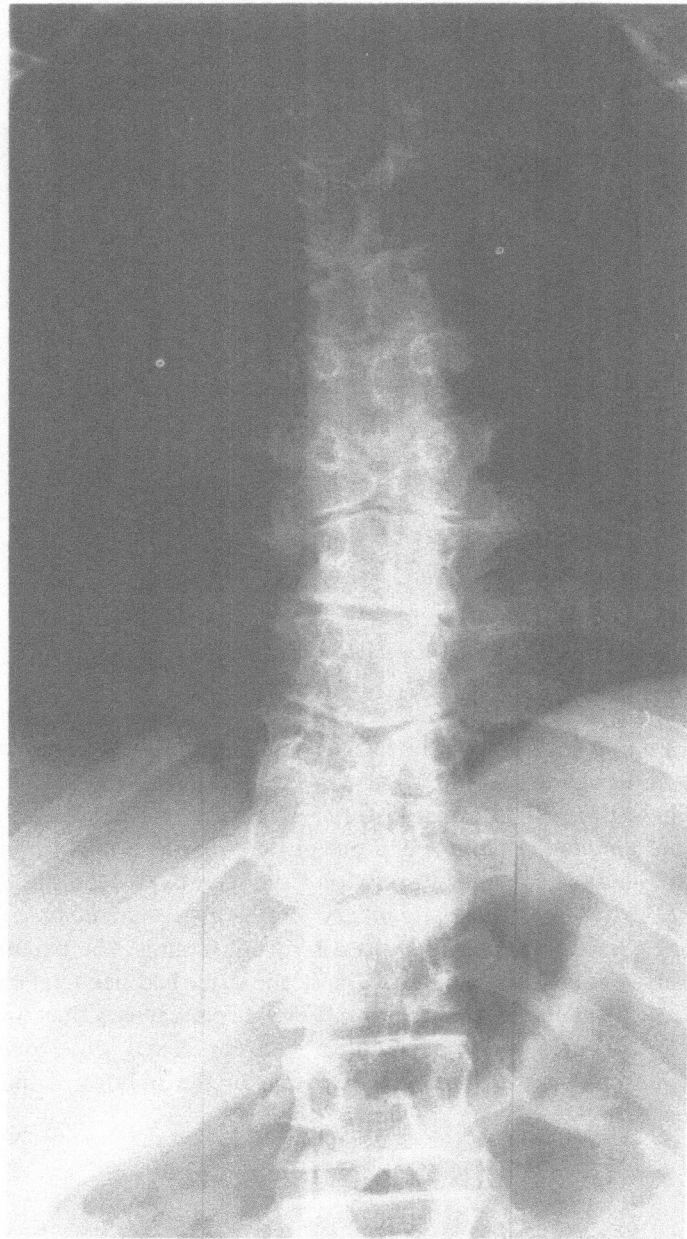

Fig. 5. Vertebral arch defects. The anterior arches of several dorsal vertebrae are not fused.

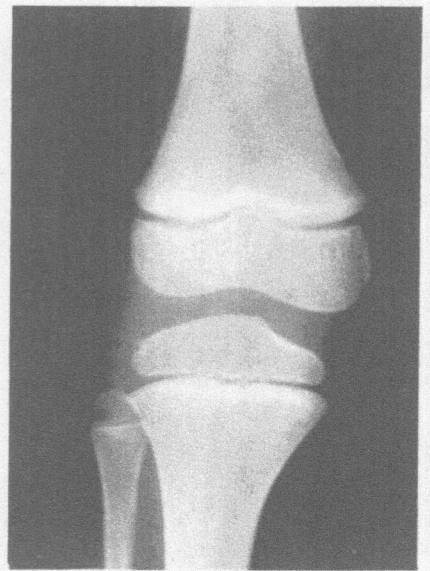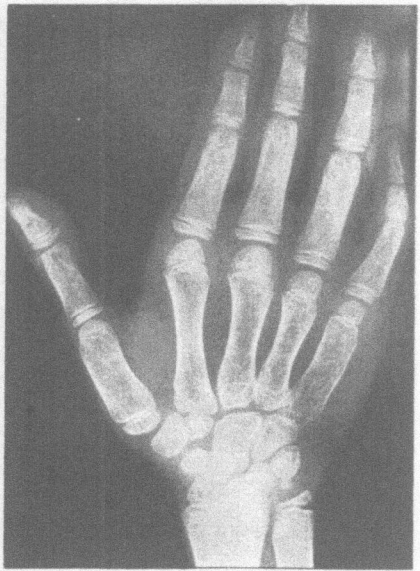

Fig. 6. Broad densification of the metaphyseal plates.
Fig. 7. Dilated medullary cavities of metacarpal and phalanges.

14 and excretion of FSH is high. One girl and one boy achieved normal puberty at the age of 12.

Familial history. The family history was positive for neonatal cholestatic conditions among the siblings of 3 out of the 19 patients (fig. 9). In 2 cases, it was possible to get some information from records of dead siblings: association of extra- or intrahepatic biliary atresia, characteristic facies, cardiac murmur, vertebral arch defects was a frequent finding. The parents of one patient are first cousins; among siblings, one sister had neonatal cholestasis until her death at 20 months: at surgery, extrahepatic biliary duct was patent. It was not possible to get any information concerning other defects. No systolic murmur was heard in either parent or the siblings of the families examined.

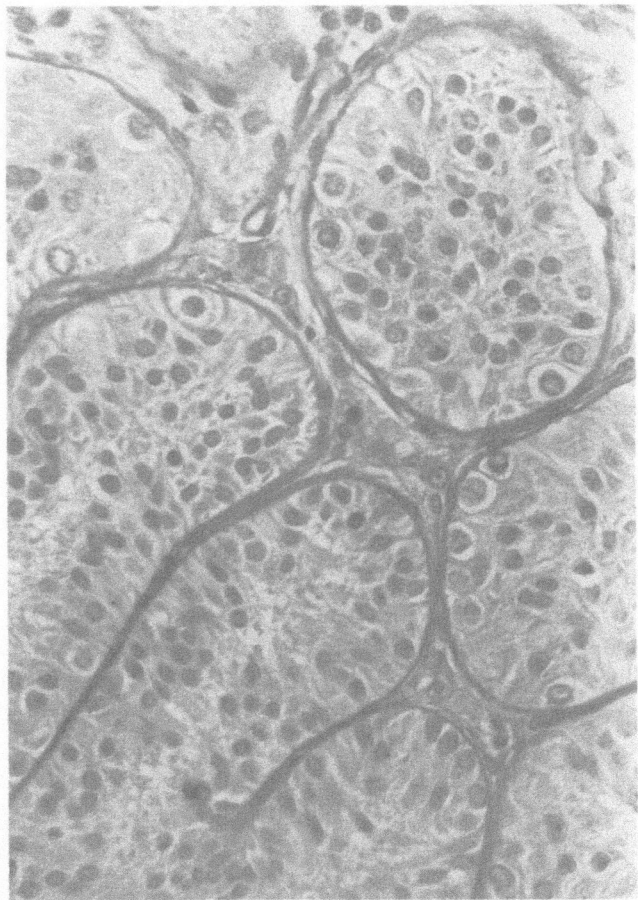

Fig. 8. Biopsy of testis (× 278). Patient at 17 years of age. Spermatogenic cells are almost completely absent.

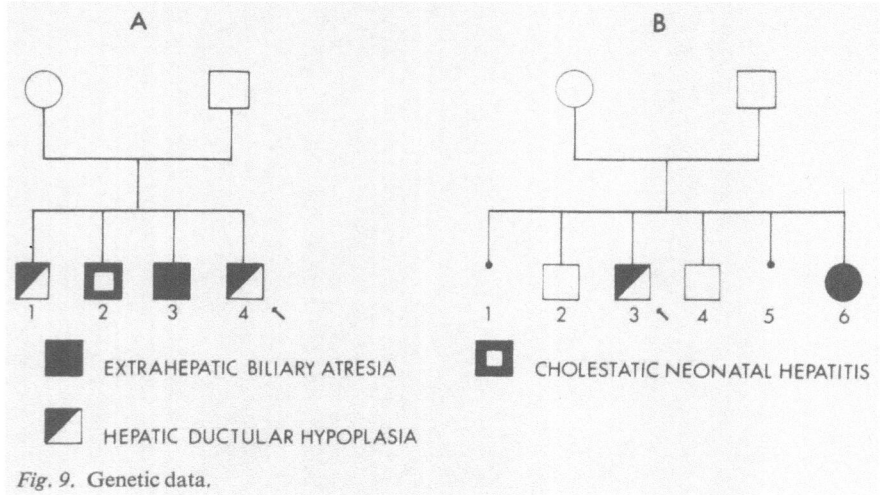

Fig. 9. Genetic data.

DISCUSSION

Defective development of hepatic bile ducts was originally described by MacMahon in 1949 (14) and histologically well studied in 1951 (2) and 1952 (3). A variety of lesions involving the interlobular bile ducts and ductules has since been recognized, reflected in terms such as 'hypoplasia of intrahepatic bile ducts', 'paucity of intrahepatic bile ducts', and 'intrahepatic biliary atresia' (13, 15). The abnormalities have been poorly classified, and their causes remain obscure. While most of these lesions are apparently congenital, the abnormal development of intrahepatic bile ducts may occasionally begin post-natally. The association of hypoplastic bile ducts with developmental abnormalities in other organs has not been previously noted. The group of 15 such patients reported here comprises approximately half the cases of intrahepatic biliary hypoplasia observed over a period of 18 years at a major center devoted exclusively to liver disease in infants and children.

Recognition of characteristic facial abnormalities has made this 'syndrome' relatively easy to diagnose and follow (5, 6). Examination of follow-up data indicated that this disorder carries a better prognosis compared with other types of intrahepatic cholestasis (1, 9). Many of these children have become relatively symptom-free, most have survived the first decade, and only 2 have died, without liver failure. However, two siblings died with extrahepatic biliary atresia and apparently normal intrahepatic biliary ducts; they had some of the associated abnormalities. These abnormalities, i.e. vertebral, cardiac and facial, can be diagnosed at birth and are not secondary to the chronic liver disease: growth retardation is only seen in association with vertebral defects and not correlated with cholestasis or other abnormalities. The cause of all these abnormalities in unclear. One can only compare the abnormal densification of the metaphyseal bands and of the skull base, the calcifications of falx cerebri associated with mental retardation and pulmonary stenosis, to those which are observed in patients with 'idiopathic hypercalcemia'.

The frequency with which similar abnormalities are present in siblings of the 15 affected children suggests a genetic disorder (2). Chromosomal and dermatoglyphic studies in these patients have yielded normal results. Infections or toxic agents, transmitted in utero from mother to one or more offspring, may also produce the teratogenic effects observed; this possibility was not studied extensively in our series.

Watson and Miller (17) reported a group of 16 patients under the term 'arteriohepatic dysplasia'. Peculiar facies, liver disease, growth retardation and vertebral defects were also noted in their series. No mention was made of mental retardation and hypogonadism. They emphasized the cardiovascular aspects; however, 11 of these 16 patients had liver diseases of various types, 3 of them hepatic ductular hypoplasia. These cases appear similar in most respects to those we first reported in the French literature (5, 6). Prospective clinical and biochemical studies of such patients and their family members may contribute towards an understanding of the etiology and pathogenesis of this collection of 'birth defects'.

REFERENCES

1. Aagenaes, Ø., C. B. van der Hagen and S. Refsum, Hereditary recurrent intrahepatic cholestasis from birth. *Arch. Dis. Childh. 43*: 646-657 (1968).
2. Ahrens, E. H., R. C. Harris and H. E. MacMahon, Atresia of the intrahepatic bile ducts. *Pediatrics 8*: 628-647 (1951).
3. Alagille, D., J. Borde, E. C. Habib, Z. Joannides, N. Thomassin et L. Kremp, Ictères cholestatiques familiaux. *Rev. int. Hépat. 8*: 701-783 (1968).
4. Alagille, D., J. Borde, E. C. Habib et N. Thomassin, Tentatives chirurgicales au cours des atrésies des voies biliaires intrahépatiques avec voie biliaire extrahépatique perméable. *Arch. franç Pédiat. 26*: 51-71 (1969).
5. Alagille, D., E. C. Habib et N. Thomassin, L'atrésie des voies biliaires intrahépatiques avec voies biliaires extrahépatiques perméables chez l'enfant. *Jour. paris. Pédiat.* 1969, pp. 301-318 (Flammarion, Paris).
6. Alagille, D., M. Odièvre, M. Gautier and J. P. Dommergues, Hepatic ductular hypo-

plasia associated with characteristic facies, vertebral malformations, retarded physical, mental and sexual development, and cardiac murmur. *J. Pediat.* *86*: 63-71 (1975).

7. Desbuquois, B., P. Tron et D. Alagille, Etude de l'excrétion fécale et urinaire de Rose Bengale marqué par l'iode radioactif au cours des ictères obstructifs du nouveau-né et du nourrisson. *Arch. franç. Pédiat. 25*: 379-391 (1968).

8. Burr, I. M., P. C. Sizonenko, S. L. Kaplan and M. M. Grumbach, Hormonal changes in puberty. Correlation of serum luteinizing hormone and follicle stimulating hormone with stages of puberty testicular size, bone age in normal boys. *Pediat. Res. 4*: 25-35 (1970).

9. Clayton, R. J., F. L. Iber, B. H. Ruebner and V. A. McKusick, Byler's disease: fatal familial intrahepatic cholestasis in an Amish kindred. *J. Pediat. 67*: 1025-1028 (1965).

10. Courtecuisse, V., J. P. Dommergues, F. Girard and J. M. Limal, *Statural growth, skeletal and endocrine abnormalities in hepatic ductular hypoplasia.* Submitted.

11. Elredge, W. J., J. B. Tingelstad, L. W. Robertson, H. P. Mauck and C. M. McCue, Observations on the natural history of pulmonary artery coarctation. *Circulation 45*: 404-409 (1972).

12. Gautier, M., D. Alagille, G. H. Watson et A. Devloo-Blancquaert, Sténose de l'artère pulmonaire et de ses branches avec hypoplasie des voies biliaires interlobulaires (un nouveau syndrome). 13th Annu. Meeting of the Association of European Paediatric Cardiologists, Marseille, 29 April-3 May, 1975.

13. Gherardi, G. J. and H. E. McMahon, Hypoplasia of terminal bile ducts. *Amer. J. Dis. Child. 120*: 151-153 (1970).

14. MacMahon, H. E. and S. J. Thannhauser, Biliary xanthomatosis. (Xanthomatous biliary cirrhosis). *Ann. intern. Med. 30*: 121-179 (1949).

15. MacMahon, H. E. and S. J. Thanhauser, Congenital dysplasia of the interlobular bile ducts with extensive skin xanthomatosis: congenital acholangic biliary cirrhosis. *Gastroenterology 21*: 488-506 (1952).

16. Saez, J. and J. Bertrand, Studies on testicular function in children: plasma concentrations of testosterone, dehydroepiandrosterone and its sulfate before and after stimulation with human chorionic gonadotrophin. *Steroids 12*: 749-761 (1968).

17. Watson, G. H. and V. Miller, Arteriohepatic dysplasia: familial pulmonary arterial stenosis with neonatal liver diseases. *Arch. Dis. Childh. 48*: 459-466 (1973).

18. Zamet, P. et B. Maitrot, Lipoprotéines sériques et atrésie des voies biliaires intra-hépatiques chez l'enfant. *Arch. franç Pédiat. 28*: 711-722 (1971).

BILE ACID SULFATION AND CHOLESTASIS

WILLIAM H. ADMIRAND, M.D.

Cholestasis is a pathologic process characterized by inability to secrete compounds into bile. It may be caused by diseased states which damage the hepatic parenchymal cell, the biliary ducts or both. Regardless of the etiology or the site of the lesion, cholestasis produces profound alterations in bile acid metabolism with elevated concentrations of these compounds in peripheral blood and tissues.

Bile acids are detergents which can dissolve membrane structures. Retention of bile acids in cholestatic liver disease could result in concentrations of these compounds in body fluid and tissue adequate to produce membrane damage. For example, in vitro studies have shown that lysosomal membranes are disrupted when bile acid concentration exceeds 0.5 mM (12). This amount of bile acid is occasionally present in serum of patients with severe cholestasis. The pathophysiologic significance of increased bile acid concentrations has not yet been established. However, it is possible that accumulation of these compounds in patients with cholestasis could lead to further liver damage.

Until recently bile acids were thought to be metabolic end-products. The first indication that these compounds underwent further structural modification was observed in patients with cholelithiasis (7). In these patients significant amounts of radioactive labeled lithocholic acid in bile was converted to a more polar metabolite. This polar metabolite was identified as the 3-alpha sulfate ester of lithocholate. Subsequently, it has been shown that 40-75 percent of all lithocholate in normal bile is sulfated (9).

The metabolism of bile acid sulfates is significantly different from that of nonsulfated bile acids. In animals, the fractional intestinal absorption of conjugated lithocholate sulfate is less than that of conjugated nonsulfated lithocholate (4). Moreover, renal excretion of conjugated lithocholate sulfate is significantly greater than excretion of conjugated, nonsulfated lithocholate(8).

We first became aware that sulfation might also be important in the metabolism of other bile acids during a study of bile acid kinetics in a patient with intrahepatic cholestasis. In this patient it was found that a large portion of the orally administered radioactive bile acids were excreted in urine. Following enzymatic hydrolysis of taurine and glycine conjugated bile acids, most of the radioactivity in urine could not be extracted into ether with the free bile salt fraction. Thin-layer chromatography indicated that the non-extractable fraction was more polar than cholate or chenodeoxycholate.

We synthesized chenodeoxycholate and cholate sulfates chemically and compared their properties with the bile salt metabolites extracted from the urine of our patient. These studies showed that the further analysis of these polar metabolites were sulfate esters of cholate and chenodeoxycholate (11). It was found that approximately 75 percent of the bile acids present in urine were sulfated (table 1). Analysis of simultaneously obtained serum samples revealed only trace quantities of bile acid sulfates (table 2). Thus, the apparent renal clearance of sulfated bile acids was many times greater than the clearance of nonsulfated bile acids (table 3).

We next extended these findings to patients with alcoholic liver disease (10). These patients also excreted large amounts of bile acid sulfates in urine.

Table 1. Urinary excretion of sulfated and nonsulfated bile acids.

	Cholate (mg/24 hrs)	Chenodeoxycholate (mg/24 hrs)	Total bile acids (mg/24 hrs)
Nonsulfated	5.3 ± 1.3	0.7 ± 0.1	6.0 ± 1.1
Sulfated	8.2 ± 1.6	10.6 ± 2.6	18.8 ± 3.8
Total	13.5 ± 1.4	11.3 ± 1.4	24.8 ± 2.4

All values represent the mean of duplicate determinations on 5 consecutive days ± SEM.

Table 2. Serum concentrations of sulfated and nonsulfated bile acids.

	Cholate (μg/ml)	Chenodeoxycholate (μg/ml)	Total bile acids (μg/ml)
Nonsulfated	98.8 ± 8.1	33.1 ± 2.5	131.9 ± 10.7
Sulfated	1.2 ± 0.1	5.5 ± 0.4	6.7 ± 0.5
Total	100.0 ± 4.1	38.6 ± 1.5	138.6 ± 5.8

All values represent the mean of duplicate determinations on 5 consecutive days ±SEM.

Table 3. Renal clearance of sulfated and nonsulfated bile acids.

	Cholate (ml/24 hrs)	Chenodeoxycholate (ml/24 hrs)	Total bile acids (ml/24 hrs)
Nonsulfated	54	21	45
Sulfated	6800	1900	2800

The apparent renal clearance of bile acid sulfates was again several hundred-fold higher than that of nonsulfated bile acids (table 4). On the basis of

Table 4. Renal bile acid clearance.

	Deoxycholate	Chenodeoxycholate	Cholate
Patient 1			
Bile acid	77	29	234
Bile acid sulfate	2,000	5,625	5,250
Patient 2			
Bile acid	59	73	279
Bile acid sulfate	4,000	14,375	14,600

findings in the patient with intrahepatic cholestasis and the patients with alcoholic liver disease it appeared that sulfation was an important metabolic process which could lead to extensive urinary and fecal excretion of bile acids. Despite the potential pathophysiologic significance of bile acid sulfation, the site and mechanism by which these sulfates are formed was unknown. We therefore undertook a study to isolate and characterize an enzyme or group of enzymes capable of catalyzing the formation of bile acid sulfates. Utilizing a reaction mixture containing buffer, taurolithocholate, and 3' phosphoadenosine 5' phosphosulfate (PAPS*), we examined a number of tissue extracts for enzyme activity. When the supernatant fraction from rat liver and kidney were placed in the incubation media a radioactive product was formed which was more polar than taurolithocholate. This product was subsequently identified as the 3-alpha sulfate ester of taurolithocholate. The relative enzyme activities in the various tissues are shown in table 5.

The enzyme was further purified by Sephadex gel-filtration. It was found that the rate of taurolithocholate sulfation was linear with respect to enzyme concentration and to time of incubation. Enzyme activity could readily be

Table 5. Cholylsulfokinase activity in the supernatant preparations of various rat tissues.

Tissue	Units/g protein $\times$ 10^{-2}	Units/g tissue $\times$ 10^{-2}
Brain	0	0
Heart	0	0
Kidney	1.8	94
Liver	3.7	136
Spleen	0	0
Intestinal Mucosa	0	0

* PAPS is a natural product formed from adenosine triphosphate which serves as a sulfate donor in a number of biological sulfations.

detected with a protein concentration of 10 micrograms of cytoplasmic protein. Lineweaver-Burk plots of reaction rates with various concentrations of taurolithocholate and PAPS indicated that the km for taurolithocholate was 5×10^{-5}M. and for PAPS 8×10^{-6}M.

We next determined the effect of enzyme inhibitors on cholylsulfokinase activity (table 6). Enzyme activity was completely inhibited by 1 mM para-

Table 6. Effect of enzyme inhibitors on cholylsulfokinase activity. Inhibition of bile acid sulfation is expressed as percent of control.

Inhibitors (mM)	Inhibition (%)
Parachloromercuribenzoate	100
3′ Phosphoadenosine 5′ Phosphate	100
Adenosine Triphosphate	45
Ethylenediamine Tetraacetic Acid	28
Sodium Azide	33
Sodium Fluoride	27

chloromercuribenzoate and by PAPS. In contrast, the other general enzyme inhibitors tested showed only partial inhibition at concentrations of 1 mM. Inhibition of the reaction by parachloromercuribenzoate indicates the requirement of free thiol groups for enzyme activity. The requirement of a sulfhydryl group to achieve full activity seems to be a general property of sulfokinases and has previously been demonstrated with estrogen sulfokinases and choline sulfokinase (1, 6).

The requirement of metal ions for sulfokinases has been a matter of controversy. Some investigators have shown increased estrogen sulfokinase activity in the presence of magnesium, whereas other studies have failed to show this effect (1, 3). This discrepancy may be due to differences in the degree of enzyme purification in these studies. Although an absolute requirement for metal ions was not demonstrated in our study, the bile salt sulfating enzyme (cholylsulfokinase) was partially inhibited by the chelating agent ethylenediamine tetraacetic acid.

It has been established that there are several sulfokinases specific for the formation of different steroid sulfates. At least 3 such enzymes have been identified in rabbit liver (5). It remains to be determined whether the enzyme responsible for bile salt sulfation is a single entity or a related group of enzymes. However, cholylsulfokinase appears to be distinct from the hepatic enzyme which sulfate phenol and estrogen. Cholylsulfokinase has a molecular weight of approximately 130,000 while the enzyme of enzymes responsible for estrogen and phenol sulfation have molecular weights of approximately 76,000. Moreover, it is likely that cholylsulfokinase is different from previously described steroid sulfokinases in view of the difference in the stereo-configuration of bile acids as compared to neutral steroids.

It has been generally accepted that sulfation of steroids occurs predominantly in liver, although sulfation of neutral steroids in intestinal wall as well as adrenal gland has been demonstrated (2). In our studies a survey of rat tissues revealed that cholylsulfokinase activity was present in rat liver and kidney, but it was not detected in other tissues examined. The presence of sulfokinase activity in rat kidney raises a question of whether renal excretion of bile salt sulfate is due to renal clearance or may arise in part from de novo synthesis and excretion by the kidney.

The identification and preliminary characterization of an enzyme capable of sulfating bile salts provides a tool by which we can investigate and evaluate the importance of bile salt sulfation in the overall picture of cholestatic liver disease.

REFERENCES

1. Adams, J. B. and A. Poulos, Enzymatic synthesis of steroid sulphates. 3. Isolation and properties of estrogen sulphotransferase of bovine adrenal glands. *Biochim. biophys. Acta 146*: 493-508 (1967).
2. Baulieu, E. E., C. Corpéchot, C. F. Dray et al., An adrenal secreted 'androgen': dehydroisoandrosterone sulphate. Its metabolism and a tentative generalization on the metabolism of other steroid conjugates in man. *Recent Progr. Hormone Res. 21*: 411-500 (1965).
3. Hilz, H. and F. Lipman, The enzymatic activation of sulfate. *Proc. nat. Acad. Sci. (Wash.) 41*: 880-890 (1955).
4. Low-Beer, T. S., M. P. Tyor and L. Lack, Effects of sulfation of taurolithocholic and glycolithocholic acids on their intestinal transport. *Gastroenterology 56*: 721-726 (1969).
5. Nose, Y. and F. Lipmann, Separation of steroid sulfokinase. *J. biol. Chem. 233*: 1348-1351 (1958).
6. Orsi, B. A. and B. Spencer, Choline sulphokinase (sulphotransferase). *J. Biochem. (Tokyo) 56*: 81-91 (1964).
7. Palmer, R. H., The transformation of bile acid sulfates: a new pathway of bile acid metabolism in humans. *Proc. nat. Acad. Sci. (Wash.) 58*: 1047-1050 (1967).
8. Palmer, R. H., Bile acid sulfates. 2. Formation, metabolism, and bile excretion of lithocholic acid sulfates in the rat. *J. Lipid Res. 12*: 680-687 (1971).
9. Palmer, R. H. and M. G. Bolt, Bile acid sulfates. 1. Synthesis of lithocholic acid sulfates and their identification in human bile. *J. Lipid Res. 12*: 671-679 (1971).
10. Stiehl, A., D. L. Earnest and W. H. Admirand, Sulfation and renal excretion of bile salts in patients with cirrhosis of the liver. *Gastroenterology 68*: 534-544 (1975).
11. Stiehl, A., M. M. Thaler and W. H. Admirand, Formation and excretion of bile salt sulfates: An important metabolic pathway in cholestasis. *Hormones Metab. Res. suppl. 4*: 49-51 (1974).
12. Weissmann, G., Studies of lysosomes. 6. The effect of neutral steroids and bile acids on lysosomes in vitro. *Biochem. Pharmacol. 14*: 525-535 (1965).

CONGENITAL CHOLESTASIS:
CLINICAL AND ULTRASTRUCTURAL STUDY*

WILLIAM K. SCHUBERT, M.D.,
JACQUELINE S. PARTIN, M.S., JOHN C. PARTIN, M.D.

Byler's disease is a recessively inherited form of progressive intrahepatic cholestasis first described by Clayton in an extensive Amish kindred descended from Jacob Byler born in the United States in 1799 (2). Clinical manifestations are steatorrhea, conjugated hyperbilirubinemia which is initially intermittent and later persistent, pruritus, and hepatosplenomegaly. Alkaline phosphatase is elevated but serum cholesterol is normal. Serum bile acid levels are elevated and an increased level of lithocholic acid has been described in one patient. The transport maximum (Tm) for bromsulphalein and storage capacity (S) are both reduced. The liver architecture early in the disease is normal and normal numbers of interlobular bile ducts are present (6). Progressive hepatic cirrhosis occurs; the longest survivor was 14 3/12 years of age and had severe cirrhosis and mental and physical retardation (6). Defective excretion of conjugated bile salts and bilirubin across the canalicular membrane has been postulated (2, 6).

Strictly the term Byler's disease should be reserved for blood relatives of the original family known to have the same as yet unknown genetic defect. This paper presents a case study of a girl with a similar cholestatic syndrome who is unrelated to the Byler family.

CASE REPORT

M.B. is now 17 years of age. She was the product of a full-term pregnancy and normal delivery. The mother had no liver disease and no pruritus during the pregnancy. The neonatal period was uncomplicated but at 6 months of age, large, pale colored but not acholic stools were first observed and have persisted. Pruritus without jaundice began at 9 months of age and enlargement of the liver 5 cm below the right costal margin at 18 months of age. At

* This work was supported in part by U.S. Public Health Service Grant RR-00123 from the General Clinical Research Centers Branch, National Institutes of Health.

12 months of age, jaundice was first noted. An operative cholangiogram was normal. The liver was large, soft, and smooth. The serum bilirubin was 4.8 mgm% total and 2.8 mgm% direct reacting. SGOT was 79 units and prothrombin time 13.5 seconds (75%). Additional serum chemistries are presented in table 1. Serum bilirubin levels, and transaminase levels in relation to therapy are presented in figure 1.

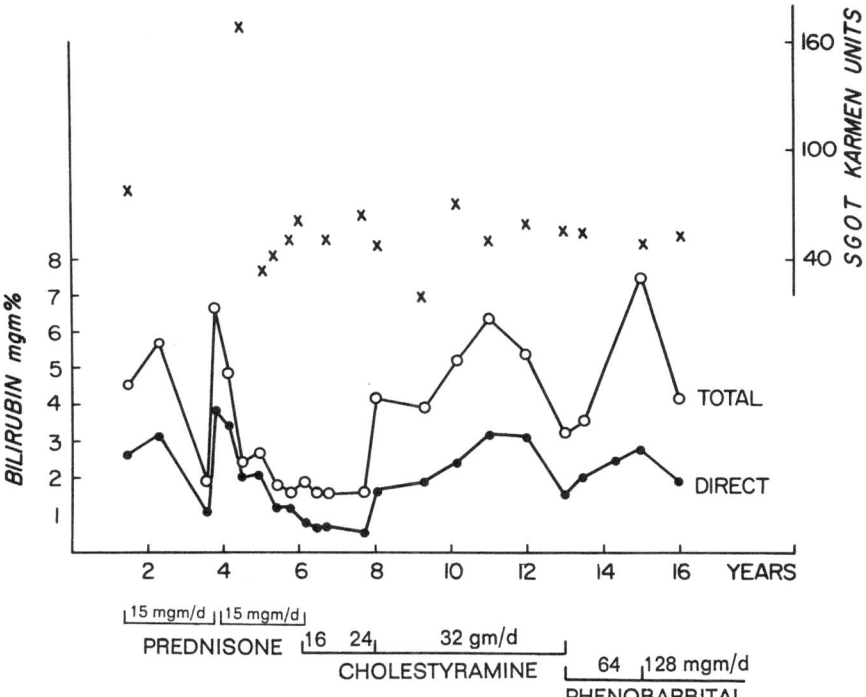

Fig. 1. Serum bilirubin and serum glutamic-oxaloacetic transaminase levels in relation to therapy during the 16 year period of observation.

When examined initially in Cincinnati Children's Hospital (age 6 years) she was cushinoid from previous steroid therapy and retarded in growth. Pruritus was severe with constant scratching and secondary thickening of the skin. The liver was enlarged 8 cm below the right costal margin. Icterus was not present. Neurologic examination and intelligence were normal. The fingers were short and stubby, and the facial features coarse. A radiopaque cholesterol gallstone was present and cholecystectomy and liver biopsy were

Table 1.

Age year	Bilirubin Total mgm %	Direct mgm %	SGOT K.units	SGPT K.units	Total protein gm %	Albumin gm %	Alkaline phosphatase Bodansky Units	Cholesterol mgm %	Triglyceride mgm %
6	1.9	.7	63	42	6.9	3.9	10.5	226	
6½	1.6	.8	45	27	7.3	3.8	23	171	190
8	4.1	1.7	48	20	7.9	3.9	11.7	208	
10	5.2	2.4	70	30	7.9	4.3	13.2		
11	6.4	3.2	50	36	6.4	3.2	15.6	160	
12	5.4	3.1	60	47	6.9	3.7	19.5	227	186
13	3.3	16.	56	32	7.5	3.6	12.8	206	
15	7.5	3.8	48	31			25.6	223	
16	5.2	2.4	51	32	8.9	9.1	18.8	251	

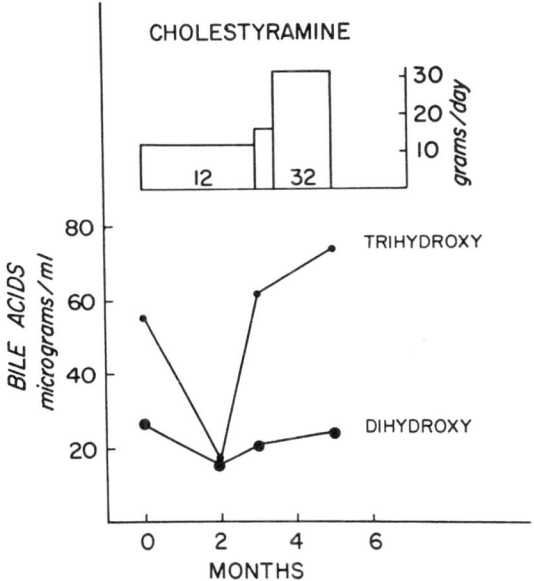

Fig. 2. Cholestyramine therapy. No significant fall in bile acid levels occurred despite large doses of cholestyramine (32 gm/day).

performed. Prednisone was stopped and cholestyramine therapy begun. Cholestyramine therapy had no effect on pruritus or serum bile acid levels (fig. 2). The liver remained enlarged 5-8 cm below the costal margin for the five years of cholestyramine therapy. Phenobarbital was then substituted for cholestyramine but with doses up to 128 mgm% daily no effect on pruritus or jaundice was noted although the liver size decreased to 2 cm below the costal margin during phenobarbital therapy.

At 10 years of age, clumsy movements were noted and at 11 years of age neurologic examination revealed bilateral ptosis, cerebellar ataxia and hyporeflexia. On repeated psychologic examination, her full scale I.Q. varied from 74-80. There was no progression of the neurologic signs from age 11 to age 16. The cerebrospinal fluid protein, cell count, colloidal gold, and chemistry were normal and the etiology of the central nervous system degeneration has not been found.

When last examined at 16 years of age, she was in the 25th percentile for height and weight. Moderate jaundice, thickened, leathery skin secondary to pruritus, enlargement of the liver 2 cm below the costal margin, bilateral ptosis, cerebellar ataxia and moderate mental retardation were the positive findings. She has never developed skin xanthoma or had significant hypercholesterolemia.

Ceruloplasmin level was 79 mgm%, alpha$_1$-antitrypsin 280 mgm%, both normal. Mild steatorrhea (15% excretion of ingested fat) was present prior to cholestyramine therapy. On cholestyramine therapy (32 gm/day), steatorrhea increased (79% of the ingested fat per day). Serum trihydroxy bile acids were 55.4 μgm/ml and dihydroxy bile acids 27.8 μgm/ml (normal 0-3.5- and 0-1.9 μgm/ml) (1). Bromsulphalein clearance measured by the method of Wheeler demonstrated a Tm of −2.60 mgm/minute and relative storage capacity (S) of 61.5 mgm/mgm% (normal Tm = 8.6±1.9 mgm/min., S = 63±25 mgm/mgm%) (9).

HISTOPATHOLOGY OF THE LIVER

Light microscopy early in the 11 year period of observation showed normal bile ducts, slight expansion of the portal areas, with minimal round cell infiltrate, minimal disruption of liver cell cords with numerous binucleate cells and bile stasis in hepatocytes and bile canaliculi. Similar findings were present in multiple liver biopsies obtained from 1964-74. Portal round cell infiltrate increased and mild septal fibrosis appeared but cirrhosis did not occur. Distorted hepatic cell cords and multinucleated hepatocytes increased in number but severe disruption of hepatic architecture did not occur. In all specimens, faintly eosinophilic inclusion bodies were present in central and midzonal hepatocytes.

ULTRASTRUCTURAL STUDY

Portions of seven liver biopsy specimens obtained during the past eight years of observation on both cholestyramine and phenobarbital therapy were studied after fixation as previously described (8). Except for a change in qualitative appearance of the canalicular bile while on phenobarbital therapy all specimens were similar in appearance with no change in relation to therapy or clinical condition. Toluidine blue stained plastic embedded sections showed thickening of the hepatocyte cell plate, normal bile ducts (fig. 3a) and bile stasis in hepatocytes and numerous peroxisomes in the centrolobular zone (fig. 3b). Hepatocytes contained numerous large lamellar arrays of smooth

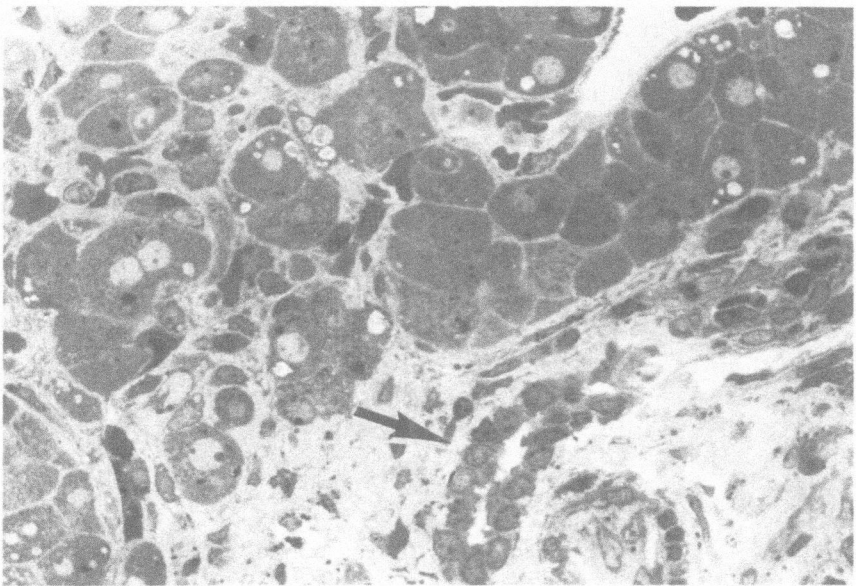

Fig. 3. a. Light micrograph of toludine blue 0 stained plastic thick section. Portal space with a normal duct (arrow). The liver cell plate is thickened and bile stasis is present in hepatocytes. (Magnification 536×)

endoplasmic reticulum (SER) along which alpha glycogen particles were regularly arranged producing a fingerprint-like pattern (fig. 4). These SER fingerprint bodies corresponded to the faintly eosinophilic inclusions visible by light microscopy with hematoxylin eosin stain and seen in the plastic embedded thick sections stained with toluidine blue (fig. 1). Numerous mitochondria had irregular vacuoles which were formed by dilatation of the intracristal space (fig. 4, 5a). The mitochondrial lesion differed from other nonspecific lesions present in cholestasis of various types such as curling of cristae and circular cristae which were also present in this patient. Other nonspecific findings, such as enlarged and abnormally shaped mitochondria with paracrystalline inclusions as illustrated by mitochondria from a patient with benign recurrent cholestasis were not observed (fig. 5b). The bile canaliculi had no thickening of the canalicular ectoplasm. The lumina were dilated and contained fine granular material while on cholestyramine therapy (fig. 6). Phenobarbital therapy was associated with a striking increase in osmophilic density of the canalicular bile plugs which were composed of curvilinear fibrillar material resembling phospholipid (fig. 7). The microvilli of the canal-

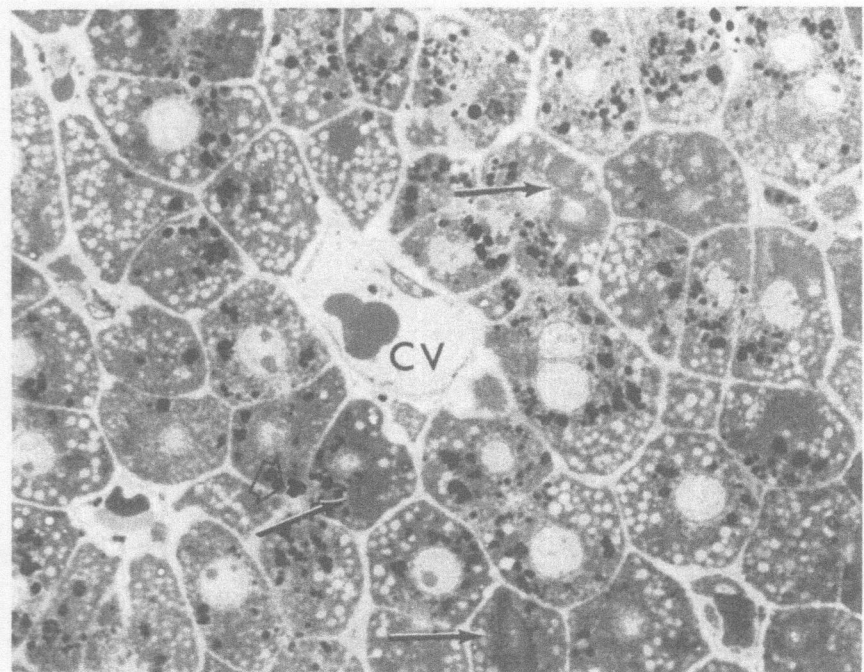

Fig. 3. *b*. **Central vein (CV) area; hepatocytes contain numerous peroxisomes (clear vacuoles) and a canalicular bile plug is visible directly below the central vein (open arrow). Smooth endoplasmic reticulum glycogen fingerprint bodies are visible (arrows). (Magnification 848 ×)**

iculi were occasionally edematous but never occluded the lumen. The Golgi apparatus was uniformly active (fig. 7). Ductular proliferation did not occur by light microscopy and was not observed by electron microscopy. The lumina of the preductular structures (Hering canals) were filled with granular material; the Hering canal cells contained a large amount of intracellular material (fig. 8). The bile duct epithelium was normal; the Hering canal cells had degenerative changes. The small bile ducts were empty and appeared histologically normal (fig. 9).

In summary, the ultrastructure of the liver showed a persistent but relatively nonprogressive lesion characterized by abnormal mitochondria not previously reported in cholestasis, dilated bile canaliculi, Hering canals filled with bile and empty normal small bile ducts all consistent with ineffective secretion of bile beyond the preductual structure. Consistent alteration in the ultrastructure of the bile appeared with phenobarbital therapy.

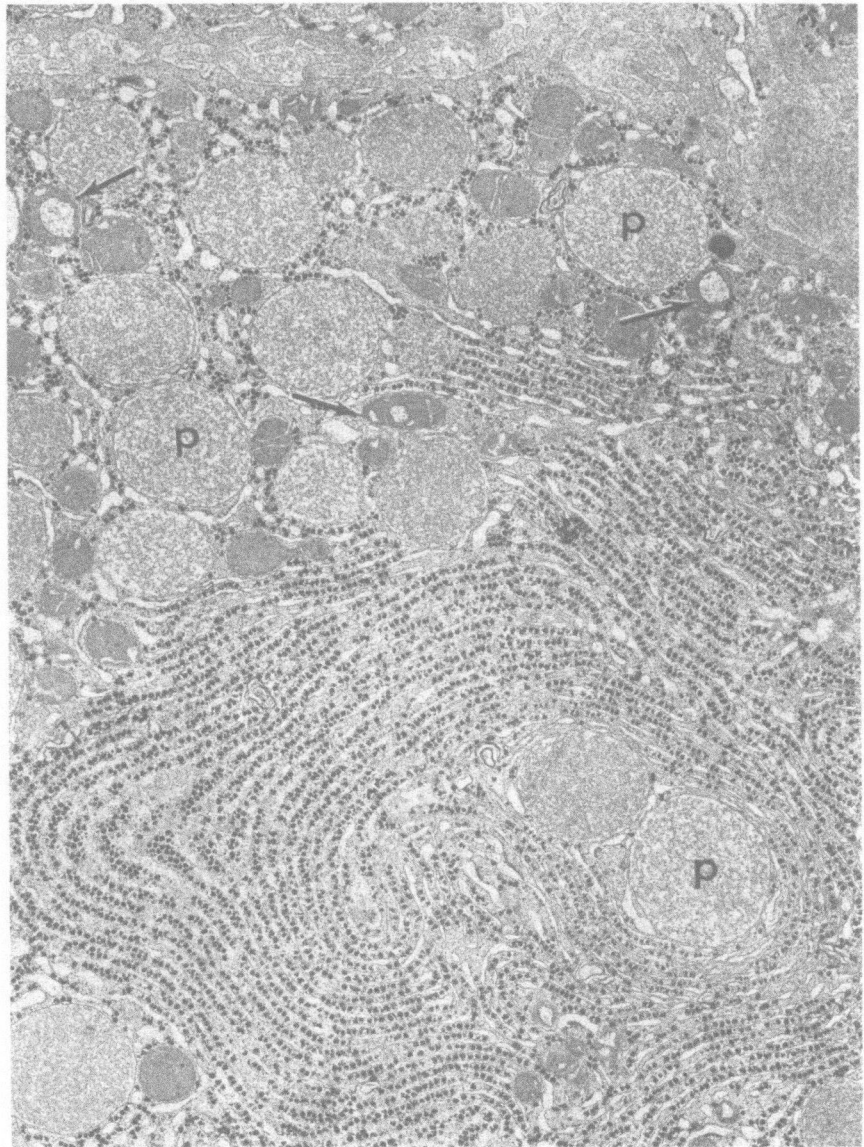

Fig. 4. Hepatocyte showing glycogen fingerprints, numerous large peroxisomes (p), and mitochondria with enlarged intracristal space (arrows). Although this specimen was taken while on phenobarbital therapy, similar findings were present in all specimens. (Magnification 12,017 ×)

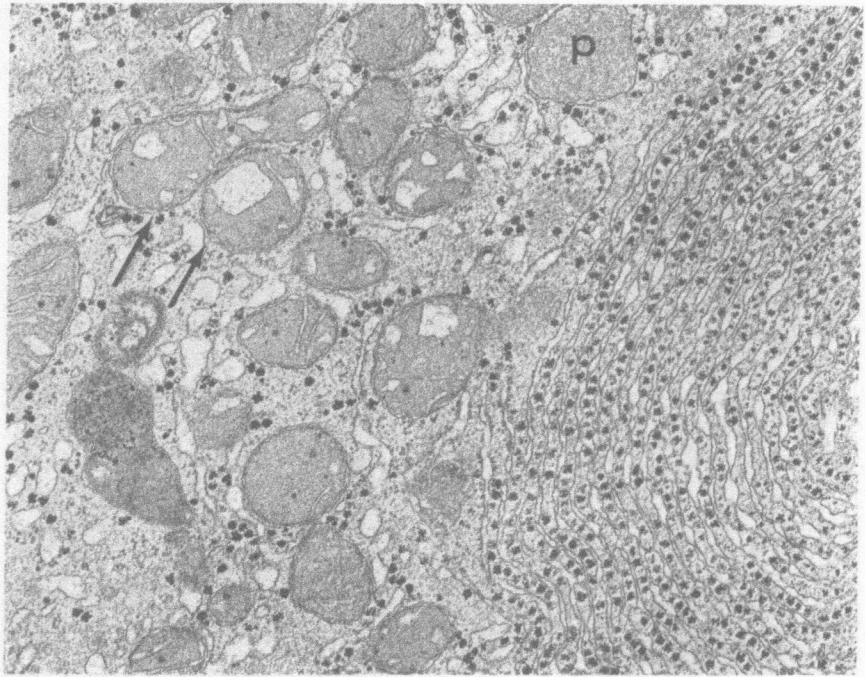

Fig. 5a. The patient M.B. Numerous mitochondria have dilated intracristal spaces containing flocculent material (arrow); p: peroxisomes. (Magnification 27,499 ×)

Several cholestatic syndromes resembling Byler's disease have been de
scribed (4, 5, 10, 3, 7). Characteristic of all of these syndromes is chronic
cholestasis, serum bile acid elevation, defective bile acid excretion with consequent steatorrhea, and growth retardation. Lithocholic acid elevation in
the serum and bile has been demonstrated in the patient described by Williams as well as in Byler's disease (6, 10). The present patient resembles the
variant described by Juberg in that mental retardation, peculiar facies and
neurologic disease were present but differs in that the level of serum cholesterol was not elevated and paucity of interlobular bile ducts has not been
observed after 17 years (5). She resembles the patients described by Williams
in that pruritus secondary to bile acid elevation preceded jaundice by 3
months and the Tm bromsulfalein was low with only moderate reduction of
storage capacity (10). She differs from all three groups in that at 17 years of
age cirrhosis is minimal. It seems likely that multiple familial cholestatic
syndromes exist associated with as yet poorly defined defects in bile acid

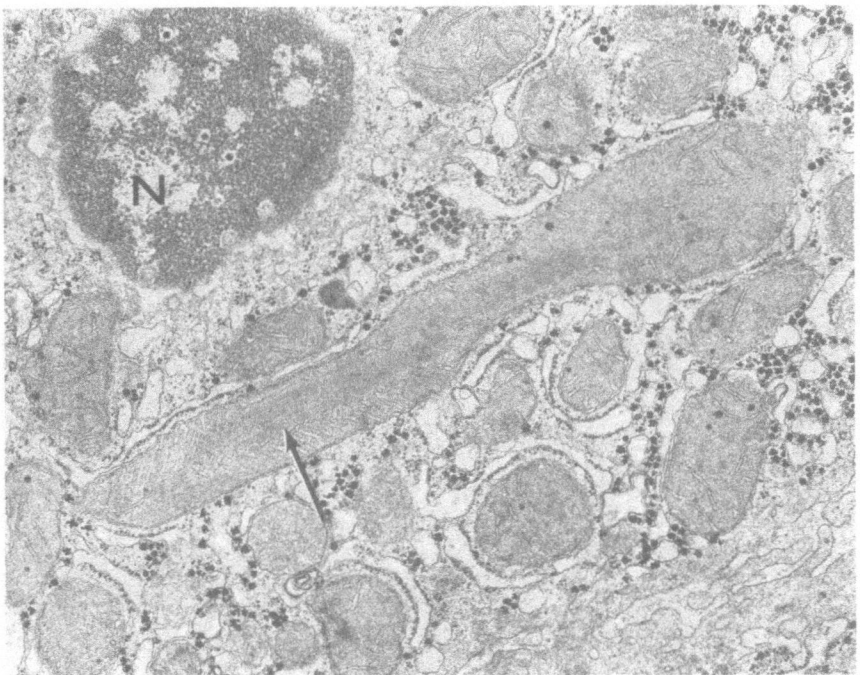

Fig. 5b. A specimen from a patient with benign recurrent cholestasis. A mitochondrion is elongated, contains long crystalline arrays and has peculiar arrangement of cristae (arrow). (Magnification 16,250 ×) N: nucleus.

metabolism. To date, the ultrastructural studies presented of these syndromes have been limited. Coarse particulate bile, thickening of canalicular ectoplasm and fusion of microvilli have been described in Byler's disease (2, 6) and similar canalicular alterations in the patient described by Williams (10). The mitochondrial lesion and the Hering canal – bile ductule abnormality observed in our patient have not been described. Although many of the ultrastructural findings of cholestasis are nonspecific, detailed and sequential electron microscopic studies of such patients may produce distinctive patterns of abnormalities which will anatomically characterize syndromes eventually to be defined by delineation of a specific biochemical defect.

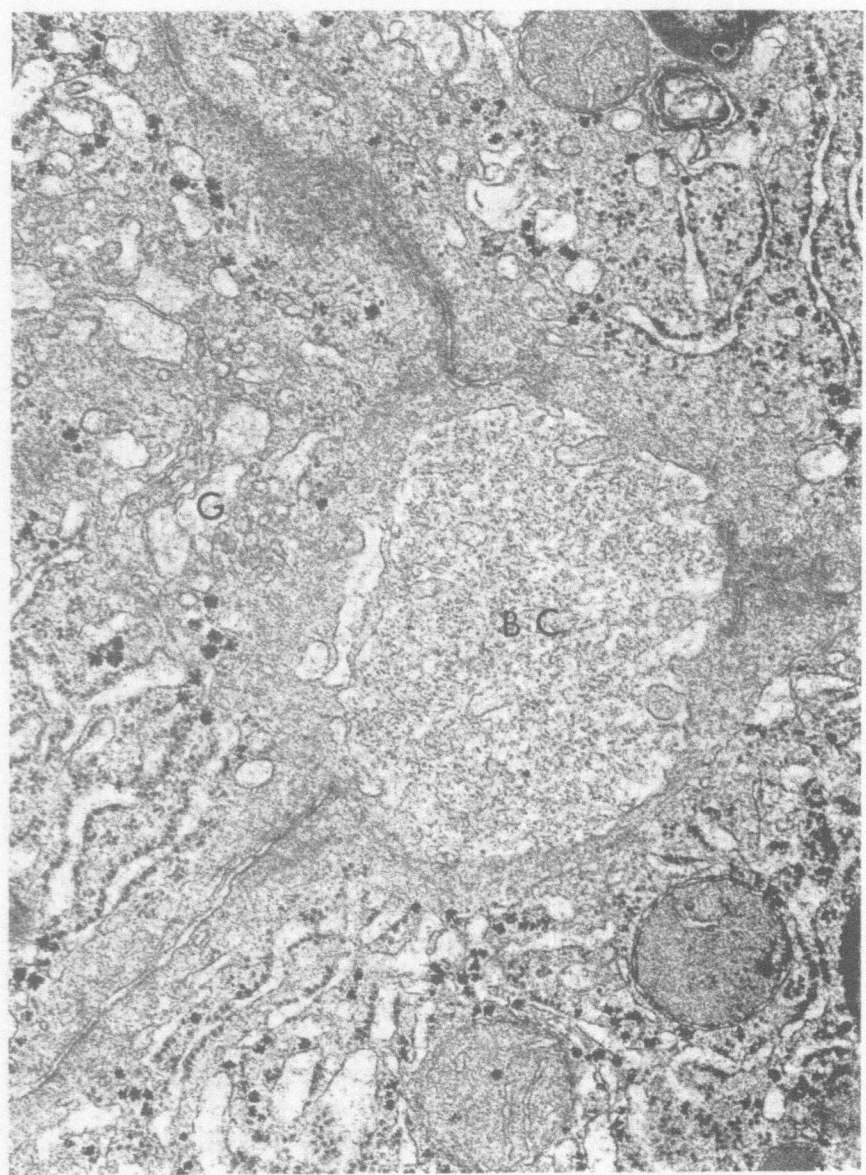

Fig. 6. Bile canaliculus (BC) while on cholestyramine. The canaliculus is dilated, the peri-canalicular ectoplasm is not thickened and the lumen contains fine granular material. The Golgi (G) is active. (Magnification 33,570 ×)

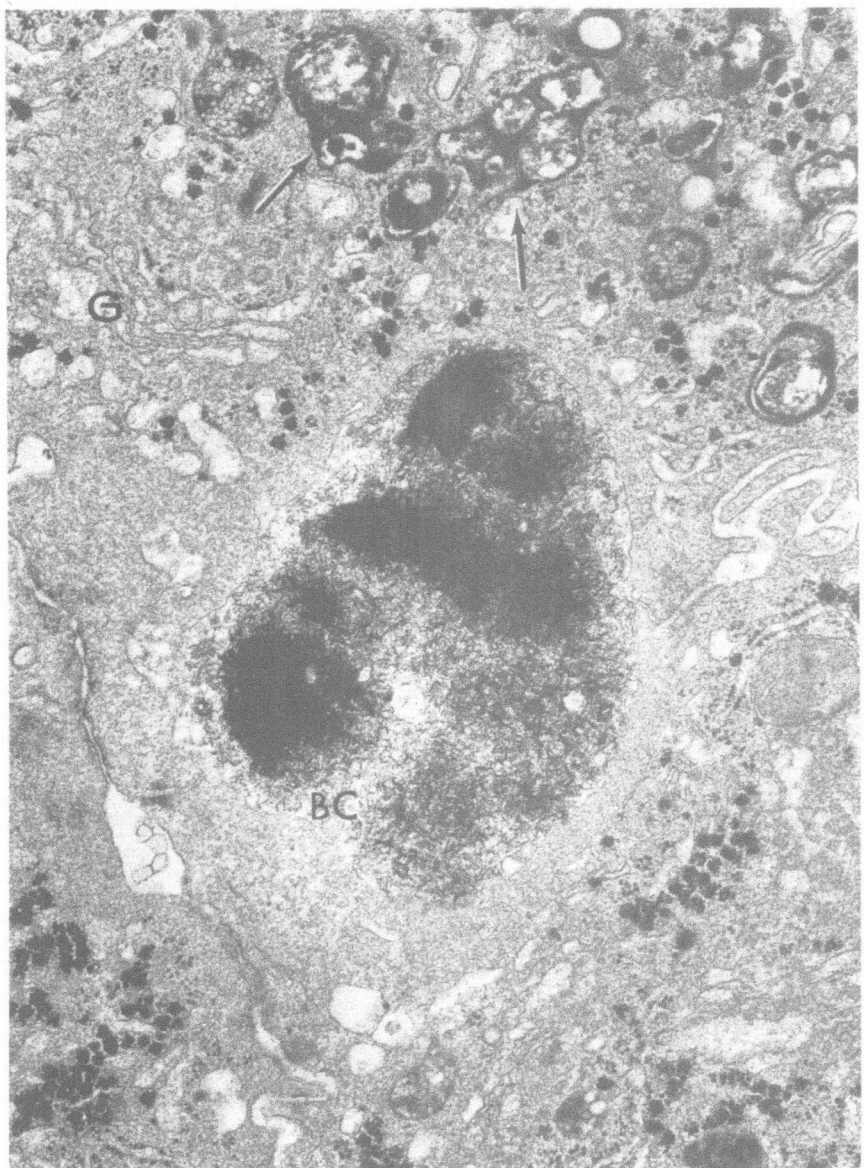

Fig. 7. Phenobarbital therapy. Bile canaliculus (BC) is filled with markedly osmophilic curvilinear material compared to figure 6. G, Golgi; arrow, lysosomes. (Magnification 29,821 ×)

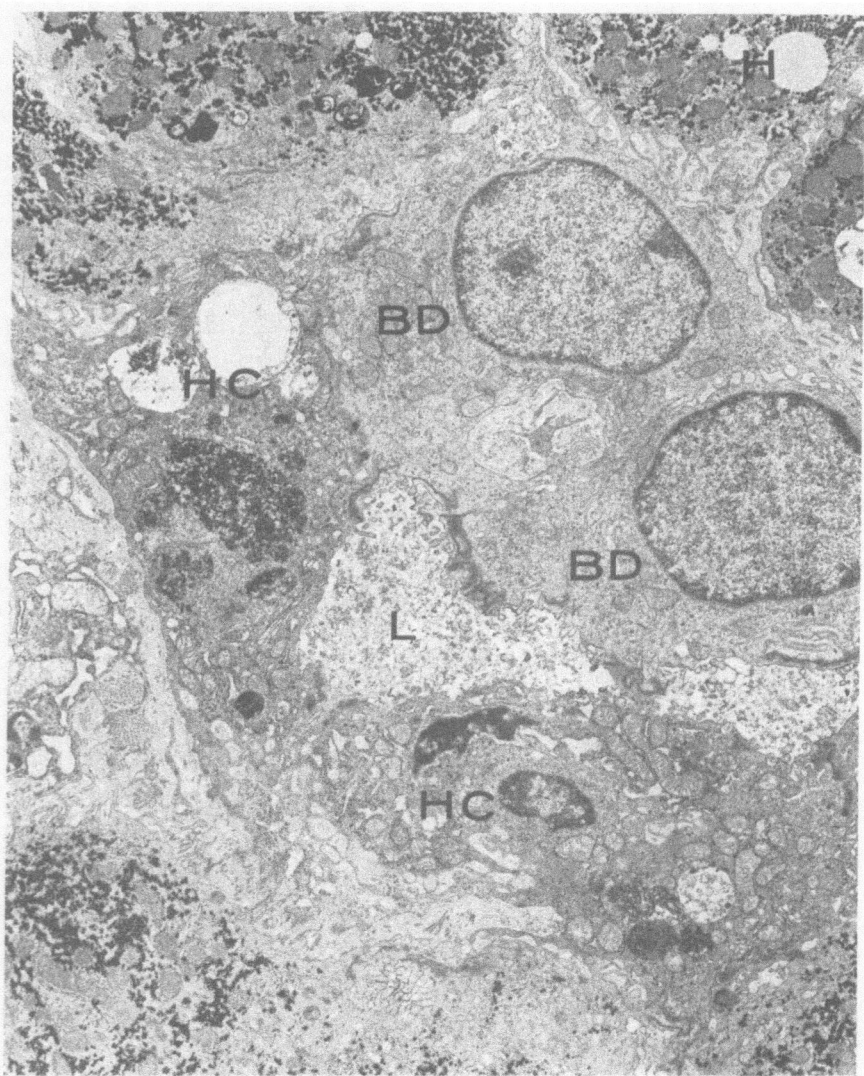

Fig. 8. Preductular structure (Canal of Hering). The lumen (L) contains much granular material which increased in osmophilic density while on phenobarbital therapy. Two Hering canal cells (HC) are shown bordering the canal lumen. Degenerative changes (vacuoles and increased intracellular material) are present in the Hering canal cells. Bile duct epithelial cells (BD) of an adjacent bile ductule are normal. H, hepatocyte. (Magnification 5,965 ×)

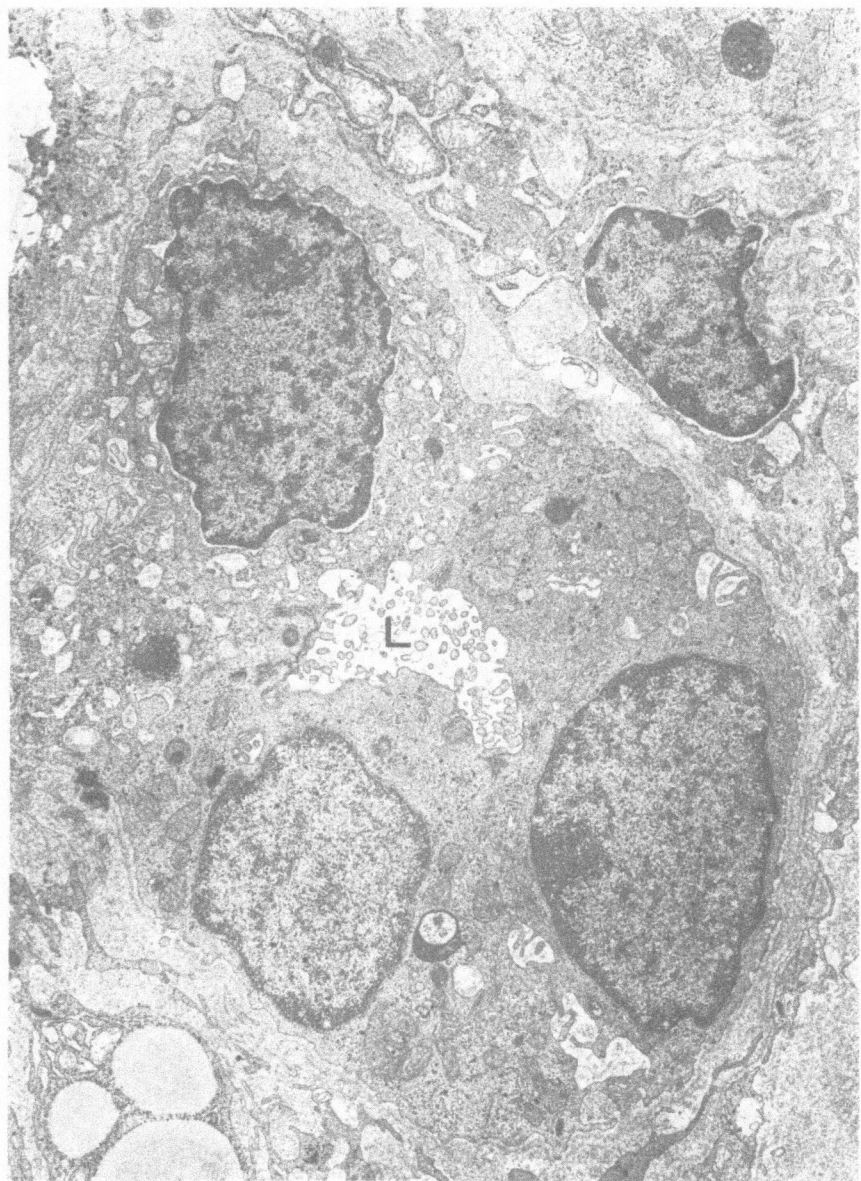

Fig. 9. Small bile duct. The lumen is relatively empty and the epithelium is normal. Similar normality of bile ducts was observed in all specimens examined. L: lumen. (Magnification 7,980 ×).

REFERENCES

1. Carey, J. B., jr., The serum trihydroxy-dihydroxy bile acid ratio in liver and biliary tract disease. *J. clin. Invest. 37*: 1494-1503 (1958).
2. Clayton, R. J., F. L. Iber, B. H. Ruebner and V. A. McKusick, Byler's disease: fatal familial intrahepatic cholestasis in an Amish kindred. *Amer. J. Dis. Child. 117*: 112-124 (1969).
3. Gray, O. P. and R. A. Saunders, Familial intrahepatic cholestatic jaundice in infancy. *Arch. Dis. Childh. 41*: 320-328 (1966).
4. Hirooka, M. and T. Ono, A case of familial intrahepatic cholestasis. *Tohoku J. exp. Med. 94*: 293-306 (1968).
5. Juberg, R. C., R. M. Holland-Moritz, K. S. Henley and C. F. Gonzalez, Familial intrahepatic cholestasis with mental and growth retardation. *Pediatrics 38*: 819-836 (1966).
6. Linarelli, L. G., C. N. Williams and M. J. Phililps, Byler's disease, fatal intrahepatic cholestasis. *J. Pediat. 81*: 484-492 (1972).
7. Odièvre, M., M. Gautier, M. Hadchouel and D. Alagille, Severe familial intrahepatic cholestasis. *Arch. Dis. Childh. 48*: 806-812 (1973).
8. Partin, J. C., W. K. Schubert and J. S. Partin, Mitochondrial ultrastructure in Reye's syndrome (Encephalopathy and fatty degeneration of the viscera). *New Engl. J. Med. 285*: 1139-1343 (1971).
9. Wheeler, H. O., J. I. Meltzer and S. E. Bradley, Biliary transport and hepatic storage of sulfobromophthalein sodium in the unanesthetized dog, in normal man, and in patients with hepatic disease. *J. clin. Invest. 39*: 1131-1144 (1960).
10. Williams, C. N., R. Kaye, L. Baker, R. Hurwitz and J. R. Senior, Progressive familial cholestatic cirrhosis and bile acid metabilosm. *J. Pediat. 81*: 493-500 (1972).

HEPATITIS B VIRUS INFECTION IN CHILDREN

FENTON SCHAFFNER, M.D.

Infection with hepatitis B virus (HBV) in children differs from that in adults in several clinical features as well as its epidemiology. Some of these differences depend on the age of the patient and some on the mode of transmission. Compared to adults the scope of the problem is probably small in children but until studies spanning more than one generation have been carried out all the implications of this infection will remain unknown.

HEPATITIS B VIRUS

The agent responsible for hepatitis B is a particle 42 nm in diameter consisting of a core containing DNA and DNA polymerase and other proteins and a coat of protein surrounding the core.

The core can be seen in the nucleus of some hepatocytes as a 27 nm ringlike particle especially in immunosuppressed persons (41, 21, 10). DNA replication or multiplication of the viral genome occurs in the nucleus as well as transcription of the genome into messenger RNA (24). The coat protein is found in the cytoplasm of hepatocytes especially in asymptomatic carriers in whom the affected hepatocytes have a bulky homogeneous acidophilic cytoplasm (ground glass cells) (36) that stains darkly with aldehyde fuchsin or orcein (77, 17). The protein is in the form of small round particles or elongated rods 22 nm in diameter within the hypertrophied profiles of the endoplasmic reticulum (ER) (81, 42, 28). The protein is synthesized in the ER because electron immunocytochemical studies show that antigenic material is in and around the ER membrane as well as in the rods and particles within the lumens of the ER profiles (28, 27). The complete virion is formed when a core particle leaves the nucleus and is surrounded by coat protein. The virion then migrates to the plasma membrane which it moves through in an unknown fashion to enter the tissue fluid and the blood stream as the Dane particle (15). This particle, the DNA polymerase, the coat or surface protein (hepatitis B surface antigen or HB$_s$Ag) and antibody to the core (HB$_c$Ab) appear in the blood a few weeks after infection and a week or two before illness begins (24). The virus or some viral induced product of the cell attaches to the hepatocellular plasma membrane where it is exposed to the immune surveillance of the host. Cellular and humoral immune responses directed against the virus or viral products on the plasma membrane, against altered plasma membrane or against liver-specific cell surface lipoprotein determine whether the cell dies, is damaged, internalizes the virus and its products or harmlessly harbors the viral core in its nucleus (24, 21, 57).

Whether naked core particles are in the serum is not clear. Fluorescent antibody studies indicate that in the prenecrotic stage of disease HB$_s$Ag is present in all hepatocytes near or on the sinusoidal membrane (67) but in the necrotic phase the antigen containing cells are eliminated (35). Children who are infected with HBV by routes other than injection eliminate few if any of the affected hepatocytes and therefore they become chronic carriers with little or no necrosis. While they produce large amounts of HB$_s$Ag, they have few Dane particles in their serum (66) except in rate instances (95) Their blood is infectious probably in transfusion amounts only. They can, however, form antibody to HB$_s$Ag and because of the antigen excess, HB$_s$A b is quickly removed from serum. Complexes of HB$_s$Ag and HB$_s$Ab along with complement can form in quantities sufficient to lower serum complement levels and may be deposited in tissues, notably in glomeruli (8), in synovia (2, 73) and in arteries (33, 82). Children seem more prone to deposit these complexes in the kidney than adults in whom arthritis with synovial complex deposition is more common.

Children who acquire HBV by parenteral means may develop typical acute viral hepatitis although the risk is less in children than in adults (74, 13). Some of these develop chronic hepatitis (13, 9) presumably because of failure to eliminate completely the cells containing virus or at least those programmed to make HB$_s$Ag (35). Indeed some or most of these cells may be incapable of making core particles, explaining why core antigen (HB$_c$Ag) and naked core particles are not often seen in nuclei in carriers.

CLINICAL HEPATITIS B

The liver disease caused by hepatitis B virus in adults is characterized by a long incubation period, a long prodrome and slowly increasing severity of an often long icteric phase (table 1). In children the onset of clinical symp-

Table 1. Clinical differences in hepatitis B in children and adults.

Clinical feature	Children	Adults
Frequency	Uncommon	Many sporadic cases
Susceptibility	High	Low
Peak incidence	Infants	Young adults
Onset	Abrupt	Gradual
GI symptoms	Often severe	Moderate
Fever	High but brief	Moderate but protracted
Duration	Short	Often protracted
Mortality	High in infants	Low except in elderly
Carrier state	Frequent	Uncommon
Chronic hepatitis	Mainly infants	Mainly elderly

toms is more abrupt and the icteric phase short (72, 93, 22). Gastrointestinal symptoms, particularly vomiting and abdominal pain are common, often with ketoacidosis while urticaria and arthritis are rare in contrast to adults. Tender hepatomegaly with splenomegaly early is the rule in children. Hepatitis B in the neonatal period is rare (46). The mortality rate is highest in infants, however, being 4-5/100,000 population under one year of age (54). In one series of hospitalized children over half died of their disease (22). Mortality drops precipitously after one year of age and rises again slowly in the later years of life reaching high levels after age 60.

While most places in the world, with the notable exception of India (52), report that acute hepatitis B is less common in children than in adults (13, 9, 37, 86), many observers have recorded a high incidence of hepatitis B among children with chronic hepatitis regardless of how the infection was acquired (13, 9). This high incidence is not universal, however, and in some series no cases were associated with HB_sAg (20).

Extrahepatic manifestations of HBV infection in children differ from those in adults in addition to the lack of arthritis and urticaria in the early stages already mentioned. Papular acrodermatitis is found mainly in children with HB_sAg not acquired by transfusions associated with lymphadenitis and mild hepatitis (31). In these children the skin disease is the major manifestation and virus particles have been identified in the skin. We have seen one young adult with persistent HB_s antigenemia and recurrent papular acrodermatitis. Glomerulonephritis is more common in children (8) than in adults (49) as a result of the deposition of antigen/antibody complexes described before. Endocapillary proliferative, membrane proliferative and membranous types of glomerulonephritis have all been associated with HB_sAg or antibody to it in serum and with immune complexes in the kidney. Bone marrow failure has been reported following hepatitis B as it has in hepatitis of other etiologies (8) in children and young adults (65).

PATHOLOGY OF HEPATITIS B

Neither the biochemical alterations in serum nor the structural alterations in the liver distinguish hepatitis B in children from that in the adult except that cholestasis in all forms of hepatitis in infants and at puberty may be prominent. Indeed the more cholestasis that is apparent, the longer the disease tends to last. The activity of alkaline phosphatase in serum is not as useful a parameter in children because of osteoblastic activity and determination of other enzymes like 5'-nucleotidase or gamma glutamyl transpeptidase may be more helpful (94). Details of the appearance of the various forms of the viral antigen and antibodies in serum have not been extensively studied in children but they probably are the same as in adults. In infants, measurement of immunoglobulins may fail to indicate the danger of transition to cirrhosis because of the not fully developed immune system although higher than normal IgM levels may indicate intrauterine infection with HBV (47). Children with HB_cAb have increased antibodies to other viral agents like influenza while those with HB_sAg do not (60). As in adults transaminase activities are useful diagnostic indicators although in infants they often do not help separate the various causes of neonatal jaundice and, as in the adult, fluctuating abnormal results may persist long after clinical disease has subsided. Asymptomatic carriers show minor fluctuating abnormalities in transaminase activities not well correlated with histologic abnormalities (43).

Too few biopsy or autopsy specimens are available in young children to appreciate if any major differences from adults exist in cases of equal severity. Furthermore insufficient data are available to answer the question whether transition to cirrhosis occurs more commonly in children than in adults. Indeed adequate data are sparse in adults, too. Spotty, bridging and massive necrosis (70) (fig. 1) have all been seen in children and the increasingly serious prognosis of these features respectively probably applies to all patients equally regardless of age. Large multinucleated hepatocellular giant cells have been seen in hepatitis B in young children (3, 46) and also at puberty (fig. 2). Portal fibrosis and transition to cirrhosis are often noted in infants with severe hepatitis (46). The morphologic indicators of cholestasis, namely bile thrombi in dilated bile canaliculi, bile staining of Kupffer cells and bile

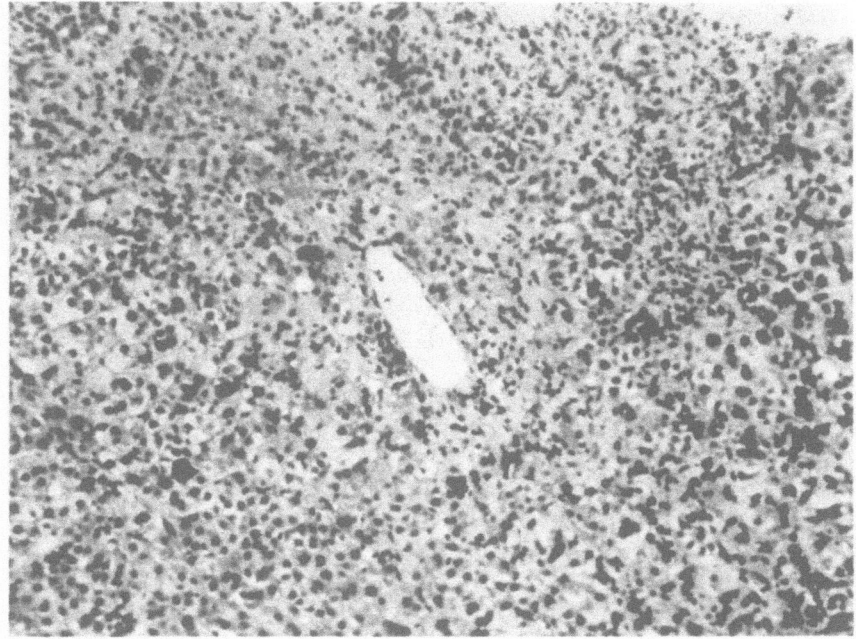

Fig. 1. Needle biopsy specimen of liver in acute hepatitis B in child with extensive spotty necrosis scattered through the lobular parenchyma, central phlebitis and two acidophilic bodies to left and slightly below the central vein. (H and E × 100).

stained vacuolated hepatocytes (feathery degeneration) may not be seen early in the course of the disease even though pruritus is present and alkaline phosphatase activity is high. When necrosis and inflammation subside cholestasis may be readily recognized (71). In the first few months of life foci of extramedullary hematopoiesis may persist from fetal life and at first glance may exaggerate the inflammation. Ground glass cells are not seen in acute hepatitis because most viral containing cells have disappeared. Even when cells with HB₈Ag are demonstrated by immunofluorescence in chronic disease, ground glass cells may not be recognized because of extensive hepatocellular injury and inflammation.

In newborn infants the differential diagnosis includes biliary atresia, neonatal giant cell hepatitis associated with viruses other than HBV, galactosemia, fructosemia and disordered metabolism of some amino acids. Later in childhood, between one year of age and adolescence, when hepatitis A is much more prominent, hepatitis B less often enters into the differential diagnosis of conditions with acute jaundice. Chronic liver disease from hepa-

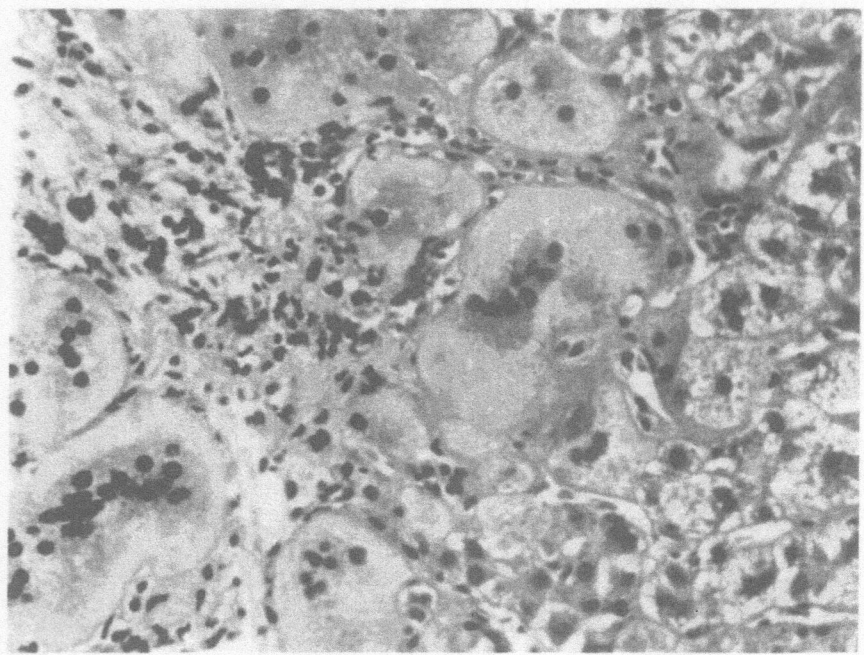

Fig. 2. Needle biopsy speciment of liver from child with acute hepatitis B showing numerous hepatocullular giant cells. (H and E ×250).

titis B may be prominent in children after one year of age and it has to be distinguished from metabolic disorders like Wilson's disease or alpha-1-antitrypsin deficiency. Most of the differential diagnoses cannot be made on pathologic grounds or on clinical grounds and therefore biochemical screening tests appropriate for the age of the patient and the type of disease must be carried out when acute or chronic hepatitis is seen histologically. In older children drug abuse has become widespread in the last decade. The disease which these adolescent addicts develop is the same as that seen in adult addicts (12, 30). In addition to the morphologic features of acute or chronic hepatitis, inflammation sometimes in the form of granulomas can develop from impurities like talc injected with the drugs (63). This inflammation superimposed on that caused by the hepatitis makes the hepatitis look more severe than it actually is. Asymptomatic carriers of HB_sAg have either normal livers or nonspecific reactive hepatitis usually with ground glass cells (fig. 3). Exceptionally chronic aggressive hepatitis with or without cirrhosis is found.

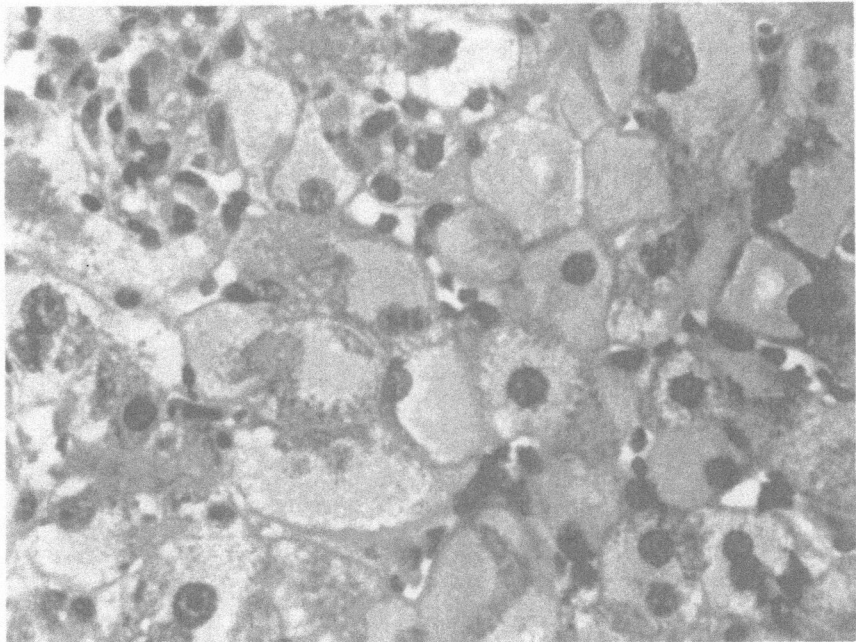

Fig. 3. Needle biopsy speciment of liver in young asymptomatic HBₛAg carrier showing enlarged hepatocytes with ground glass cytoplasm. (H and E ×443)

EPIDEMIOLOGY OF HEPATITIS B VIRUS

Infection with HBV may express itself in many different ways, the most frequent being the asymptomatic carrier (table 2). Hepatitis B antigen especially in male children has been increasing in incidenc in the United States (34). It is most common in the first year of life and the incidence rises again during adolescence (54). The carrier rate can reach adult levels in some countries like Thailand by age 5 (84). HBₛAg has been found in cord blood in some series (76, 69, 47) but not others (80, 40) and transplacental transmission does not account for the great majority of asymptomatic carriers especially in those parts of the world where the incidence is high (14). Indeed the carrier mothers and cord blood contain antibody to HBᴄ but it disappears from the serum in newborns shortly after birth (69). Rather vertical transmission via mother's milk (6), saliva (78, 91) or vaginal secretions (16) is more likely particularly via saliva (91). Thus post natal exposure accounts

Table 2. Expressions of hepatitis B infection.

Acute hepatitis	Anicteric
	Icteric
	Fulminant
Chronic hepatitis	Persistent or aggressive
	With or without cirrhosis
Extrahepatic diseases	Glomerulonephritis
	Papular acrodermatitis
	Other rashes
	Arthritis
	Vasculitis
Carrier state	Transplacental
	Post natal from mother
	Post transfusion
	Family contact
	Institutional exposure
	Immunosuppression by disease or medication
	Drug abuse

for the often delayed appearance of HB_sAg in children of HB_sAg positive mothers who are asymptomatic carriers or had hepatitis in the last trimester of pregnancy until six weeks or so post partum (79, 62). About 10 percent of children born of asymptomatic chronic carriers or of women who had hepatitis early in pregnancy had evidence of infection as did half of those whose mothers had hepatitis within two months before or after birth (75). The poorly developed immune system in the infant makes possible immune tolerance necessary for the carrier state (62) and accounts for the higher incidence of the carrier state in children infected with HBV than adults (30). Part of this tolerance may also be genetic in that family clustering of carriers especially siblings (89) is common and genetic factors may be as important (4) as ethnic origin, age and sex (25). The HB_sAg subtypes (55) are related to geographic and epidemiologic factors rather than to the type of infection (56). By contrast, the e-antigenic complex may be related to the pathological process in the host, notably the development of chronic hepatitis (61). No relation between the carrier state and histocompatibility antigens has been detected (45).

A second means of transmission in infants is via blood transfusion, often given as exchange transfusions in newborns. This type of spread is more likely to produce overt hepatitis although the carrier state can develop in this group, too.

The incidence of HB antibody in the middle class and more affluent segments of the adult population of New York is about 15 percent and that in children is about 5 percent (11, 48). These data suggest that exposure to HB virus is common in early life and factors such as visits to doctors' offices and contact with carrier family members and playmates may also play a role. Mosquitoes may also be responsible for spreading HBV since HB_sAg has been demonstrated in those caught in urban areas (18).

Transmission of HBV from one person to the next in the general population occurs. Carriers of the virus infect members of their own household or other close contacts (38). While siblings seem most susceptible (89) possibly because of the higher incidence of antibody in adults (11), family studies indicated that an index case in a family outbreak can be a child with hepatitis (3), an asymptomatic adult (44), an addict (64) or a patient on hemodialysis (26). Children were affected in all these families. The high incidence of HB_sAg carriers among patients receiving chemotherapy (92) indicates that this is another source of infection for younger family members. Children may also serve as index cases in epidemics, for example by spreading HBV to medical personnel working in specialized units like those for dialysis or chemotherapy (7).

Institutionalized children, especially those with Down's syndrome, have a high incidence of HB antigenemia with a low incidence of HB antibodies (85, 87). The closed environment of the institutional life (87) and some immunologic deficiency (85) that is part of the chromosomal abnormality account for frequently found HB_sAg in the serum of these patients. Children with Down's syndrome not in institutions and institutionalized children with other diseases do not have a high incidence of antigenemia. Furthermore HB_sAg is not more frequent in mothers who delivered infants with Down's syndrome (19).

In adolescents, drug abuse is the main means of spread of HBV but accurate estimates of the extent of this problem are difficult to obtain. As many as 80 percent of those exposed are infected with HBV. Most develop antibodies, some have overt hepatitis which may have a protracted course, some have chronic persistent or aggressive hepatitis following acute icteric hepatitis or without any acute disease and some become carriers (12, 39). In a methadone maintenance therapy program in which most of the patients were Hispanic Americans, about 40 percent per year of those who were HB_sAg positive became negative over a 4 year period (83). These data suggest that permanent immune tolerance to HB_sAg acquired later in life is less common than in infants.

The incidence of HB$_s$Ag varies in different parts of the world and under different circumstances. The incidence is highest in the islands of the South Pacific, mainly in asymptomatic carriers (5). In post transfusion hepatitis in Japanese children it was 30 percent while in hepatitis without exposure to blood it was 78 percent (13). In India where the overall HB$_s$Ag carrier rate is 4 percent, HBV was detected during hepatitis at the same rate (HB$_s$Ag 16 percent, HB$_s$Ab 5 percent) in adults as in children (52). Similar data have not been recorded anywhere else. In Thailand the adult HB$_s$Ag carrier rate of 10 percent is reached by age 5 with a male predominance (84). Malnutrition increased the incidence of antigenemia and erased the sex difference. Diseases other than Down's syndrome that affect immune responsiveness like lymphomas and lepromatous leprosy are associated with a high HB$_s$Ag carrier rate (4, 5). The same is true in patients with renal disease undergoing dialysis or after transplantation. In Germany about a third of multiply transfused children with hemophilia had evidence of HBV infection but only about a third of these had clinical hepatitis (74). Almost all susceptible children exposed to HBV parenterally in an immunization program developed HB$_s$Ag and most of these had abnormal liver function but icteric hepatitis was uncommon (53). Oral transmission was also demonstrated in these studies. Children with or without Down's syndrome had about the same incidence of circulating HB$_s$Ag years after this experimental inoculation.

PREVENTION AND TREATMENT

Antiviral chemotherapy of hepatitis B remains an elusive goal. Immunotherapy in the form of serum containing a high titer of antibody had some initial promise when given alone (32, 23) or in combination with exchange transfustion (68) or plasmapheresis (58) but it was not therapeutically useful in a larger series of patients. A nationwide controlled trial of partially purified antibody in patients with fulminant hepatitis B including many children, showed it to be of no value in reducing mortality although the amount of antibody failed to abolish antigenemia in any case (1). Serious adverse reactions did not occur in this study although in an infant we treated prior to the study, cardiac arrest followed infusion of antibody-rich serum. Antibody may be of some value in preventing infection with HBV. Newborn infants of HB$_s$Ag positive mothers given antibody did not develop antigenemia while untreated controls did (50). Children entering institutions did not become carriers when they were given antibody but half of the controls did (88).

An extensive trial of antibody is underway in the United States for prevention of hepatitis in health care personnel after 'finger sticks'. A problem with this study has been the low incidence of antigenemia in control subjects given placebos. Inoculation with inactivated antigen appears promising in prevention of institutional spread of HBV (53). Efficacy and safety must be demonstrated first in animals and then in man before such a vaccine is made available to all. Transfer factor as well as antibody has been tried in chronic hepatitis with HB_sAg but insufficient data are available to evaluate this (51). Indeed no controlled data are available regarding the effect of any therapy on chronic hepatitis caused by HBV. Uncontrolled observations suggest that the spontaneous remission rate is greater in the presence of HB_sAg than in its absence but that the response to corticosteroids is less striking.

Hepatitis B is usually a self limited disease that requires only the simplest of supportive measures such as a nutritious diet and sufficient rest. Dietary restrictions or supplementations, absolute bed rest and pharmacotherapy of any sort have no rational basis. Many physicians still employ some of these outmoded therapies and we will surely continue to see many for at least another generation. Corticosteroids should be avoided in acute hepatitis B because they are ineffective, have many adverse effects and favor persisting antigenemia. Exchange transfusions, initially felt to be useful in fulminant hepatitis especially in children (90) have been shown to be ineffective in a controlled trial. Plasmapheresis successfully removed HB_sAg from serum in patients with fulminant hepatitis B but no one survived the illness (39). Perfusion through cadaver, pig, calf and baboon livers has been tried but the effort has waned because of discouraging results. Perfusion through a charcoal column is in the process of being evaluated in fulminant hepatitis. Transplantation has also been attempted with transient but not permanent elimination of antigenemia.

This decade held the promise of providing the solution to the problem of prevention and therapy of hepatitis. The decade is half over and progress in the field of prevention has been striking, first with the development of sensitive tests for the viruses and antibodies to them and, secondly with the beginning of testing of vaccines. Progress in therapy has lagged, however, and the research effort is now being directed to the question of how HBV causes the hepatocyte to die or to malfunction. The answer will serve as the basis of rational therapy.

SUMMARY

The hepatitis B virus consists of a DNA containing core particle that replicates in the nucleus of hepatocytes and coat or surface protein made in the hepatocellular endoplasmic reticulum. Children infected with this virus may develop acute hepatitis, chronic hepatitis or an asymptomatic carrier state. Acute hepatitis B in children is uncommon and differs from that in adults by having a more abrupt onset and a shorter course. The mortality is highest in infants. Extrahepatic manifestations caused by deposition of hepatitis B antigen-antibody complexes like glomerulonephritis or papular acrodermatitis are more frequently found in children while arthritis and vasculitis are unusual. The laboratory findings and the morphological alterations are the same as in hepatitis in adults. The carrier state is associated with minimal or no disease but ground glass hepatocytes containing hepatitis B surface antigens can be seen in liver biopsy specimens. The carrier rate of hepatitis B has been increasing in the United States. Transplacental transmission accounts for only a small proportion of carriers and neonatal acquisition of the virus from the mother is mainly responsible. Family contacts, institutional contacts and drug abuse explains spread of the virus later in childhood. Males are more often infected than females all over the world. Host responsiveness and genetic factors determine the type of infection in the individual patient while viral subtypes and geographic factors are important in epidemiology. Effective therapy has not been devised but prevention by immunization has great promise.

REFERENCES

1. Acute Hepatic Failure Study Group, Specific immunotherapy of fulminant type B hepatitis. Presented during Digestive Disease Week, San Francisco, May 19-25, 1974.
2. Alpert, E., K. J. Isselbacher and P. H. Schur, The pathogenesis of arthritis associated with viral hepatitis complement-component studies. *New Engl. J. Med. 285*: 185-189 (1971).
3. Bancroft, W. H., R. L. Warkel, A. A. Talbert and P. K. Russell, Family with hepatitis-associated antigen. *J.A.M.A. 217*: 1817-1820 (1971).
4. Blumberg, B. S., A. Sutnick and W. T. London, Australia antigen as a hepatitis virus. Variation in host response. *Amer. J. Med. 48*: 1-8 (1970).
5. Blumberg, B. S., A. I. Sutnick, W. T. London and L. Melartin, Sex distribution of Australia antigen. *Arch. intern. Med. 130*: 227-231 (1972).
6. Boxall, E. H., T. H. Flewett, D. S. Dane, D. H. Cameron, F. O. MacCallum and T. W. Lee, Hepatitis B surface antigen in breast milk. *Lancet 2*: 1007 (1974).
7. Bryan, J. A., H. E. Carr and M. B. Gregg, An outbreak of nonparenterally transmitted hepatitis B. *J.A.M.A. 223*: 279-283 (1973).
8. Brzosko, W. J., K. Krawczynski, T. Nazarewicz, M. Morzycka and A. Nowoslawski,

Glomerulonephritis associated with hepatitis B surface antigen immune complex in children *Lancet 2*: 477-482 (1974).

9. Brzosko, W. J., B. E. Mikulska, R. Biedrzychka, K. Roszkowka, A. Rudkowski, C. Rabenda, H. Oziemska-Lozinska and R. Debski, Hepatitis B in children. *Lancet 2*: 259 (1973).
10. Caramia, F., C. Debac and G. Ficci, Virus-like particles within hepatocytes of Australia antigen carriers. *Amer. J. Dis. Child. 123*: 309-311 (1972).
11. Cherubin, C. E. ,R. H. Purcell, J. J. Lander, T. G. McGinn and L. A. Cone, Acquisition of antibody to hepatitis B antigen in three socioeconomically different medical populations. *Lancet 2*: 149-151 (1972).
12. Cherubin, C. E. W. Rosenthal, R. Stenger, A. Prince, T. McGinn, M. Baden, S. Kane, D. Weinberger and S. Strauss, Chronic liver disease in asymptomatic narcotic addicts. *Ann. intern. Med. 76*: 39-396 (1972).
13. Chiba, S., T. Fujiwara, H. Shiono and T. Nakao, Frequency of Australia antigen detected by radioimmunoassay in hepatitis in children. *Tohoku J. exp. Med. 109*: 307-308 (1973).
14. Cossart, Y. E., F. D. Hargreaves and S. P. March, Australia antigen and the human fetus. *Amer. J. Dis. Child. 123*: 376-378 (1972).
15. Dane, D. S., C. H. Cameron and M. Briggs, Virus-like particles in serum of patients with Australia-antigen-associated hepatitis. *Lancet 1*: 695-698 (1970).
16. Darani, M. and M. Gerber, Hepatitis B antigen in vaginal secretions. *Lancet 2*: 1008 (1974).
17. Deodhar, K. P., E. Tapp and P. J. Scheuer, Orcein staining of hepatitis B antigen in paraffin sections of liver biopsies. *J. clin. Path. 28*: 60-70 (1975).
18. Dick, S. J., D. H. Tamburro and C. M. Leevy, Hepatitis B antigen in urban caught mosquitoes. *J.A.M.A. 229*: 1627-1629 (1974).
19. Dietzman, D. E., E. B. Matthew, D. L. Madden, J. L. Sever, M. Rostafinski, S. M. Bouton and B. Nagler, The occurrence of epidemic infectious hepatitis in chronic carriers of Autralia antigen. *Pediatrics 80*: 577-582 (1972).
20. Dubois, R. S., A. Silverman and T. L. Slovis, Chronic active hepatitis in children. *Amer. J. Dig. Dis. 17*: 575-582 (1972).
21. Dudley, F. J., R. A. Fox and S. Sherlock, Cellular immunity and hepatitis-associated, Australia antigen liver disease. *Lancet 1*: 723-726 (1972).
22. Dupuy, J. M., D. Frommel and D. Alagille, Severe viral hepatitis type B in infancy. *Lancet 1*: 191-194 (1975).
23. Dupuy, J. M., J. L. Virelizier and D. Frommel, Fulminant hepatitis-virus B in a three months old infant: Therapeutic trial with specific anti-HB globulins in antibody excess. *Infection 1*: 62-64 (1973).
24. Edington, T. S. and F. V. Chisari, Immunological aspects of virus B infection. *Amer. J. Med. sci. 270*: 213-227 (1975).
25. Feinman, S. V., N. Cooter, J. C. Sinclair, D. M. Wrobel and B. Berris, Clinical and epidemiological significance of the HB$_S$Ag (Australia antigen): carrier state. *Gastroenterology 78*: 113-120 (1975).
26. Garibaldi, R. A., F. E. Hatch, A. L. Bisno, M. H. Hatch and M. B. Gregg, Nonparenteral serum hepatitis. Report of an outbreak. *J.A.M.A. 220*: 963-966 (1972).
27. Gerber, M. A. and S. Hadziyannis, Immunoelectron microscopy and histochemistry of HB Ag. *New Engl. J. Med. 291*: 532-533 (1974).
28. Gerber, M. A., S. Hadziyannis, C. Vissoulis, F. Schaffner and H. Popper, Electron microscopy and immunoelectron microscopy of cytoplasmic hepatitis B antigen in hepatocytes. *Amer. J. Pathol. 75* 489-502 (1974).
29. Gerber, M. A., F. Schaffner and F. Paronetto, Immunoelectron microscopy of hepatitis B antigen in liver, *Proc. Soc. exp. Biol. Med. 140*: 1334-1339 (1972).   ·

30. Gerety, R. M., J. A. Hoofnagle, J. A. Markenson and L. F. Barker, Exposure to hepatitis B virus and development of chronic HB Ag carrier state in children. *J. Pediat. 84* :661-665 (1974).
31. Gianotti, F., Papular acrodermatitis of childhood. An Australia antigen disease. *Arch. Dis. Childh. 48*: 794-799 (1973).
32. Gocke, D. J., Fulminant hepatitis treated with serum containing antibody to Australia antigen. *New Engl. J. Med. 284*: 919 (1971).
33. Gocke, D. J., K. Hsu, C. Morgan, S. Bombardier, M. Lockshin and C. L. Christian, Vasculitis in association with Australia antigen. *J. exp. Med. 134*: 330-336 (1971).
34. Gregg, M. D., The changing epidemiology of viral hepatitis in the United States. *Amer. J. Dis. Child. 123*: 350-354 (1972).
35. Gudat, F., L. Bianchi, W. Sonnabend, G. Thiel, W. Aenishaenslin and G. A. Stalder, Pattern of core and surface expression in liver tissue reffects state of specific immune response in hepatitis B. *Lab. Invest. 32*: 1-9 (1975).
36. Hadiyannis, S., M. A. Gerber, C. Vissoulis and H. Popper, Cytoplasmic hepatitis B antigen in 'ground-glass' hepatocytes of carriers. *Arch. Path. 96*: 327-330 (1973).
37. Hadziyannis, S., B. Haralambides, A. Giustozi, G. Karvountzis and G. Merikas, Epidemiologic aspects of viral hepatitis in Greece. *Amer. J. Dis. Child. 123*: 356-357 (1972).
38. Heathcote, J., P. Gateau and S. Sherlock, Role of hepatitis B antigen carriers in non-parenteral transmission of hepatitis B virus. *Lancet 2*: 370-372 (1974).
39. Heilmann, K., P. Hinhart and A. Weizel, Morphological aspects of liver damage in drug addiction and misuse. *Dtsch. Med. Wschr. 96*: 453-457 (1971).
40. Holzbach, R. T., Australia antigen hepatitis in pregnancy. *Arch. intern. Med. 130*: 234-236 (1972).
41. Huang, S. N., Hepatitis-associated antigen hepatitis. An electron microscopic study of virus-like particles in liver cells. *Amer. J. Path. 64*: 483-500 (1971).
42. Huang, S. N., V. Groh, J. G. Beaudoin, W. D. Dauphinee, R. D. Guttmann, D. D. Morehouse, A. Aronoff and H. Gault, A study of the relationship of virus-like particles and Australia antigen in liver. *Hum. Path. 5*: 209-222 (1974).
43. Ichida, F., H. Sasaki, T. Sekine and T. Inagaki, Clinico-pathological studies of the liver in asymptomatic carriers of Australia antigen (HBAg). *Acta. hepat. gastroent. 22*: 13-21 (1975).
44. Irwin, G. R., A. M. Allen, W. H. Bancroft, J. J. Karwacki, R. H. Pinkerton and P. K. Russell, Hepatitis B antigen and antibody. Occurrence in families of asymptomatic HBAg carriers. *J.A.M.A. 227*: 1042-1043 (1974).
45. Jeannet, M. and J. J. Farquet, HL-A antigens in asymptomatic chronic HBA g carriers. *Lancet 2*: 1383-1384 (1974).
46. Kattamis, C. A., D. Demetrios and N. S. Matsaniotis, Australia antigen and neonatal hepatitis syndrome. *Pediatrics 54*: 157-164 (1974).
47. Keys, T. F., J. L. Sever, W. L. Hewitt and G. L. Gitnick, Hepatitis-associated antigen in selected mothers and newborn infants. *J. Pediat. 80*: 650-653 (1972).
48. Kofman, S., Hepatitis B. *A physician's guide to the disease and its associated hepatitis B (Australia) antigen*, pp. 20 (Abbott Laboratories, North Chicago 1974).
49. Kohler, P. F., R. E. Cronin, W. S. Hammond, D. Olin and R. I. Carr, Chronic membranous glomerulonephritis caused by hepatitis B antigen-antibody complexes. *Ann. intern. Med. 81*: 448-451 (1974).
50. Kohler, P. F., R. S. Dubois, D. A. Merrill ànd W. A. Bowes, Prevention of chronic neonatal hepatitis B virus infection with antibody to hepatitis B surgace antigen. *New Engl. J. Med. 291*: 1378-1380 (1974).
51. Kohler, P. F., J. Trembath, D. A. Merrill, J. W. Singleton and R. S. Dubois, Immuno-

therapy with antibody, lymphocytes and transfer factor in chronic hepatitis B. *Clin. Immunol. Immunopath. 2*: 465-471 (1974).
52. Kotwal, S. E. and S. S. Kelkar, Hepatitis B antigen in endemic hepatitis at Aurangabad. *Indian J. Med. Sci.* 855-860 (1973).
53. Krugman, S., J. P. Giles, Viral hepatitis, type B (MS-2-Strain): Further observations on natural history and prevention. *New Engl. J. Med. 288*: 755-760 (1973).
54. Kurylowicz, W., Epidemiology of viral hepatitis and its long term sequelae in Poland. *Amer. J. Dis. Child. 123*- 335:340 (1972).
55. Le Bouvier, G. L., The heterogeneity of Australia antigen. *J. infect. Dis. 123*: 671-675 (1971).
56. Le Bouvier, G. L., Subtypes of hepatitis B antigen: Clinical relevance? *Ann. intern. Med. 79*: 894-896 (1973).
57. Lee, W. M., W. D. Reed, C. G. Mitchell, R. M. Galbraith, A. L. W. F. Eddleston, A. J. Zuckerman and R. Williams, Cellular and humoral immunity to hepatitis-B surface antigen in active chronic hepatitis. *Brit. med. J. 1*: 705-708 (1975).
58. Lepore, M. J., P. J. McKenna, D. B. Martinez, L. J. Stotman, C. A. Bonanno, E. F. Conklin and J. G. Robilotti jr., Fulminant hepatitis with coma successfully treated by plasmapheresis and hyperimmune Australia antibody-rich plasma. *Amer. J. Gastroenterology 58*: 381-389 (1972).
59. Lepore, M. J., L. J. Stumann, C. A. Bonanno, E. F. Conklin, J. G. Robilotti jr. and P. J. McKenna, Plasmapheresis with plasma exchange in hepatic coma. II. Fulminant viral hepatitis as a systemic disease. *Arch. intern. Med. 129*: 900-907 (1972).
60. Lozovskaya, L. S., M. A. Kasavina, L. L. Nisevich, V. D. Sobloeva, O. M. Shigina, L. V. Chistova, A. A. Yakovleva and K. N. Krasnova, Hepatitis-related Australia antigen and specific antiviral immunity in children with chronic disease. *Sovetsk. Med. 5*: 7-12 (1973).
61. Magnius, L. O. and J. A. Espmark, New specificities in Australia antigen positive sera distinct from the Le Bouvier determinants. *J. Immunol. 109*: 1017-1021 (1972).
62. Merrill, D. A., R. S. Dubois and P. F. Kohler, Neonatal onset of the hepatitis associated carrier state. *New Engl. J. Med. 287*: 1280-1282 (1972).
63. Min, K. W., F. Gyorkey and D. Cain, Talc granulomata in liver disease in narcotic addicts. *Arch. Path. 98*- 331-335 (1974).
64. Mitch, W. E., J. R. Wands and W. C. Maddrey, Hepatitis B transmission in a family. *J.A.M.A. 227*: 1043-1044 (1974).
65. Nagaraju, M., S. Weitzman and G. Baumann, Viral hepatitis and agranulocytosis. *Amer. J. Dig. Dis. 18*: 247-252 (1973).
66. Nielsen, J. O., M. H. Neilsen and P. Elling, Differential distribution of Australia-antigen-associated particles in patients with liver diseases and normal carriers. *New Engl. J. Med. 288*: 484-487 (1973).
67. Nowoslawski, A., K. Krawizynski and W. J. Brzoski, Tissue localization of Australia antigen immune complexes in acute and chronic hepatitis and liver cirrhosis. *Amer. J. Path. 68*: 31-56 (1972).
68. Opolon, P., P. Gateau and C. Salmon, Passive immunotherapy in HB Ag positive fulminant hepatitis. Preliminary results (abstr.). *Gastroenterology 66*: 891 (1974).
69. Papaevangelou, G., J. Hoofnagle and J. Kremastinou, Transplacental transmission of hepatitis B virus by symptom-free chronic carrier mothers. *Lancet 2*: 746-749 (1974).
70. Popper, H., Clinical pathological correlation in viral hepatitis. The effect of the virus on the liver. *Fed. Proc.* In press.
71. Popper, H., The pathology of viral hepatitis. *Canad. med. Ass. J. 106*: 447-452 (1972).
72. Rossi, E. A., Clinical aspects of acute forms of viral hepatitis. *Amer. J. Dis. Child. 123*: 277-281 (1972).
73. Schumacher, H. R. and E. P. Gall, Arthritis in acute hepatitis and chronic active

hepatitis. Pathology of the synovial membrane with evidence for the presence of Australia antigen in synovial membranes. *Amer. J. Med. 57*: 655-664 (1974).

74. Schwartz, B. und G. Landbeck, Australia/SH-Antigen und Antikörper nach mehrfachtransfusionen bei Kindern und Jugendlichen mit schwerer und mittelschwerer Hämophilie. *Dtsch. Med. Wschr. 98*: 2016-2019 (1973).

75. Schweitzer, I. L., J. W. Mosley, M. Ashcaval, V. M. Edwards and L. B. Overby, Factors influencing neonatal infection by hepatitis B virus. *Gastroenterology 65*: 277-283 (1973).

76. Schweitzer, I. L., A. Wing, C. McPeak and R. L. Spears, Hepatitis and hepatitis-associated antigen in 56 mother-infant pairs. *J.A.M.A. 220*: 1092-1095 (1972).

77. Shikata, T., T. Uzawa, N. Yoshiwara, T. Akatwuka and S. Yamazaki, Staining methods of Australia antigen in paraffin section. Detection of cytoplasmic inclusion bodies. *Japan. J. exp. Med. 44*: 35-36 (1974).

78. Shirachi, R., H. Shiraishi, S. Matsumoto, S. Matsuda, and N. Ishida Hepatitis B antigen in saliva. *Tohoku J. exp. Med. 104*: 201-202 (1973).

79. Skinhøj, P., H. Sardemann, J. Cohn, M. Mikkelsen and H. Olesen, Hepatitis associated antigen (HAA) in pregnant women and their newborn infants. *Amer. J. Dis. Child. 123*: 380-381 (1972).

80. Smithwick, E. M. and S. C. Go, Hepatitis-associated antigen in cord and maternal sera. *Lancet 2*: 1080-1081 (1970).

81. Stein, O., M. Fainary and Y. Stein, Visualization of virus-like particles in endoplasmic reticulum of hepatocytes of Australia antigen carriers. *Lab. Invest. 26*: 262-269 (1972).

82. Stevens, D. P., J. Walker, E. Crum, H. P. Roth and R. W. Moskowitz, Anicteric hepatitis presenting as polyarthritis. *J.A.M.A. 220*: 687-689 (1972).

83. Stimmel, B., S. J. Vernace and F. Schaffner, Hepatitis B surface antigen and antibody in asymptomatic drug users: A prospective study. *J.A.M.A. 234*: 1135-1138 (1975).

84. Suskind, R. M., L. C. Olson and R. E. Olson, Protein calorie malnutrition and infection with hepatitis-associated antigen. *Pediatrics 51*: 525-530 (1973).

85. Sutnick, A. I., W. T. London and B. S. Blumberg, Effects of host and environment on immunoglobulins in Down's syndrome. *Arch. intern. Med. 124*: 722-725 (1969).

86. Szmuness, W., A. M. Prince, G. Diebolt, L. Leblanc, R. Baylet, R. Masseyeff and J. Linhard, The epidemiology of hepatitis B infections in Africa: Results of a pilot survey in the Republic of Senegal. *Amer. J. Epidem. 98*: 104-110 (1973).

87. Szmuness, W., A. M. Prince, G. F. Etling and R. Pick, Development and distribution of hemagglutinating antibody against the hepatitis B antigen in institutionalized populations. *J. infect. Dis. 126*: 498-506 (1972).

88. Szmuness, W., A. M. Prince, M. Goodman, C. Ehrich, R. Pick and M. Ansari, Hepatitis B immune serum globulin in prevention of nonparenterally transmitted hepatitis B. *New Engl. J. Med. 290*: 701-706 (1974).

89. Szmuness, W., A. M. Prince, R. L. Hirsch and B. Brotman, Familial clustering of hepatitis B infection. *New Engl. J. Med. 289*: 1162-1166 (1973).

90. Trey, C., D. G. Burns and S. L. Saunders, Treatment of hepatic coma by exchange blood transfusion. *New Engl. J. Med. 274*: 473-481 (1966).

91. Villarejos, V. M., K. A. Visona, A. Gutierrez and A. Rodriguez, Role of saliva, urine and feces in the transmission of type B hepatitis. *New. Engl. J. Med. 291*: 1375-1378 (1974).

92. Wands, J. R., C. M. Chuba, F. J. Roll and W. C. Maddrey, Serial studies of hepatitis-associated antigen and antibody in patients receiving antitumor chemotherapy for myeloproliferative and lymphoproliferative disorders. *Gastroenterology 68*: 105-112 (1975).

93. Wewalka, F. G., Protracted and recurrent forms of viral hepatitis. *Amer. J. Dis. Child. 123*: 283-286 (1972).
94. Whitfield, J. B., R. E. Pounder, G. Neale and D. W. Moss, Serum γ-glutamyl transpeptidase activity in liver disease. *Gut 13*: 702-708 (1972).
95. Yamada, G. and K. Kosaka, Intranuclear virus-like particles in hepatocytes of an asymptomatic hepatitis B antigen carrier with Dane particles in the serum. *Gastroenterology 68*: 270-373 (1975).

TRANSMISSION OF HEPATITIS B TO FETUS AND INFANT

Y. E. COSSART, M.D. AND B. J. COHEN, B.SC.

There are now numerous reports of the transmission of hepatitis B from mother to child (27, 28, 15, 3, 8) but it is still not clear how often it occurs nor by which route infection is transferred. Nor is the course of hepatitis B in infants well understood.

Table 1. Prospective studies of hepatitis B in pregnancy.

Country	Reference	Number of mothers	Number cord bloods HBsAg+	Number follow up bloods HBsAg+
U.S.A.	Holzbach	2	0	0
U.S.A.	Schweitzer et al.	23	2/19	13
U.S.A.	Merrill et al.	5	1	4
England	Cossart	6	0	3

Prospective studies, table 1 (9, 23, 16, 5) show that there is a substantial risk to babies whose mothers contract hepatitis B near term, and most workers have found a much lower risk for babies whose mothers are chronic carriers or develop hepatitis early in pregnancy, tables 2 and 3 (23, 24, 2, 18). However in a large study in Taiwan (26) the risk to babies of carriers was comparable with that of babies born in Europe or North America to mothers with hepatitis.

It is uncertain whether infection occurs in utero or during delivery. On the one hand cord blood is usually negative (25, 23) but antigenaemia tends to appear before the sixth week of life (10, 5). This allows only a very short incubation period if the infants have been infected at birth. Babies readily contract hepatitis B if they are inadvertently transfused with HBsAg positive blood (6) and it is hard to envisage how an infant can escape exposure to its mother's blood during delivery. It therefore seems probable that some feature of the maternal infection determines whether the baby becomes infected.

Table 2. Transmission of hepatitis B from carrier mothers to their infants.

Country	Reference	Number of mothers	Number cord bloods HBsAg+	Number follow up bloods HBsAg+
Denmark	Skinhøj	53	0	0
Pakistan	Aziz et al.	17	0	0
Greece	Papaevagelou et al.	11	2	0
U.S.A.	Schweitzer et al.	21	0	1
Taiwan	Stevens et al.	158	21/103	63

Table 3. Maternal history for HBsAg positive infants.

Mother acute hepatitis B ± 4 weeks delivery (4, Merrill, 1, Turner, 1, Wright, 1, Gillespie, 13, Schweitzer, 3, Cossart)	23
Mother acute hepatitis B in early pregnancy (2, Schweitzer)	2
Mother carrier (3, Merrill, 1, McCarthy, 2, Papaevangelou, 1, Buchholz)	7

There are few longitudinal studies of the course of hepatitis B in infants. Both prolonged antigenaemia with few signs of hepatitic injury (23, 12) and rapid progression to cirrhosis (28, 5) and death have been reported. Acute hepatitis does not seem to occur, presumably because of the immaturity of the immunologic response of the infants.

A study has therefore been undertaken in the hope of defining a test which could be used to predict which infants born to HBsAg positive mothers would become infected so that they could be given hyperimmune globulin soon after birth.

METHODS

An attempt was made to follow women who were HBsAg positive during pregnancy whether they were carriers or developed acute hepatitis. A formal survey of antenatal patients was not undertaken.

All blood samples were examined by electrophoresis (20) passive haemagglutination (21, 4) and radioimmunoassay (11). Electronmicroscopy was performed by a conventional technique (1) and the presence of Dane particles assessed over ten grid squares. Subtyping was performed by electrophoretic titration of the antigens against absorbed 'monospecific' antisera, and by electrophoretic mobility (7).

All the results in the tables refer to maternal sera taken at or about the time of delivery.

RESULTS

Not all specimens were available in sufficient quantity to be tested by all methods, the actual numbers examined are indicated in each table.

The best indicator that transmission to the infant was likely was a maternal history of hepatitis near term (table 4). However some babies of carriers were

Table 4. Transmission of hepatitis B from mother to child.

	Transmission (i.e. baby's blood HBsAg positive)	No transmission
Acute hepatitis B ± 4 weeks of delivery	4	2
HBsAg carrier in pregnancy	4	18

infected, and some babies escaped although their mothers had hepatitis.

The titre of maternal antigen tended to be higher in the hepatitis patients than in the carriers, figure 1, and there is a secondary correlation with transmission, figure 2. However some mothers with low titres transmitted and some with high titres did not.

Similarly although 3 of the 5 mothers with ay antigen transmitted, compared with only 4 of 14 with ad antigen (table 5) this finding reflects the predominance of ad subtype in carriers and ay in acute hepatitis (table 6) in London.

The presence of Dane particles did not correlate well with transmission (table 7). Little difficulty was experienced in categorising the samples as double shelled particles were either very numerous or almost absent.

All 29 cord bloods were negative by electrophoresis, but HBsAg could be detected by passive haemagglutination and radioimmunoassay in three. The

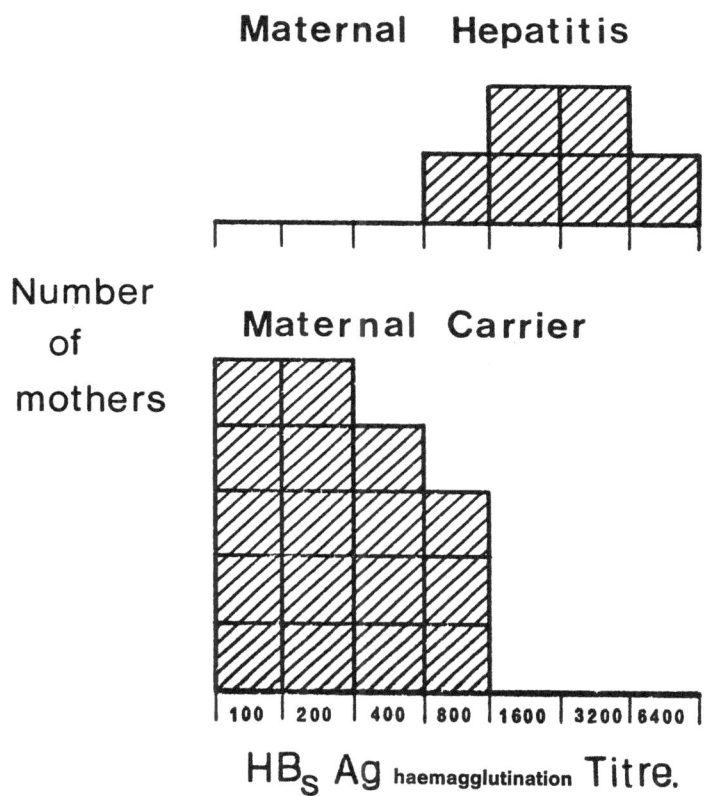

Maternal Hepatitis

Number of mothers

Maternal Carrier

HB$_S$ Ag haemagglutination Titre.

Fig. 1.

titre of maternal antigen in these three instances were 1/200, 1/400 and 1/800 by passive haemagglutination, so it is unlikely that the presence of antigen in the cord blood merely reflects the height of the titre in the mother's blood. Follow-up samples from the babies were obtained when they were between three and twelve months of age. All the positive samples (table 8), reacted by electrophoresis as well as by the more sensitive tests.

Specific immunoglobulin (250 mg) was given, soon after delivery, to the infants of 2 women who went into labour during the acute phase of hepatitis B. One mother delivered twins who were separated from her at birth and subsequently adopted into separate households. One twin became HBsAg positive during the sixth month of life, the other remains negative. The third baby developed antigenaemia during the fifth month of life.

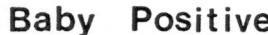

Baby Positive

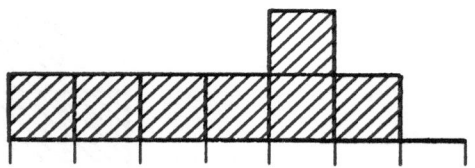

Number
of
mothers

Baby Negative

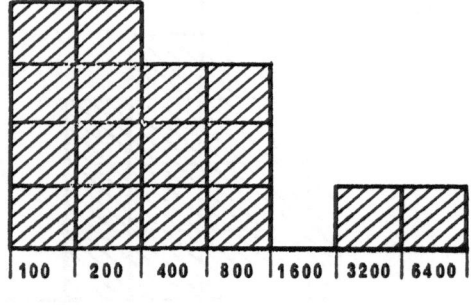

| 100 | 200 | 400 | 800 | 1600 | 3200 | 6400 |

HB$_S$ Ag haemagglutination Titre.

Fig. 2.

Table 5. Effect of HBsAg subtype on transmission from mother to child.

Mothers Ag.	Transmission	No transmission
ad	4	10
ay	3	2

Table 6. Subtypes of HBsAg in pregnant women in London.

	Carriers	Acute hepatitis
ad	12	0
ay	0	5

Table 7. Morphology of maternal HBsAg related to transmission of hepatitis B.

Dane particles	Transmission occurred	No transmission
Present	1	2
Absent	2	9

Table 8. HBsAg in babies.

Cord blood	Later blood	
Negative 26	Negative 20 Positive 6	
Positive 3	Negative 1 Positive 2	

DISCUSSION

It was already known (22) that acute hepatitis near term was more dangerous than the carrier state, and our study suggests that clinical information is a better guide to the likely outcome than any of the laboratory tests.

The effect of titre and subtype seem to be related to the presence or absence of hepatitis. Stevens et al. (26) found that babies in Taiwan were more likely to be affected if the maternal antigen titre was high, but they used a very sensitive test for screening antenatal sera. HBsAg could be detected by electrophoresis in all the sera from the mothers in this study so the divergence in results is even more striking than might appear from table 1. The ad subtype predominates in the Far East as it does in Denmark, England and the United States, while in Greece carriers are usually of ay subtype. This suggests that subtype cannot be important in determining whether transmission will occur, and this impression is confirmed by our findings. We have not tested for w/r subtypes in our material as the r specificity is very rare in England. Although r predominates in Taiwan there is no other reason to suppose that the minor antigens determinants of HBsAg are useful markers of congenital transmission.

It was thought that the presence of e antigen (14) in the mother's serum might be related to the probability that transplacental infection would occur. However as the e antigen is unstable (13) it was not possible to test this hypothesis by examining sera which had been sent to the laboratory by post and subsequently stored for long periods. The morphology of the maternal antigen was used as an index of this factor since a close correlation has been reported between the presence of double shelled particles and detection of e antigen serologically (17). Our results do not show that this test is useful in predicting congenital infection with hepatitis B. However there were more pregnant carriers with double shelled particles than was expected on the basis of experience with blood donors. This might suggest that some of the asymptomatic pregnant 'carriers' had significant liver disease. This might in turn be responsible for the occasional transmission by 'carrier' mothers. Chronic HBsAg positive hepatitis and cirrhosis are common in the Far East where congenital infection is also common while several of the carrier mothers who have transmitted in the United States have an antecedent history of acute hepatitis B or were drug abusers (23).

Most carriers have high titres of anti HB core antibody circulating and it has been suggested that this antibody might cross the placenta and protect the infant when it was exposed during delivery (5). In the study by Papaevangelou et al. (18) the anti HB core antibody titres in cord bloods were found to be only slightly below the maternal level, but a protective effect could not be found.

The small amounts of HBsAg found in some cord blood samples is likely to result from maternal/fetal transfusion. Despite this clear evidence of exposure the infants frequently procedure no further evidence of hepatitis B infection (19).

All the babies who developed 'late' antigenaemia became persistent carriers but so far none has developed serious liver disease. It is probable that some will clear the antigen as their immune systems mature, but others seem to have been rendered specifically tolerant. An unknown number develop chronic active hepatitis or cirrhosis and although the proportion is less than was suggested by early reports it would undoubtedly be desirable to prevent infection of the babies. It has been suggested that the administration of specific 'hyperimmune' globulin soon after birth might be effective if exposure took place during delivery.

Our experience is not encouraging. The incubation periods for both affected babies were very long (5 and 6 months) compared with average of 5 weeks for the untreated cases. This suggests that some attenuation of hepatitis B had occurred and that larger doses of immunoglobulin might be effective.

REFERENCES

1. Almeida, J. D., A. J. Zuckerman, P. E. Taylor and A. P. Waterson, Immune electron-microscopy of the Australia-SH (serum hepatitis) antigen. *Microbios. 2*: 117-123 (1969).
2. Aziz, M. A., G. Khan, T. Khanum and A. R. Siddiqui, Transplacental and postnatal transmission of the hepatitis-associated antigen. *J. infect. Dis. 127*: 110 (1973).
3. Buchholz, H. M., G. G. Frosner and G. B. Ziegler, HBAg carrier state in an infant delivered by caesarean section. *Lancet 2*: 343 (1974).
4. Cayzer, I., D. S. Dane, C. H. Cameron and J. V. Denning, A rapid haemagglutination test for hepatitis B antigen. *Lancet 1*: 947-949 (1974).
5. Cossart, Y. E., Acquisition of hepatitis B antigen in the newborn period. *Postgrad. Med. 50*: 334-337 (1974).
6. Embil, J. A., S. A. Bustamante and K. E. Scott, Transmission of hepatitis type B by exchange transfusion in newborn infants. *Canad. J. Publ. Hlth. 66*: 44-47 (1975).
7. Gibson, P. E. and Y. E. Cossart, The relation between electrophoretic mobility and serological subtype of HBsAg. In Proc. 1st int. Workshop on HBs subtypes. Paris, April 1975, Courouc\u00e9, Holland, Muller, and Soulier (eds.). *Bibl. haemat. (Basel) 42*: 11-14 (1976).
8. Gillespie, A., D. Dorman, J. A. Walker-Smith and J. S. Yu, Neonatal hepatitis and Australia antigen. *Lancet 2*: 1081 (1970).
9. Holzbach, R. T., Australia antigen hepatitis in pregnancy. Evidence against trans-placental transmission of Australia antigen in early and late pregnancy. *Arch. intern. Med. 130*: 234-236 (1972).
10. Kohler, P. F., R. S. Dubois, D. A. Merrill and W. A. Bowes, Prevention of chronic neonatal hepatitis B virus infection with antibody to the hepatitis B surface antigen. *New Engl. J. Med. 291*: 1378-1380 (1974).
11. Ling, C. M. and L. R. Overby, Prevalence of Hepatitis B virus antigen as revealed by direct radioimmune assay with ^{125}I-antibody. *J. Immunol. 109*: 834-841 (1972).
12. McCarthy, J. W., Hepatitis B antigen (HB Ag) positive chronic aggressive hepatitis and cirrhosis in an 8 month old infant: A case report. *J. Pediat. 83*: 638-639 (1973).
13. Magnius, L. O., Characterization of a new antigen-antibody system associated with hepatitis B. *Clin. exp. Immunol. 20*: 209-216 (1975).
14. Magnius, L. O., A. Lindholm, P. Lundin and S. Iwarson, A new antigen-antibody system: clinical significance in long term carriers of hepatitis B surface antigen. *J. Amer. med. Ass. 231*: 356-359 (1975).
15. Marshall, W. and J. A. Dudgeon, Australia Antigen in a child with congenital mal-formation and in his mother. *Amer. J. Dis. Child. 123*: 378-379 (1972).
16. Merrill, D. A., R. S. Dubois and P. F. Kohler, Neonatal onset of the hepatitis-associated-antigen carrier state. *New. Engl. J. Med. 287*: 1280-1282 (1972).
17. Nielsen, J. O., O. Dietrichson and E. Juhl, Incidence and meaning of the 'e' determi-nant among hepatitis B antigen positive patients with acute and chronic liver diseases. *Lancet 2*: 913-915 (1974).
18. Papaevangelou, G., J. Hoofnagle and J. Kremastinou, Transplacental transmission of hepatitis B virus by symptom-free chronic carrier mothers. *Lancet 2*: 746-748 (1974).
19. Papaevangelou, G., T. Kremastinou, C. Prevedourskis and D. Kaskarelis, Hepatitis B antigen and antibody in maternal blood, cord blood and amniotic fluid. *Arch. Dis. Childh. 49*: 936-939 (1974).
20. Pesendorfer, F., O. Krassnitsky and F. Wewalka, Immunelektrophoretischer Nach-weis von Hepatitis associated antigen. *Klin. Wschr. 48*: 58-59 (1970).
21. Reesnick, H. W., W. J. Duimel and H. G. Brummelhuis, Evaluation of a new haemag-glutination technique for the demonstration of Hepatitis-B antigen. *Lancet 2*: 1351-1353 (1973).

22. Schweitzer, I. L., J. W. Mosley, M. Ashcaval, V. M. Edwards and L. B. Overby, Liver Physiology and Disease. *Gastroenterology 65*: 277-283 (1973).
23. Schweitzer, I. L., A. Wing, C. McPeak and R. L. Spears, Hepatitis and Hepatitis-Associated antigen in 56 mother-infant pairs. *J. Amer. med. Ass. 220*: 1092-1095 (1972).
24. Skinhøj, P., H. Olesen, J. Cohn and M. Mikkelsen, Hepatitis-associated antigen in pregnant women. *Acta path. microbiol. scand. Sect. B. 80*: 362-366 (1972).
25. Smithwick, E. M. and S. C. Go, Hepatitis associated antigen in cord and maternal sera. *Lancet 2*: 1080 (1970).
26. Stevens, C. E., R. P. Beasley, J. Tsui and W. C. Lee, Vertical transmission of hepatitis B in Taiwan. *New Engl. J. Med. 292*: 771-774 (1975).
27. Turner, G. C., A. M. Field, R. M. Lasheen, R. Mcl. Todd, G. B. B. White and A. A. Porter, SH (Australia) antigen in early life. *Arch. Dis. Childh. 46*: 616-672 (1971).
28. Wright, R., J. R. Perkins and D. Bouch, Cirrhosis associated with Australia antigen in an infant who acquired hepatitis from its mother. *Brit. med. J. 4*: 719-721 (1970).

NEONATAL SUSCEPTIBILITY
TO MHV3 INFECTION IN MICE*

E. LEVY-LEBLOND, M.D., AND JEAN-MARIE DUPUY, M.D.

Neonatal susceptibility to viral infections and increasing resistance with age is frequently observed but poorly understood (6). In human newborns, for example, several viral infections – e.g. herpes virus – lead to the development of severe disease contrasting with the benign form presented by normal adults. In addition, for reasons which are still unknown, newborns often developed persistent viral infections. In mice, it has been shown that age-dependent resistance to Sindbis virus might be related to several factors including cellular immunity (4, 6). Hirch et al. (3) showed that resistance to herpes simplex virus in suckling mice can be achieved by transfer of adult macrophages. A progression from susceptibility to complete resistance was demonstrated with MHV2 in the C3H strain of mice (2). Liver macrophage cultures from C3H mice of various ages showed a parallel increasing resistance (2).

In the case of infection with mouse hepatitis virus type 3 (MHV3) we found that mice of the A strain were resistant when tested at adult age but were highly susceptible during the first 2 weeks of life (5). It was also shown that resistance to MHV3 implied a normal mature cell-mediated immune system (1, 5). Therefore, MHV3 susceptibility of newborns of the resistant A strain of mice was used as a model for studying the mechanisms involved in such a susceptibility.

When A strain mice, immunologically depressed either by neonatal thymectomy or by long term administration of antilymphocytic serum, were challenged at 6 weeks of age with MHV3, they appeared to be highly susceptible (table 1). Control animals of the same age, either sham thymectomized or treated with normal rabbit serum behaved as non treated mice and resisted the virus challenge (table 1). It was likely, then, that cell mediated immunity was involved in the resistance mechanism against MHV3 infection.

Since protection of susceptible animals was not achieved by passive ad-

* This study was supported by I.N.S.E.R.M. ATP 29, and by the University Paris-Sud.

Table 1. Effect of neonatal thymectomy and long term ALS treatment on resistance of mice to MHV3 infection.

Treatment	No. dead/No. tested[3]
Thymectomy[1]	10/10
Sham thymectomy	0/10
ALS[2]	10/10
NRS	1/11
O	0/20

1. Thymectomy was performed during the first 12 hours after birth.
2. ALS and NRS were prepared in rabbits which were injected subcutaneously twice a week from birth up to 6 weeks of age. Each mouse received a total volume of 2.15 ml.
3. 2×10^3 LD_{50} of MHV3 was injected IP into 6 week old mice.
ALS = antilymphocytic serum.
NRS = normal rabbit serum.

Table 2. Role of passive administration or transfer of MHV3 antibody in protection of susceptible animals.

Origin of MHV3-antibody	Recipients No. dead/No. tested
Immune serum[1]	23/30
Normal serum	28/30
Immunized mothers[2]	15/15
Non-immunized mothers	19/19

1. One to 3 ml of serum from MHV3 immunized or normal A strain mice were injected I.P. into susceptible DBA/2 mice before challenge with MHV3 virus.
2. MHV3 virus was injected in 1 to 3 day old animals born either to non-immunized or to mothers immunized with 6 injections of virulent virus, 3 of them given during pregnancy.

ministration or transplacental transfer of anti MHV3 antibody (table 2), we studied the effect of cell transfer from isogenic adult animals. Table 3 shows the results of various experiments in which 3 to 6 day old A strain mice were injected with or without various types of spleen cells from isologous adult donors and challenged with MHV3. Good protection was obtained when the animals were injected with 15 million spleen cells (76% survival). Cell separation by means of adherence to plastic for 4 hours revealed that neither the non adherent nor the adherent cells injected separately had any protective capacity. When both populations however were first separated then reconstituted and injected, a good protection was again obtained with 76% survival.

In order to further analyze the involvement of T cells, whole spleen cells and non adherent cells were treated by anti theta-antiserum or by CBA

Table 3. Effect of whole or separated spleen cells from adult A strain mice on neonatal sensitivity to MHV3 infection.

| Donor spleen cells | | | Recipients[3] |
Type[1]	Treatment[2]	No. ($\times 10^6$)	No. dead/No. tested
None	. .	. .	36/36
Whole	. .	15	7/29
Adherent	. .	26	7/ 7
Non-adherent	. .	30	10/10
Adherent	. .	15	
+			6/25
Non-adherent	. .	15	
Whole	anti-θ	28	9/ 9
Whole	CBA serum	25	2/ 7
Adherent	. .	15	
Non-adherent	anti-θ	15	19/19
Adherent	. .	15	
Non-adherent	CBA serum	15	2/16

1. Separation of spleen cells was obtained by means of adherence as non-adherence to plastic.
2. Anti-theta antiserum was prepared by immunization of CBA mice with AKR thymocytes. Treatment of spleen cells with anti-theta antiserum and guinea pig complement decreased the cell viability from 95% to 60%.
3. 3 to 6 day old A strain animals were injected I.P. with 100 LD$_{50}$ of MHV3.

control serum and complement before injection in newborns. Non adherent treated cells were injected with non treated-adherent cells. As shown in table 3, treatment with anti theta-antiserum and complement entirely suppressed the protective effect against MHV3 infection. In addition, when adherent cells were injected with purified T cells, all the animals survived. In a similar attempt of better characterization, spleen macrophages were collected after 24 hours of culture in plastic flasks and were characterized by phagocytic functions and acid phosphatase labelling. When such macrophages were injected with non adherent cells, none of the recipients died after MHV3 infection. No protection however was obtained when purified T cells or macrophages were injected separately.

From the results presented here, several points can be outlined. 1. Newborn mice from the resistant A strain are susceptible to MHV3 infection up to 3 weeks of age but can be well protected against virus challenge by transfer of adult isologous spleen cells. 2. Cell separation by means of plastic adherence property revealed that at least 2 types of cells were involved and that injection of both populations was required to achieve a transfer of resistance to MHV3. 3. Treatment of cells with anti theta antiserum as well as purification and characterization of T cells and macrophages showed that both populations are likely to be involved in the transfer of resistance. 4. Therefore, the state of neonatal susceptibility to MHV3 infection in mice is probably due to a delayed maturation of cell mediated immunity and of the macrophage population. Synergy between T cells and macrophages is certainly required to achieve a resistant state against MHV3 infection. However, the type of interaction is still unknown.

REFERENCES

1. Dupuy, J. M., E. Levy-Leblond and C. Le Prevost, Immunopathology of mouse hepatitis virus type 3 infection. Effect of immunosuppression in resistant mice. *J. Immunol.* *114*: 226-230 (1975).
2. Gallily, R., A. Warwick and F. B. Bang, Ontogeny of macrophage resistance to mouse hepatitis in vivo and in vitro. *J. exp. Med.* *125*: 537-548 (1967).
3. Hirch, M. S., B. Zisman and A. C. Allison, Macrophages and age-dependent resistance to herpes simplex virus in mice. *J. Immunol.* *104*: 1160-1165 (1970).
4. Johnson, R. T., H. F. McFarland and S. E. Levy, Age-dependent resistance to viral encephalitis: Studies of infections due to Sindbis virus in mice. *J. infect. Dis.* *125*: 257-262 (1972).
5. Le Prevost, C., E. Levy-Leblond, J. L. Virelizier and J. M. Dupuy, Immunopathology of mouse hepatitis virus type 3 infection. Role of humoral and cell-mediated immunity in resistance mechanisms. *J. Immunol.* *114*: 221-225 (1975).
6. Reinarz, A. B. G., M. G. Broome and B. P. Sagik, Age-dependent resistance of mice to Sindbis virus infection: Viral replication as a function of host age. *Infect. Immun.* *3*: 268-273 (1971).

HEPATITIS B VACCINES

ARIE J. ZUCKERMAN, M.D., D.SC., DIP. BACT.

The repeated failure to pass hepatitis B virus serially in tissue or organ cultures (16) has hampered progress towards the development of a safe and effective vaccine. Attention has therefore been directed recently towards the use of other preparations for active immunization against hepatitis B (17, 18).

Active immunization has been attempted (6, 7, 5) using as the immunogen a known infective human serum (MS-2 serum) that contains hepatitis B virus. The serum was diluted 1 in 10 in distilled water and heated at 98° C for one minute. The serum treated in this manner was not infective and it successfully prevented or modified hepatitis B in 69% of susceptible persons inoculated with the heated serum and challenged with the original infective serum 4-8 months later. The results with the heat-inactivated serum were essentially the same after one, two or three inoculations. However, this is a crude way of inducing immunity and it is unlikely to be accepted for general use. This work, nevertheless, laid the foundations for unconventional immunogens that could be used as vaccines.

SUBUNIT HEPATITIS B VACCINES

Isolated viral coat protein challenges the immune mechanism of the body in the same way as the intact infectious agent and the possibility of using purified spherical 22 nm hepatitis B surface antigen particles (fig. 1), which are free of detectable nucleic acid, seems attractive. Such experimental vaccines have been prepared and a limited number of susceptible chimpanzees have been shown to be protected by such immunogens. It is expected that cautious preliminary trials in man will be undertaken in the near future.

However, a variable amount of host protein, and perhaps carbohydrate, may be complexed with hepatitis B viral protein. These host proteins may include various pre-existing structures of the liver cell and may thus induce undesirable immunologic reactions (13). Recently, Neurath et al. (12)

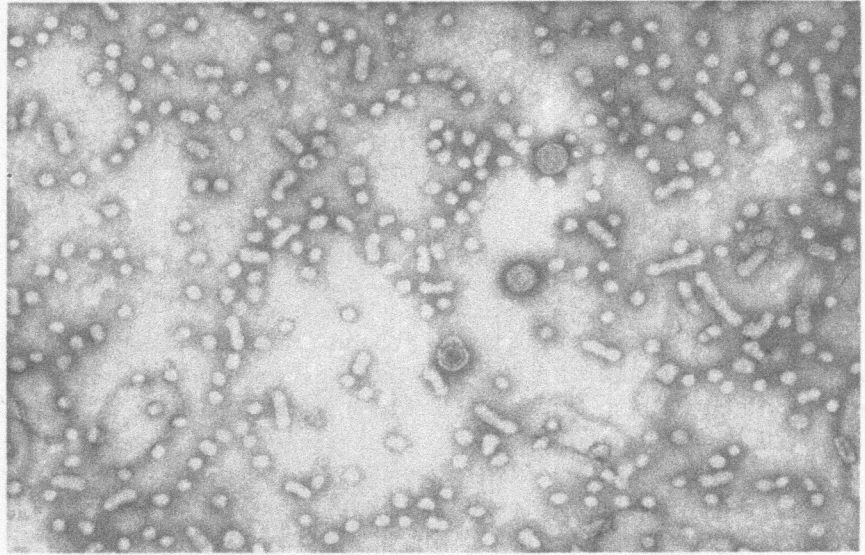

Fig. 1. Low power electron micrograph showing the three morphological forms of hepatitis B antigen: the small pleomorphic 20-25nm spherical forms, tubular forms and the 42nm double-shelled (Dane) particles. The small particles generally predominate. ($\times$86,301) (Electron micrograph reproduced with permission from *Human Viral Hepatitis*, A. J. Zuckerman. North Holland Publishing Co., Amsterdam, 1975).

reported that antigenic determinants related to human plasma proteins are constituents of hepatitis B surface antigen. These determinants appear to be related to antigenic specificities on prealbumin, albumin, apolipoproteins C and D, and the gamma chain of immunoglobulin G. Other studies indicated that the larger polypeptides of purified surface antigen are probably adsorbed serum proteins which are necessary for the preservation of antigenic activity. Finally, the close association of the surface antigen with normal serum components has been an acknowledged difficulty in developing purification techniques for separation of the antigen.

HOST ANTIGENS AND IMMUNIZATION

Burrell et al. (1) found demonstrable and significant levels of carbohydrate in purified fractions of the surface antigen. The total carbohydrate content of purified small antigen particles is reported as 3.6-6.5%. Three glycoproteins have also been found as well as a glycolipid and three major phospholipids

(3, 2, 14). The carbohydrate may be necessary for maintaining the structure and functional integrity of the antigenic determinants, or the carbohydrate itself may constitute a major antigenic determinant. The carbohydrate might have a novel haptenic specificity which is either virus-coded or virus-induced host cell-coded. Alternatively, the carbohydrate, and some lipoprotein components, might simply be derived from the host cell membranes as the mature virus particles are released. There may be some similarity between such a carbohydrate hapten, or the lipoprotein components, and those carbohydrate and lipoprotein antigens of normal cell surfaces, leading to a degree of tolerance because of a close antigenic resemblance between hepatitis B surface antigen and 'self' antigens. Alternatively, an autoimmune reaction may be initiated.

An autoimmune reaction might also be induced by hepatitis B infection because of a change in antigenicity of the hepatocyte cell membranes, due to alteration of existing antigens or the appearance of viral determinants. T lymphocytes responsive to such new antigenic determinants could promote a B cell response to unaltered 'self' antigens. The synthesis and release of the resulting autoantibody is subject in turn to control by suppressor T cells. These complex interactions between T and B cells, could be of fundamental importance in the pathogenesis of chronic liver disease.

The development of cell-mediated immunity to hepatitis B virus antigens during the acute stage of the disease, its persistence during convalescence and its disappearance after recovery, and its absence in persistent asymptomatic carriage of the surface antigen is consistent with the hypothesis that cell-mediated immunity may be involved in terminating viral infection and, under certain circumstances, in promoting hepatocellular damage.

Liver-specific lipoprotein is a macrolipoprotein which is thought to be a normal constituent of the hepatocyte plasma membrane (4). The isolation of two organ-specific proteins from human liver (10) was followed by the demonstration of organ-specific antibodies in the sera of a proportion of patients with active chronic hepatitis (11). In addition, active chronic hepatitis has been induced in rabbits by repeated immunization with extracts containing the liver-specific proteins (9). Cellular hypersensitivity, as measured by leucocyte migration inhibition to these proteins was found in 69% of 16 patients with active chronic hepatitis, and 50% of 12 patients with primary biliary cirrhosis (8). More recently, evidence was found of cell-mediated sensitization to hepatitis B surface antigen in all patients with acute hepatitis B and transitory sensitization to liver-specific lipoprotein was detected in many of the patients.

These findings are consistent with the hypothesis that a cell-mediated immune response to hepatitis B antigen, present early on at the onset of acute hepatitis, is the cause of acute liver damage by a cytotoxic effect on virus-infected cells. If the response to liver-specific lipoproteins persisted, it could be responsible for progression to chronic liver damage. It is also postulated that the progressive liver damage of active chronic hepatitis is due to an autoimmune reaction directed against an hepatocyte surface lipoprotein which is initiated in most cases by infection with hepatitis B virus. Lee et al. (8) found evidence of cell-mediated immunity to HBsAg in 62% of patients with antigen-negative chronic hepatitis, suggesting a high frequency of previous infection with hepatitis B virus. A cellular response to the antigen was found in the majority of hepatitis B antigen-positive patients. Evidence of sensitization to liver-specific lipoprotein was found in more than half of the patients, with a similar frequency in the two groups. These results are consistent with the hypothesis that infection with hepatitis B virus is important in initiating the disease in many cases of active chronic hepatitis and that sensitization to the liver cell membrane antigen is responsible for the perpetuation of the liver injury. Thomson et al. (15) demonstrated the killing of isolated rabbit hepatocytes in vitro when incubated with lymphocytes from 20 out of 22 patients with untreated active chronic hepatitis. Blocking experiments strongly suggest that the cytotoxicity is due to an immunological reaction directed at a cell surface antigen.

All these observations indicate that immunologic mechanisms and the presence of antibodies reacting with various tissue components may well be involved in the pathogenesis of liver damage. It may therefore be undesirable to employ preparations of HBsAg which contain host cell components for immunization against this infection.

ANTIGENIC POLYPEPTIDES

Subunits of the surface antigen, in the form of polypeptides, on the other hand, offer an attractive proposition as immunogens. Such preparations would exclude genes of viral and cellular origin and could not be infectious. Analysis of the proteins of the surface antigen by polyacrylamide gel electrophoresis has shown that the antigen contains between five and nine polypeptides ranging in molecular weight from approximately 15,000 to 120,000. Work is currently in progress to determine if such preparations can be used as vaccines.

SYNTHETIC HEPATITIS B VACCINE

The primary sequence of the haptenic peptide of the surface antigen may also provide an approach for the development of a synthetic peptide, which when coupled to a macromolecular carrier could serve as a suitable immunogen. Once detailed data are available on the protein, peptide and aminoacid composition of the surface antigen, it should be possible to define by animal immunization the moiety responsible for the antigenic activity.

SUMMARY

Experimental hepatitis B vaccines consisting of purified spherical 22nm surface antigen particles have been tested in a limited number of susceptible chimpanzees. A variable amount of host protein and other components may be complexed with hepatitis B viral protein and such host antigens may induce undesirable immunologic reactions. There are indications that humoral immunologic mechanisms and cell-mediated immune responses may well be involved in the pathogenesis of liver damage.

Subunits of the surface antigen, in the form of polypeptides, offer an attractive proposition as immunogens.

ACKNOWLEDGEMENTS

The work in progress at the London School of Hygiene and Tropical Medicine is supported by generous grants from the Medical Research Council, the World Health Organization and the Department of Health and Social Security, and the Wellcome Trust.

REFERENCES

1. Burrell, C. J., E. Proudfoot, G. A. Keen and B. P. Marmion, Carbohydrates in hepatitis B antigen. *Nature new Biol.* *243*: 260-262 (1973).
2. Chairez, R., B. Hollinger, J. L. Melnick and G. R. Dreesman, Biophysical properties of purified morphologic forms of hepatitis B antigen. *Intervirology 3*: 129-140 (1974).
3. Chairez, R., S. Steiner, J. L. Melnick and G. R. Dreesman, Glycoproteins associated with hepatitis B antigen. *Intervirology 1*: 224-228 (1973).
4. Hopf, U., K. H. Meyer zum Buschenfelde and J. Freudenberg, Liver-specific antigens of different species. II. Localization of a membrane antigen at cell surface of isolated hepatocytes. *Clin. exp. Immunol. 16*: 117-124 (1974).

5. Krugman, S. and J. P. Giles, Viral hepatitis type B (MS-2 strain): Further observations on natural history and prevention. *New Engl. J. Med. 228*: 755-760 (1973).
6. Krugman, S., J. P. Giles and J. Hammond, Hepatitis virus: Effect of heat on the infectivity and antigenicity of the MS-1 and MS-2 strains. *J. infect. Dis. 122*: 432-436 (1970).
7. Krugman, S., J. P. Giles and J. Hammond, Viral hepatitis type B (MS-2 strain). Studies on active immunization. *J. Amer. med. Ass. 217*: 41-45 (1971).
8. Lee, W. M., W. D. Reed, C. G. Mitchell, R. M. Galbraith, A. L. W. F. Eddleston, A. J. Zuckerman and R. Williams, Cellular and humoral immunity to hepatitis B surface antigen in active chronic hepatitis. *Brit. med. J. 1*: 705-708 (1975).
9. Meyer zum Buschenfelde, K. H., F. K. Kossling and P. A. Miescher, Experimental chronic active hepatitis in rabbits following immunization with human liver proteins. *Clin. exp. Immunol. 11*: 99-108 (1972).
10. Meyer zum Buschenfelde, K. H. and P. A. Miescher, Liver specific antigens; purification and characterization. *Clin. exp. Immunol. 10*: 89-102 (1972).
11. Miller, J. G., M. G. M. Smith, C. G. Mitchell, A. L. W. F. Eddleston, W. D. Reed and R. Williams, Cell-mediated immunity to a human liver specific antigen in patients with active chronic hepatitis and primary biliary cirrhosis. *Lancet 2*: 296-297 (1972).
12. Neurath, A. R., A. M. Prince and A. Lippin, Hepatitis B antigen: antigenic sites related to human serum proteins revealed by affinity chromatography. *Proc. nat. Acad. Sci.* (Wash.) *71*: 2663-2667 (1974).
13. Popper, H. and I. R. Mackay, Relation between Australia antigen and autoimmune hepatitis. *Lancet 1*: 1161-1164 (1974).
14. Steiner, S., M. T. Huebner and G. R. Dreesman, Major polar lipids of hepatitis B antigen preparations: Evidence for the presence of a glycosphingolipid. *J. Virol. 14*: 572-577 (1974).
15. Thomson, A. D., M. A. G. Cochrane, I. G. McFarlane, A. L. W. F. Eddleston and R. Williams, Lymphocyte cytotoxicity to isolated hepatocytes in chronic active hepatitis. *Nature 252*: 721-722 (1974).
16. Zuckerman, A. J. and P. M. Earl, Tissue and organ culture studies of hepatitis type B. *Vox Sang.* (Suppl.) *24*: 123-128 (1973).
17. Zuckerman, A. J. and C. R. Howard, Prospects for hepatitis B vaccines. *Nature 246*: 445-447 (1973).
18. Zuckerman, A. J. and C. R. Howard, Toward hepatitis B vaccines. *Bull. N.Y. Acad. Med. 51*: 491-500 (1975).

HEREDITARY NEONATAL CHOLESTASIS COMBINED WITH VASCULAR MALFORMATIONS

ØYSTEIN AAGENAES, M.D., TOM HENRIKSEN, M.D., SVEIN SØRLAND, M.D.*

In the recent years Alagille and coworkers (3) and Watson & Miller (7) have described a condition with cholestasis and hepatic ductular hypoplasia combined with peripheral pulmonary stenosis and some other malformations of which a characteristic facies and columnar malformations were the most consistent.

Aagenaes and colleagues (1) described in 1968 a hereditary cholestasis with giant cell transformation combined with lymph vessel hypoplasia and lymphedema in later childhood.

At the Pediatric department, Rikshospitalet, National Hospital of Oslo, we have studied each of these conditions in recent years. Below is a short summary of our findings.

We have studied 6 patients with the first mentioned condition, also called arterio-hepatic dysplasia, which include one father and his daughter.

Figure 1 shows a picture of patient A.H., with the typical appearance, hypertelorism, low nose bridge and a large forehead.

The birth weights and birth lengths of 5 of the patients are shown on table 1. We can see that they are all small for gestational age, with an average birth weight of 2,610 g, and an average birth length of 47 cm. Three of the 5 studied had a columnar anomaly and all 6 had peripheral pulmonary stenosis.

Table 2 shows the clinical course in these patients. Jaundice was of short duration, while pruritis frequently was of relatively long duration, persisting in many of them until about 10-12 years of age. Two children showed transient growth retardation; and one had permanent growth retardation. Only one child showed mental retardation.

Figure 2 shows the growth curve of one of the children with transient growth retardation. After age 2 growth was higher than normal average, and at 10 year of age height was normal.

---

* From the Department of Pediatrics, Rikshospitalet, University Hospital Oslo, Norway.

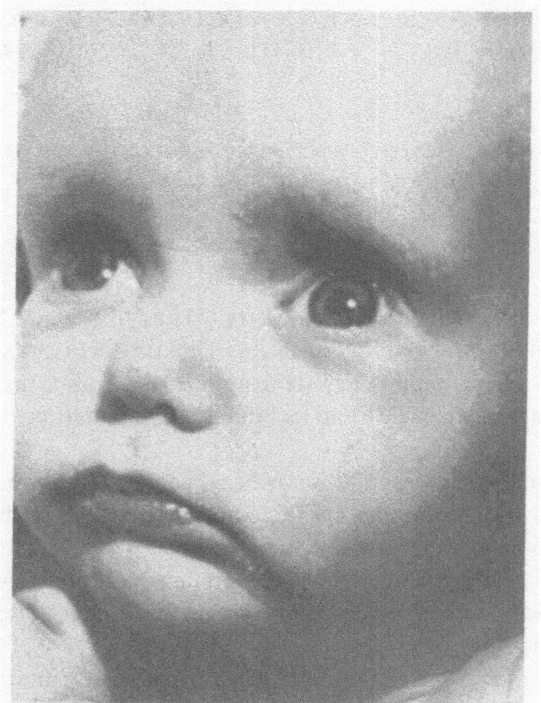

Fig. 1.

Table 1. Birth weight, birth length, columnar anomaly and peripheral pulmonary stenosis in our 6 patients.

Arteriohepatic dysplasia

	Age years	Birth weight	Birth length	Columnar anomaly	Peripheral pulmonary stenosis
T.R.	30	?	?	?	+
J.H.	12	3140 g	51 cm	(+)	+
T.O.	11	3080 g	48 cm	+	+
C.H.	10	2310 g	45 cm	+	+
A.H.	3½	2020 g	46 cm	0	+
A.K.R.	3	2500 g	47 cm	+	+

Table 2. Duration of jaundice and pruritus, growth and mental development in our patients.

Arteriohepatic dysplasia - clinical course

	Age years	Jaundice/ duration	Pruritus/ duration	Growth	Mental development
T.R.	30	short	childhood	N?	N
J.H.	12	0	persists	(R)	N
T.O.	11	short	persists	N	N
C.H.	10	short	few years	(R)	N
A.H.	3½	persists	persists	R	R
A.K.R.	3	short	(persists)	N	N

N = normal
R = retarded
(R) = transiently retarded

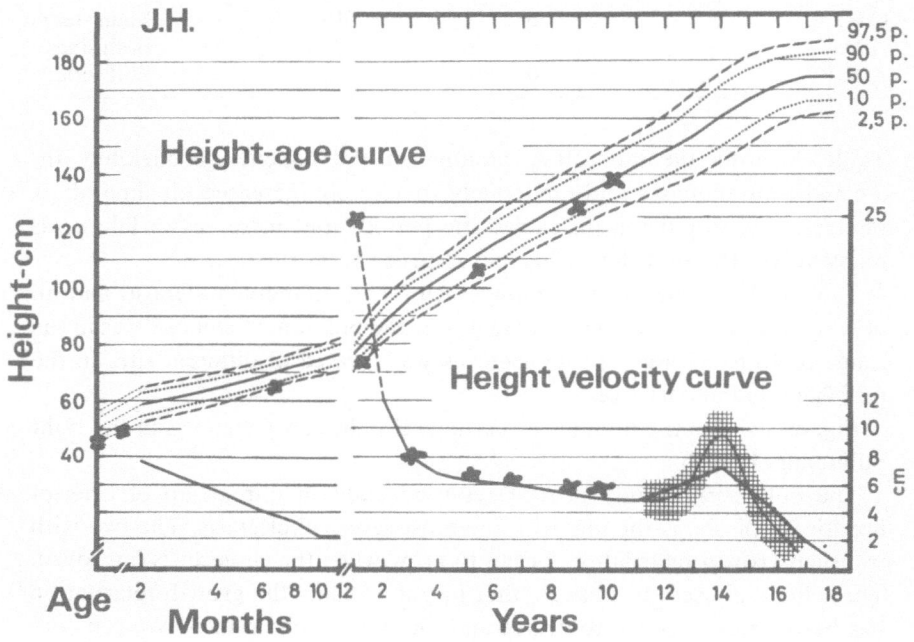

Fig. 2.

Table 3. Laboratory findings in our patients, in infancy and at follow up.
Arteriohepatic dysplasia - laboratory findings

Increased	Transaminases	Alk. phosphatases	Lipids	Bile acids
T.R.	+	+ +	Not now	+
J.H.	+	+	+	+
T.O.	+	+ +	Not now	+
C.H.	+→(+)	+ +→+	+ +→+	?
A.H.	+ + +→+	+ + + +→+ +	+ + + +→+ +	+
A.K.R.	+→+	+ +→+ +	+	+

Table 4. Degree and location of pulmonary stenosis in our patients.
Arteriohepatic dysplasia - cardiac findings

	Peripheral pulm. sten.	Other cardiac findings	Gradient/mm	Side
T.R.	+	0	20	?
J.H.	+	0	15	Left
T.O.	+	0	not cat.	?
C.H.	+	0	10	Main stem
A.H.	+	0	25	Both sides
A.K.R.	+	0	35	Both sides

Table 3 shows the laboratory findings in the patients. Moderately increased transaminases and moderately to severely increased alkaline phosphatases, hyperlipidemia in cholestatic periods and increases in bile acids many years after bilirubin levels had returned to normal.

Table 4 shows the cardiac findings. All 6 had pulmonary stenosis and no other cardiac anomalies. The gradient over the pulmonary stenosis was in the range of 10 to 35 mm and the stenosis was located at different sites in the peripheral pulmonary tree.

Figure 3 shows the findings of peripheral pulmonary stenosis in the right pulmonary branch.

The only permanently growth retarded child in our group of arteriohepatic dysplasia, is the one with the most severe cholestasis. The two with transient growth retardation, began to grow when the cholestasis improved. These findings seem to indicate that in our patients the growth retardation has been directly related to degree and duration of cholestasis. We can confirm the finding of Courtecuisse et al. (4), who has reported extremely high growth hormone-values in their growth retarded children with hepatic duc-

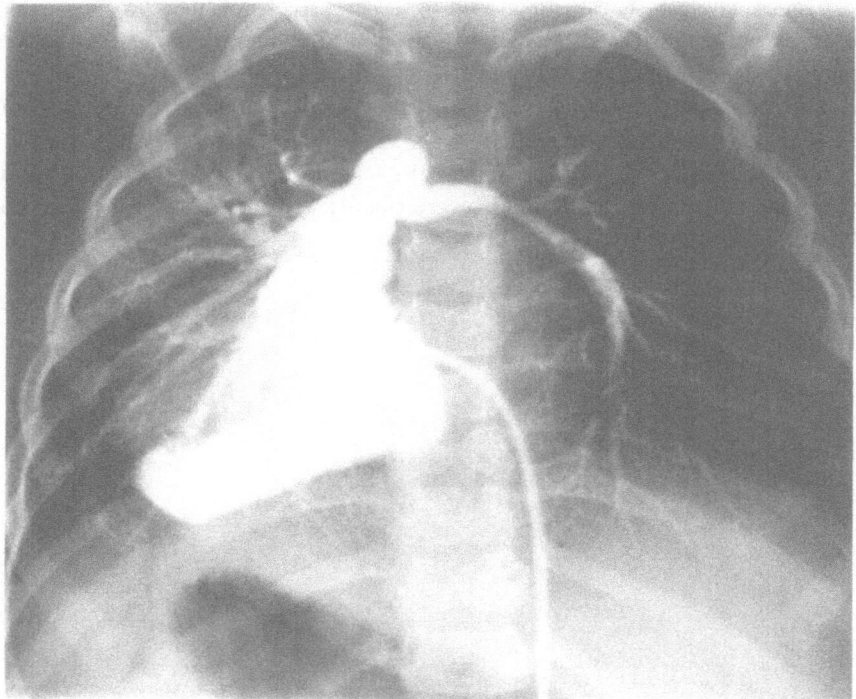

Fig. 3.

tular hypoplasia. Growth hormone level in the one patient we studied was in the range usually found in acromegalic patients.

Studies of gonadal function are not yet complete. So far we can say that our adult with the syndrome, is the father of a daughter with the same disease, which speaks against severe hypogonadism. Our other boys are still prepubertal. The size of their testes seems to be normal for prepubertal boys.

The other condition, which has been described in papers from Norway (1, 2, 6) and from Minnesota (5), is also characterized by intrahepatic neonatal cholestasis. Sixteen patients with this condition were found in a large Norwegian family with a high frequency of inbreeding. Two other small families with the condition are described later; in one family 3 siblings were affected, in the other there was consanguinity between the parents (2).

These infants had high normal birth weights. The average birth weight in 10 of the children for whom we have the birth weights is 3,750 g.

Clinical cholestasis was diagnosed in the first weeks of life; the cholestasis was severe. In all infants on whom a liver biopsy was done, a pronouncde giant cell transformation was found.

The duration of the cholestasis was sometimes less than a year. In many of the patients it lasted for years.

In later childhood lymphedema of the legs developed, and in adulthood this lymphedema was sometimes severe (fig. 4). Lymphangiography showed lymph vessel hypoplasia.

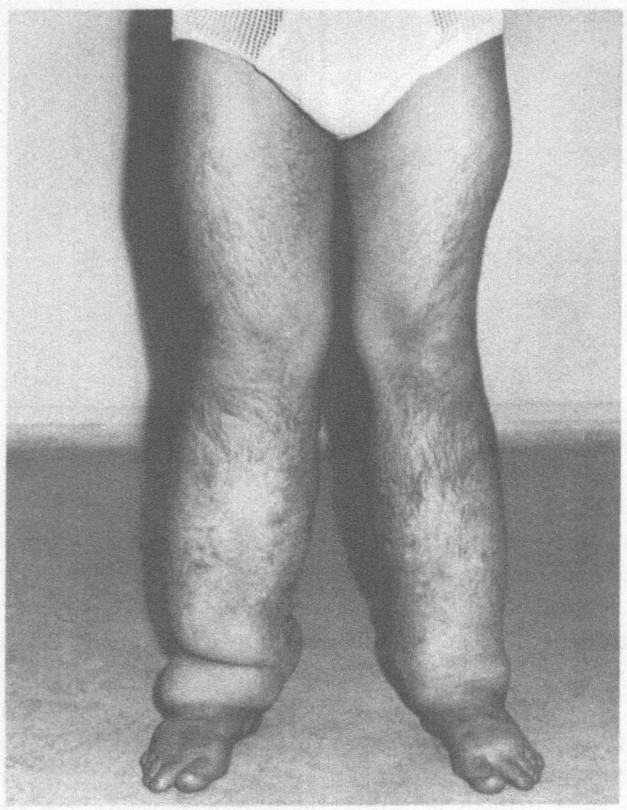

Fig. 4. Lymphedema.

The prognosis in this condition was poor in the period before vitamin K (table 5). Nearly all children born before vitamin K was regularly used, died in infancy.

Table 5. Hereditary giant cell transformation - cholestasis + lymphoedema.

Prognosis:	
Death in infancy (before vitamin K)	9/11
Death in childhood - progressive liver disease	1/11
Severe liver cirrhosis - age 9 years	1/11
Living - age 9-40 years - no severe cirrhosis	9/11
Recurrent cholestasis in adulthood	4/6

Those surviving infancy, mainly those born after 1942, often had a good prognosis. One of 11 died in liver failure (no autopsy performed); another is currently in very poor condition at 9 years of age, with progressive liver cirrhosis. The liver condition of the rest of the patients is good at the moment.

We have now 6 adult patients with this condition, 4 female and 2 male. All the females have had more or less recurrent cholestasis. One of the females has had 3 pregnancies, all accompanied by jaundices. The others have not been pregnant, but have had periods of cholestasis after puberty. None of the two males has had a recurrence of cholestasis.

DISCUSSION

These two conditions have some similarities and some differences. They are both hereditary. In the first condition the mode of inheritance seems to be a dominant inheritance with varying penetrance, while in the second condition an autosomal recessive mode of inheritance seems pretty certain.

In the first condition the liver pathology is dominated by bile duct hypoplasia, while in the second condition the liver pathology is dominated by giant cell transformation.

The vascular malformation in the first condition is a peripheral pulmonary stenosis, while in the other condition it appears to be lymph vessel hypoplasia.

No biochemical abnormalities have been found within the bile acids in these conditions. A developmental morphologic type of malformation therefore seems to be the most probable pathogenesis in both conditions. At present it seems to be a popular hypothesis that a common unitarian pathogenesis lies behind both intrahepatic and extra-hepatic obstructive jaundice. I think we have convincing evidence that common pathogenesis in some infants may give both intrahepatic and extrahepatic obstruction. On the other hand we have some convincing evidence that many etiologies and many pathogeneses may give intrahepatic cholestasis. The great difference in the frequence of heredity in the extrahepatic and intrahepatic obstructions seems to indicate that in most instances both etiology and pathogenesis are different in the two conditions.

REFERENCES

1. Aagenaes, Ø., C. B. van der Hagen and S. Refsum, Hereditary recurrent intrahepatic cholestasis from birth. *Arch. Dis. Childh. 43*: 646-657 (1968).
2. Aagenaes, Ø., Hereditary recurrent cholestasis with lymphoedema – two new families. *Acta paediat. scand. 63*: 465-471 (1974).
3. Alagille, D., M. Odièvre, M. Gautier and J. P. Dommergues, Hepatic ductular hypo-plasia associated with characteristic facies, vertebral malformations, retarded physical, mental, and sexual development, and cardiac murmur. *J. Pediat. 86*: 63-71 (1975).
4. Courtecuisse, V., F. Girard, J. M. Limai and J. P. Dommergues, Statural growth, skeletal and endocrine abnormalities in hepatic ductular hypoplasia in children. Sub-mitted to publication.
5. Sharp, H. and W. Krivit, Hereditary lymphoedema and obstructive jaundice. *J. Pediat. 78*: 491-496 (1971).
6. Sigstad, H., Ø. Aagenaes, R. W. Bjørn-Hansen and K. Rootwelt, Primary lymphoedema combined with hereditary recurrent intrahepatic cholestasis. *Acta med. scand. 188*: 213-219 (1970).
7. Watson, G. H. and V. Miller, Arteriohepatic dysplasia. Familial pulmonary arterial stenosis with neonatal liver disease. *Arch. Dis. Childh. 48*: 459-466 (1973).

PORTAL HYPERTENSION IN EARLY CHILDHOOD: ETIOLOGY AND DIAGNOSTIC PROCEDURES

SYDNEY S. GELLIS, M.D.

This report is confined to children with portal hypertension secondary to extrahepatic disease, consisting essentially of portal vein thrombosis, since space limitations exclude any discussion of children with portal hypertension resulting from primary hepatic disease. It seems appropriate to limit the discussion in this manner since other sections of this book are concerned with the surgical aspects of portal hypertension and most of the surgical experience is with portal hypertension secondary to portal vein thrombosis. Although there are infants and children with portal hypertension resulting from primary hepatic disease who have had shunting procedures, their numbers are limited, because the majority of such children succumb to their liver disease and not to the complications of their hypertension. It should be emphasized, however, that far more children present today with portal hypertension secondary to liver diseases such as cirrhosis, cystic fibrosis, chronic hepatitis, etc., than with portal hypertension resulting from portal vein thrombosis. Since 1948 I have seen 38 patients with extrahepatic portal hypertension whereas a total of 82 patients with portal hypertension secondary to primary liver disease has come to my attention during the same period.

I shall compare our findings with those reported by Drs. Fonkalsrud, Myers, and Robinson (1), chiefly because theirs is not only a large series of patients, but also because they have the largest series of patients who have not been treated surgically and whose follow-up is important since it offers the opportunity to examine the natural course of the disorder. In addition, their series is the most recently published, in 1974.

In our series the age at which the diagnosis of portal hypertension secondary to portal vein thrombosis was made corresponds closely with Fonkalsrud's series. By age 6 years, 80 per cent of his series had been diagnosed; 14 per cent were diagnosed between birth and 1 year, 23 per cent between 1-3 years, and 18 per cent from 3-6 years. Six per cent were diagnosed at 6-10 years and 8 per cent from 10-14 years. In our series of 38 patients, 92 per cent were diagnosed before the 6th birthday and 30 per cent were diagnosed before the first birthday. I do not know why we have a higher incidence of earlier diagnosis. I can only theorize that since the majority of our patients were from high economic levels, frequent examination was regularly performed. This may account for recognition of physical findings at an earlier age.

In the Fonkalsrud study the most frequent initial clinical manifestation was variceal bleeding, occurring in 57 per cent of his patients. Asymptomatic splenomegaly was the second most common manifestation, occurring in 26 of the 69 patients. In contrast, splenic enlargement was the first manifestation in 70 per cent of our patients and bleeding from varices in the remainder.

In contrast to Fonkalsrud's patients, of whom 22 per cent had a definite history of neonatal infection, most commonly peri-umbilical, history of neonatal infection in our series has been very low – 2 patients. Another of our patients has had a history of umbilical vein catheterization and a second received several exchange transfusions. I cannot account for this striking difference. In Fonkalsrud's series umbilical vein catheterization could not be associated with portal vein thrombosis.

More than half of Fonkalsrud's patients had radiographically demonstrated esophageal varices and in 19 of these, variceal bleeding subsequently developed. It was uncommon for us to demonstrate varices radiographically until bleeding had occurred. Esophagoscopy was not performed on our patients.

Thus in our series, the usual clinical picture of an infant or young child with portal hypertension secondary to extrahepatic disease is one of an infant who has had a normal delivery following a normal gestation and birth. They had no history of neonatal infection such as skin infection, gastroenteritis, omphalitis or respiratory disease, and had a normal neonatal course, free of catheterization procedures or transfusions. During the first few years of life they gained and grew normally. Between the ages of 6 months to 3 years routine examination showed splenic enlargement. The spleen has quite regularly been noted to be firm. The liver is not enlarged. Liver function tests are normal but the hematocrit may be below normal, white blood count low and platelets low. Barium swallow usually shows no varices.

Essentially, then, in our experience the majority of patients present solely with splenic enlargement. The physician must investigate all possible causes of splenomegaly. Once esophageal bleeding occurs in a patient with splenomegaly and normal liver function tests, the diagnosis is straightforward.

Prior to hemorrhage, the major disorders which require investigation are hemolytic disorders, malignancy and storage diseases. Since fever is not present, infectious causes of splenomegaly or rheumatoid arthritis without joint involvement are very unlikely. At this stage of the disorder, hematologic and bone marrow studies are most important. The most troublesome possibility in the afebrile child with splenomegaly, and without esophageal bleeding, with normal liver function tests and normal barium swallow, low platelets, white count and hematocrit is a malignancy, especially aleukemic leukemia. A normal bone marrow examination does not necessarily eliminate this diagnosis. Normal long bones and radiographically normal-sized kidneys are reassuring, but the diagnosis must still trouble the physician. Repeated normal bone marrow examinations will finally eliminate leukemia, or the demonstration of a narrowing or block in the portal vein or its tributaries will permit the conclusive diagnosis of portal vein thrombosis with portal hypertension.

The best method for this demonstration is portal venography, far superior to any technic aimed at measuring portal vein pressure. The majority of our patients have had percutaneous splenic portovenography, a small number have had operative mesenteric venography with excellent visualization of the portal venous system. Indirect photography via injection of contrast material into the celiac artery has been used increasingly in the past few years and has permitted excellent visualization of the splenic and portal veins.

I see no great benefit from measurement of portal vein pressure. In our series it has varied tremendously and has not proved satisfactory to me as a means of determining the need for a shunt or the likelihood of its remaining patent when one has been done. I believe it is the size of the vessels which are shunted which determine patency.

I am avoiding discussion of the management of portal hypertension by shunting procedures, leaving this aspect of the problem to the surgeons. From the medical point of view two recommendations can be stressed: First, the importance of avoiding aspirin in the management of the usual febrile illnesses which these infants and children will encounter. All too frequently severe hemorrhage from esophageal varices follows an upper respiratory infection. It is not clear from available data whether infection has been the trigger for hemorrhage or whether it has been due to aspirin, used so freely in the past because its effects on clotting mechanism were not well recognized. Second, the threat to these children of severe pneumococcal infection owing to hypofunctioning of the spleen must be recognized.

Children with splenectomy performed for hemolytic disorders or storage disease are at highest risk of overwhelming bacteremia; children splenectomized because of trauma appear to be at much lower risk. The infants and children with splenomegaly secondary to portal hypertension have engorgement of the spleen which results in hyposplenism – as evidenced by the increased numbers of Heinz bodies and Howell-Jolly bodies in their red blood cells, inclusion bodies which are removed or culled by the normally functioning spleen. Hence these children also have an increased risk from bacterial infections, especially the pneumococcus. It may be wise to keep them on prophylactic penicillin pending the demonstration of the effectiveness or lack of value of such prophylaxis. If this is not done, it is important for the physician to be aware of the child's increased risk. He or she must treat promptly and with large doses of penicillin any child with splenomegaly who suddenly develops high fever without an obvious reason for the fever.

I am troubled by two areas of the extrahepatic portal hypertension problem. Although the thrombosis and narrowing of the portal vein system is found in these children at the time of exploration and shunting, relatively few give a clear-cut history of infection in the early weeks of life which could account for a thrombophlebitis of the portal vein or its tributaries. The striking increase in umbilical vein catheterization during the past few years does not seem to have increased the frequency of portal vein thrombosis followed by portal hypertension. Are there additional factors of which we are presently unaware which produce clotting of blood within the portal vein?

Similarly I am troubled by the general acceptance that shunting procedures are responsible for the subsequent decline in variceal hemorrhage. The Fonkalsrud series indicates that a limited number of children who have managed to escape a shunting operation tend to have fewer bleeding episodes as they grow older. It seems to me that pediatric surgeons must not go on operating on every child who develops esophageal hemorrhage, but must, by combined hospital studies, develop controlled series of patients to determine if risk of hemorrhage is truly reduced by surgery. At the present time surgeons are debating the optimum time for surgery and appear to have overlooked the possibility that surgery may not be required.

REFERENCE

1. Fonkalsrud, E. W., N. A. Myers and M. J. Robinson, Management of extrahepatic portal hypertension in children. *Ann. Surg. 180*: 487-493 (1974).

PORTAL HYPERTENSION IN EARLY CHILDHOOD:
SURGICAL PROBLEMS

WILLIAM P. LONGMIRE JR., M.D. AND ERIC W. FONKALSRUD, M.D.

Reports from different centers comparing the incidence of intrahepatic and extrahepatic portal hypertension have varied widely. In several recent accounts (7, 9, 10, 18) the conditions have been reported to occur with about equal frequency, as has been the case in our center. In other reports, however, extrahepatic obstruction has been much more common (5, 15, 16).

Since the management and the prognosis of portal hypertension vary considerably, depending upon the nature of the underlying pathologic process, it is essential that the type of obstruction be determined as accurately as possible before therapy is instituted. In most instances, the differentiation of intra- from extrahepatic portal hypertension is not difficult.

David Hsia and Sidney Gellis (9) have described the distinguishing features of intrahepatic and extrahepatic block. Extrahepatic block is suggested by 1. history of omphalitis or severe infection; 2. a negative history prior to onset of portal hypertension; 3. hematemesis or splenomegaly as a presenting complaint; 4. no prior evidence of jaundice or liver disease; and 5. normal liver function tests. Intrahepatic block is suggested by a. previous history of jaundice or liver enlargement; b. hepatomegaly or tenderness prior to splenomegaly; c. ascites or other evidence of liver failure; and d. impaired liver function tests.

In a recently reported series (5) of 47 cases of extrahepatic portal hypertension, 13 patients (28%) had a history consistent with omphalitis neonatally, and three patients (6%) had a neonatal history of diarrhea and fever. In the remaining two-thirds of the patients, no apparent etiological factor was involved in the thrombosis. An increasing number of cases of thrombosis in the portal system are being reported after exchange transfusions (17) or administration of hypertonic solutions (20) through the umbilical vein in newborn infants.

Transient ascites has been mentioned as one of the first signs of extrahepatic portal obstruction (13). Clatworthy and Boles (3) suggested that portal occlusion occurring during infancy is accompanied by a very high portal pressure at a time when minimal collateral circulation has developed. This results in the formation of ascites which then resolves as collateral circulation is established, only to be followed some months or years later by massive hemorrhage from a ruptured varix or symptoms and signs of hypersplenism.

The 12 cases of intrahepatic portal hypertension in children reported by Keighley et al. (10) were classified as portal cirrhosis (nonspecific), 5 cases; congenital hepatic fibrosis, 5 cases; and postnecrotic scarring, 2 cases. A high incidence of pancytopenia with signs of liver failure occurred in the patients with cirrhosis. The features of hepatocellular failure were absent in the children with congenital hepatic fibrosis. Pancytopenia was frequent in patients with postnecrotic scarring.

It has been noted that portal hypertension due to intrahepatic block carries a much less favorable outlook than does extrahepatic obstruction because of the serious and often progressive nature of the primary hepatic disease (6). Intrahepatic portal obstruction is almost always a sequela of cirrhosis of the liver which may either follow neonatal hepatitis or exposure to toxic agents or be associated with congenital hepatic fibrosis, fibrocystic disease, or congenital biliary atresia. Periportal fibrosis, regardless of the cause, may produce portal venous hypertension.

CLINICAL MATERIAL

Forty children with evidence of portal hypertension have been treated at the UCLA Hospital during the past 20 years. Intrahepatic portal hypertension was diagnosed in 28 patients, extrahepatic portal hypertension in ten, and posthepatic portal hypertension in two. Twenty-six operations for portal hypertension have been performed in the ten patients with extrahepatic obstruction, 16 such procedures in the 28 patients with intrahepatic obstruction, and one operation each in the two patients with posthepatic block. At the time of the review, nine patients with extrahepatic obstruction were alive, and one was dead. In the intrahepatic disease group, 14 were alive, 12 were dead, and two were lost to follow-up. One patient with posthepatic obstruction was alive. Symptoms related to portal hypertension were present in all of these patients before the age of six years.

SURGICAL PROBLEMS IN INTRAHEPATIC DISEASE

The surgical management of intrahepatic portal hypertension is, in large part, determined by the prognosis of the hepatic disease. Hepatic function was moderately to severely depressed in most of our patients with intrahepatic obstruction; however, three of the five patients with cystic fibrosis (mucoviscidosis) had normal or near normal liver function tests.

Portal hypertension was a significant clinical factor in five patients with biliary atresia, but no specific vascular surgical treatment was instituted, as the biliary anomaly was uncorrectable (table 1). Miyata and associates (14) reported that in 15 of 51 patients who underwent hepatic portoenterostomy for biliary atresia, the jaundice cleared completely. However, in seven of these patients, clinical signs of portal hypertension subsequently developed, and four died. They attributed the frequent development of portal hypertension to the transient episodes of retrograde hepatic cholangitis that occurred in 71% of the jaundice-free patients. A side-to-side portacaval shunt was utilized in one patient with biliary hypoplasia with good results for more than three years.

Signs of portal hypertension accompanied biliary cirrhosis in two patients with recurrent cholangitis due to abnormalities of the biliary tract. Correction of bile stasis and concomitant splenorenal shunt provided relief in one of these patients who had bled from large esophageal varices.

Three of the six patients with intrahepatic obstruction due to posthepatic cirrhosis were not treated surgically. One died of liver failure, and the other two did not return to the hospital and are presumed to be dead. Portacaval shunts were performed in two patients: one died of liver failure in the early postoperative period, and the other did well until his accidental death 12 years after operation. The final patient had an esophagogastrectomy after the failure of splenectomy and mesocaval anastomosis to control bleeding. One year after operation, the patient has general nutritional problems but has had no further bleeding.

Two patients with neonatal hepatitis died within the first 18 months of life without operation. Signs of portal hypertension disappeared with steroid therapy in a patient with plasma cell hepatitis. Portal hypertension has been successfully relieved for six years in one patient with a cavernous hemangioma and cirrhosis who underwent end-to-side splenorenal anastomosis. Two other patients with cirrhosis, one following heavy chemotherapy and the other after combined chemotherapy and radiation therapy administered for mal-

Table 1. Intrahepatic obstruction (28 patients).

Etiology	No. of patients	Treatment	Age at treatment	Results
Biliary atresia	5	None for PH	—	Died
Biliary hyperplasia	3	None for PH (2 cases)	—	Died
		PCA, SS (1 case)	6 year	Well - 9 year
Cystic fibrosis	5	PCA, SS, Sp	6 year	Died - hepatic failure 7 yr postoperatively
		PCA, ES, Sp	13 year	Well - 6½ year
		No operation (3 cases)	—	Hepatospleno-megaly
Recurrent cholangitis	2	Duct repair	6 year	Well
		SRA and duct repair	11 year	Well
Posthepatic cirrhosis	6	No operation (3 cases)	—	Died - hepatic failure (1 case) Lost 2 cases
		PCA (2 cases)	2½ year 3 year	Well - 12 yr (1 case) Died postoperatively (1 case)
		Sp MCA (1 case) EsGa	5 year 6 year 8 year	Continued bleeding No further bleeding, edema and ascites 1 year
Neonatal hepatitis	2	No operation	—	Died hepatic failure 8 months Died hepatic failure 1½ year
Wilson's disease	1	No operation	—	Improved
Plasma cell hepatitis	—	No operation (steroids)	—	Improved
Hemangioma with cirrhosis	1	SRA, ES	15 year	Well - 6 year

Table 1. (continued)

Etiology	No. of patients	Treatment	Age at treatment	Results
Post-chemotherapy	2	SP	4 year	Continued bleeding
		LV (1 case)	7 year	Continued bleeding
		PCA, ES	8 year	Well - 11 year
+ X-ray therapy		PCA, SS (1 case)	16 year	Well - 2 year

PH	= portal hypertension	SRA = splenorenal anastomosis
PCA	= portacaval anastomosis	MCA = mesocaval anastomosis
SS	= side-to-side anastomosis	EsGa esophagogastrectomy
ES	= end-to-side anastomosis	LV = ligation varices
Sp	= splenectomy	

ignant tumors, lived for 11 years and 2 years, respectively, after end-to-side and side-to-side portacaval anastomoses.

Portacaval and splenorenal shunts successfully relieved portal hypertension in eight of the nine patients in whom the operations were used (table 2). Splenectomy and transesophageal ligation of esophageal varices provided only temporary relief of hemorrhage. One technically difficult mesocaval shunt was followed by recurrent bleeding. Subsequent esophagogastrectomy has controlled bleeding successfully but has produced moderately severe nutritional problems. Five of the portacaval-type shunts were performed in

Table 2. Intrahepatic obstruction.

Treatment	No of patients	Result
Splenectomy	4	Continued bleeding
Ligation varices	1	Continued bleeding
Portacaval shunt	7	5 patients alive from $6\frac{1}{2}$-12 year
		1 death liver failure
		7 year postoperatively
		1 death after operation
Splenorenal shunt	2	Well - 6 and 12 year
Mesocaval shunt	1	Continued bleeding
Esophagogastrectomy	1	No bleeding, poor nutrition
Steroids	1	Improved
No operation	16	10 died of primary disease
		6 living, improved

Lost to followup – 2 patients.

Table 3. Intrahepatic obstruction.

No. of patients	Age at operation	Type of shunt	Result
1	2½ year	PCA, ES	Well - 12 year
1	3 year	PCA, ES	Died postoperatively
3	6 year	PCS, ES	Well - 9 year
		PCA, SS	Died 7 years postoperatively hepatic failure
		MCA	Bleeding
1	8 year	PCA, ES	Well - 11 year
1	11 year	SRA, ES	Well - 11 year
1	13 year	PCA, ES	Well - 6½ year
1	15 year	SRA, ES	Well - 6 year
1	16 year	PCA, SS	Well - 2 year

PCA = portacaval anastomosis   SRA = splenorenal anastomosis
ES = end-to-side anastomosis   SS = side-to-side anastomosis
MCA = mesocaval anastomosis

children less than six years of age (table 3). A successful shunt was performed on a 2½-year old child, and a technically adequate anastomosis was accomplished in a 3 year old who died of hepatic failure after operation. In three 6 year old children, two end-to-side portacaval shunts were successfull and one mesocaval shunt failed. The five shunts in children from 8 to 16 years of age have functioned satisfactorily.

The surgical treatment of intrahepatic portal hypertension associated with incurable hepatic disease, such as biliary atresia or severe neonatal or posthepatic hepatitis, offers little hope of even palliative benefit. However, in a wide variety of disease processes that produce intrahepatic scarring and fibrosis and subsequent portal hypertension, substantial, if not permanent, benefit can be achieved with portacaval-type operations. In our series, end-to-side portacaval anastomosis has been used most frequently. The portal vein in a child 2½ to 3 years of age is of sufficient size to allow the construction of a shunt that is not unusually prone to postoperative thrombosis. Temporizing measures, such as splenectomy, variceal ligation, or injection, are probably unnecessary. Unless the prognosis of the hepatic disease is hopeless, consideration should be given to the elective creation of a portacaval shunt in intrahepatic portal hypertension, even in the infant two to three years of age. The prognosis when intrahepatic conditions cause severe symptoms of portal hypertension before this age is usually quite grave.

SURGICAL PROBLEMS IN EXTRAHEPATIC PORTAL VEIN OBSTRUCTION

The ten patients in the present series with signs of extrahepatic portal hypertension in early childhood underwent 26 surgical procedures (table 4). Three of these patients have had no recurrence of bleeding more than two years after their last operation. Two of the five patients with mesocaval anastomosis and one with a portacaval shunt had not rebled at the time of our review. In one patient with a makeshift shunt, more than three years transpired before bleeding recurred.

Table 4. Extrahepatic obstruction (10 patients).

Treatment	No. of cases	Results
Splenectomy	8	Rebled
Ligation	5	Rebled
Total gastrectomy	1	Rebled
SRA	1	Rebled
Partial gastrectomy	2	Rebled
PCA	1	Well - 10 year
MCA	5	3 rebled
		2 well over 2 year
Makeshift shunt	2	1 rebled
		1 well - 3 year
Colon interposition	1	No bleeding, anastomotic stricture, living - 6 year
Varix injections	2	Rebled
No surgical treatment	1	Severe respiratory infections Repeat minor hemorrhages

SRA = splenorenal anastomosis
PCA = portocaval anastomosis
MCA = mesocaval anastomosis

All patients who underwent splenectomy alone, variceal ligation or injection, partial or total gastrectomy, or makeshift shunts have eventually rebled, and, as has been previously emphasized (8), once operative management was undertaken, subsequent operations were frequently necessary.

Arcari and Lynn (1) designated the portal vein as the site of the thrombosis in 25 patients in whom the exact site of the block was determined. Martin (12) has reported that in nine consecutive operations for extrahepatic portal hypertension, the thrombus was confined to that portion of the portal vein adjacent to the liver; thus, after a retropancreatic dissection and division of the portal vein, a 1 to 2 cm segment of the intestinal end was available for a successful anastomosis to the cava or left renal vein. In our experience, as well as that of others (2), the thrombotic process frequently extends more widely in the portal system and involves more than the hepatic end of the portal vein. The identifiable site of obstruction in the 25 cases of Arcari and Lynn (1) were: cavernous portal vein, 12 cases; stenosis of portal vein, 5 cases; thrombus of portal vein, 5 cases; and thrombus of splenic vein, 3 cases.

Except by actual operative dissection and exploration, the true extent of the thrombosis can probably be accurately determined only by operative portogram performed through a branch of the superior mesenteric vein. Important information concerning the patency of the system may be gained, however, by splenoportogram, selective injection of the superior mesenteric artery, or both, and visualization of the superior mesenteric and portal veins. The extent of thrombosis within the portal system is a vitally important consideration in the planning of a shunt operation, for if the occlusion extends down the superior mesenteric vein below the junction with the splenic and coronary veins, esophageal and gastric varices will not be decompressed by shunting that portion of the superior mesenteric bed that drains the small intestine (7).

Ten of the 18 patients with extrahepatic block reported by Mikkelsen (13) had symptoms at or before two years of age. Spontaneous cessation of recurrent varix bleeding was noted in these patients.

In a review of 75 children reported to have bleeding from esophageal varices, 88% of whom had extrahepatic obstruction, 25.3% had their first bleeding episode during the first two years of life and 72% before the seventh year (1). None of the patients died during the first hemorrhage, and of 42 patients followed from the time of the first until the second hemorrhage without operation, only one patient died during the second hemorrhage. The death occurred six years after the first bleeding episode. Three of every four patients who underwent emergency operation for bleeding died.

Clatworthy and de Lorimier (4) enumerated five conditions that they considered to be essential to achievement of a successful shunt in an infant or young child: 1. the veins to be used in the anastomosis must be free of active thrombophlebitis; 2. the shunt must be of sufficient size to decompress the portal system; 3. the shunt must grow as the child grows; 4. the entire portal system must be drained; and 5. the shunt must remain patent.

The frequent thrombosis of shunts in young patients with extrahepatic obstruction and the knowledge that nearly all early hemorrhages in infants and young children can be managed successfully by nonoperative treatment have led to the general acceptance of a plan of management that delays operation until the eighth to the tenth year or until the patient weighs about 60 pounds. At this age the branches of the portal system generally used are of sufficient size to render the shunt less susceptible to thrombosis. Although rebleeding has occurred in three of the five patients treated by mesocaval anastomosis in the present series, this procedure has produced the best results of any of the shunt procedures in several reported series (8, 10, 11, 18). Non-operative management consists of bed rest, sedation, transfusion, and administration of systemic pitressin. In the rare case of the infant or young child in whom bleeding cannot be controlled, transesophageal ligation of varices may provide an opportunity to evaluate the possible effectiveness of elective shunting procedure. Fonkalsrud et al. (8), in a report of 69 patients with extrahepatic portal hypertension, found emergency operation rarely necessary to control bleeding. Sixteen patients were alive without having undergone any operative procedure, and they noted that bleeding episodes became less frequent as the patients increased in age. Their review supports the concept that many patients with portal vein thrombosis can be managed continuously without operation and that operation should be reserved for those patients with repeated, truly life-threatening hemorrhage. Further, if a shunt operation is to be performed on an elective basis, appropriate pre-operative diagnostic studies are essential to indicate the optimum site for the creation of a portacaval shunt.

SURGICAL PROBLEMS IN POSTHEPATIC PORTAL HYPERTENSION

Two patients with posthepatic portal hypertension have been treated (table 5). One boy had onset of vague abdominal pains when five to six years of

Table 5. Posthepatic obstruction (2 patients).

Cause	Age	Symptoms	Treatment	Result
Thrombosis IVC, hepatic veins	8 year	Leg ulcers, GI bleeding	Splenic veindistal pulmonary artery bypass graft	Improved 2 yr. Died - thrombosed graft
Obstruction hepatic veins	5 year	Ascites	PCA, SS	External drainage, peritoneal fluid

PCA = portacaval anastomosis
SS   = side-to-side anastomosis

age. Thoracotomy and subsequent exploratory laparotomy revealed sclerosing mediastinitis and retroperitoneal fibrosis with obstruction of the superior vena cava and the inferior vena cava in the region of the hepatic veins. Repeated gastrointestinal hemorrhages and chronic leg ulcers were alleviated for two years by splenectomy and placement of a teflon graft between the proximal end of the splenic vein and the distal end of the pulmonary artery to the right lower pulmonary lobe. At the time of his death following recurrence of the symptoms approximately two years after operation, the graft was found to be thrombosed.

Intractable life-threatening ascites occurred in a 5 year old boy with hepatic vein obstruction, the exact nature of which has not been identified but possibly caused by some congenital abnormality. He was treated by side-to-side portacaval anastomosis. Persistent external drainage of large amounts of ascitic fluid made management of the early postoperative course exceedingly difficult.

A 25 year old woman with portal hypertension, massive ascites, obstruction of the inferior vena cava just below the right atrium, partial hepatic vein obstruction, probably due to superimposed thrombus, and an anomalous hepatic vein drainage recently has been treated by placement of a graft between the inferior vena cava distal to the obstruction and the right atrium.*

Ascites was the predominant symptom in two of these three patients. Improvement in one patient occurred coincident with the placement of a bypass graft about the obstructed vena cava and hepatic outflow. Result of the portacaval shunt in the other patient cannot be evaluated at this time.

SUMMARY

A variety of intrahepatic conditions may produce signs of portal hypertension early in life. The prognosis is directly related to the primary hepatic disease process. Some conditions, such as noncorrectable biliary atresia, are uniformly fatal, and treatment of portal hypertension per se is not indicated. Patients with other conditions, such as congenital hepatic fibrosis, may have an excellent prognosis. Portacaval anastomosis, either end-to-side or side-to-side, is effective treatment and may be successfully performed within the first two years of life.

The majority of intrahepatic conditions with portal hypertension amenable

* Patient of Dr. Donald G. Mulder.

to surgical treatment becomes significantly symptomatic at a later period, five to 14 years of age, and treatment by portacaval shunt may be indicated. Long-term deleterious neurological effects of portacaval shunt, as reported by Voorhees et al. (19) have not been seen.

Evidence of portal hypertension associated with extrahepatic obstruction of the portal venous system frequently appears in the first two to three years of life. With appropriate medical therapy, variceal hemorrhage is rarely fatal, and emergency operations are generally contraindicated.

Since hemorrhage becomes less frequent and less severe as the patients become older, since delay of operation until eight to ten years of age is generally recommended, and since thrombosed and ineffective shunts occur even in older patients with extrahepatic blocks, continuation of nonoperative management into adult life should be considered, although each patient must be individually evaluated.

Demonstration, preferably before operation, that the site of the proposed shunt will effectively decompress the variceal portion of the portal bed is an important consideration in the decision to perform a shunt operation.

Posthepatic block in early childhood is associated with severe ascites. Limited experience would suggest treatment by side-to-side portacaval anastomosis.

REFERENCES

1. Arcari, F. A. and H. B. Lynn, Bleeding esophageal varices in children. *Surg. Gynec. Obstet. 112*: 101-105 (1961).
2. Boles, T., Discussion of reference 12 (below). *J. pediat. Surg. 7*: 563 (1972).
3. Clatworthy, H. W., jr. and E. T. Boles jr., Extrahepatic portal bed block in children *Ann. Surg. 150*: 371-383 (1959).
4. Clatworthy, H. W., jr. and A. A. de Lorimier, Portal decompression procedures in children. *Amer. J. Surg. 107*: 447-451 (1964).
5. Ehrlich, F., S. Pipatanagul, W. K. Sieber and W. B. Kiesewetter, Portal hypertension: Surgical management in infants and children. *J. pediat. Surg. 9*: 283-287 (1974).
6. Fonkalsrud, E. W., Portal hypertension in children. In: *Current Problems in Surgery*. W. P. Longmire jr. (ed.) (Year Book Medical Publishers, Chicago 1966).
7. Fonkalsrud, E. W. and W. P. Longmire jr., Reassessment of operative procedures for portal hypertension in infants and children. *Amer. J. Surg. 118*: 148-157 (1969).
8. Fonkalsrud, E. W., N. A. Myers and M. J. Robinson, Management of extraheptaic portal hypertension in children. *Ann. Surg. 180*: 487-493 (1974).
9. Hsia, D. Y. and S. S. Gellis, Portal hypertension in infants and children. *Amer. J. Dis. Child. 90*: 290-298 (1955).
10. Keighley, M. R. B., R. W. Girdwood, G. H. Wooler and M. I. Ionescu, Long-term results of surgical treatment for bleeding oesophageal varices in children with portal hypertension. *Brit. J. Surg. 60*: 641-646 (1973).
11. Lambert, M. J., III, E. S. Tank and J. G. Turcotte, Late sequelae of mesocaval shunts in children. *Amer. J. Surg. 127*: 19-24 (1974).

12. Martin, L. W., Changing concepts of management of portal hypertension in children. *J. pediat. Surg.* 7: 559-564 (1972).
13. Mikkelsen, W. P., Extrahepatic portal hypertension in children. *Amer. J. Surg. 111*: 333-340 (1966).
14. Miyata, M., M. Satani, T. Ueda and E. Okamoto, Long term results of hepatic porto-enterostomy for biliary atresia: Special reference to postoperative portal hypertension. *Surgery 76*: 234-237 (1974).
15. O'Donnell, B. and M. A. Moloney, Development and course of extrahepatic portal obstruction in children. *Lancet 1*: 789-791 (1968).
16. Pinkerton, J. A., G. W. Holcomb jr. and J. H. Foster, Portal hypertension in childhood. *Ann. Surg. 175*: 870-886 (1972).
17. Shaldon, S. and S. Sherlock, Obstruction to the extrahepatic portal system in childhood. *Lancet 1*: 63-67 (1962).
18. Tank, E. S., V. W. Wallin jr., J. G. Turcotte and C. G. Child, III, Surgical management of bleeding gastroesophageal varices in children. *Arch. Surg. 98*: 451-456 (1969).
19. Voorhees, A. B., jr., E. Chaitman, S. Schneider, J. F. Nicholson, D. S. Kornfeld and J. B. Price jr., Portal-systemic encephalopathy in the noncirrhotic patient. *Arch. Surg. 107*: 659-663 (1973).
20. Vos, L. J. M., V. Potocky, F. H. L. Bröker, J. A. de Vries, L. Postoma and E. Edens, Splenic vein thrombosis with esophageal varices: A late complication of umbilical vein catheterization. *Ann. Surg. 180*: 152-156 (1974).

MANAGEMENT OF PORTAL HYPERTENSION IN YOUNG CHILDREN BY PORTAL SYSTEMIC SHUNTS

H. BISMUTH, M.D. AND D. FRANCO, M.D.

In a recent report of the 1974 meeting of the American Surgical Association on the management of extra-hepatic portal hypertension in children and in the following discussion (6) the general consensus was in favor of conservative measures and against portal-systemic shunts in children less than 8 years and on veins less than 8 mm diameter. This attitude derived from the following items: 1. bleeding episodes were not life-threatening, at least in extra hepatic portal hypertension; 2. direct attack of varices was fraught with a high rate of recurrent bleeding and 3. thrombosis frequently occurred after portal-systemic shunts when the vein was narrow.

Our experience with portal derivation in 23 children less than 6 years was not in accordance with these conclusions. The purpose of this work was to study the risks and efficacy of portal-systemic shunts in young children with portal hypertension.

MATERIAL AND METHODS

From December 1970 to May 1975, 23 children under 6 years of age underwent a portal systemic shunt for portal hypertension.

Age ranged from 18 months to 5 11/12 years (table 1). Mean age was 46 ± 14 months. The cause of portal hypertension was extrahepatic in 14 cases and intrahepatic in 9 cases. In 4 patients, extrahepatic portal hypertension was due to thrombosis of the portal vein secondary to catheterization of the umbilical vein at birth. The cause of cavernomatous transformation was not found in the others. Intrahepatic portal hypertension was due to various liver diseases: secondary biliary cirrhosis – 3, cirrhosis with alpha-antitrypsin deficiency – 2, cirrhosis of unknown origin – 3, congenital hepatic fibrosis – 1. All patients with cirrhosis were of the type A of Child's classification (2).

There were 18 therapeutic and 5 prophylactic shunts. The number of

Table 1. 23 children with portal hypertension treated by portal diversion.

	Number of patients	Age (m ± 1 s.d.)	Number of bleeding episodes per child	Size of the veins used (m ± 1 s.d.)	Type of shunts
Extrahepatic	14	3 yrs 8 m. ±20 m.	2	8 ± 0.6 mm	13 SRA* 1 MCA**
Intrahepatic	9	5 yrs 1 m. ±15 m.	0.5	5 ± 1.9 mm	7 SRA* 2 PCA***

```
  * SRA  = splenorenal anastomosis
 ** MCA  = mesocaval anastomosis
*** PCA  = portacaval anastomosis
    m    = month
```

bleeding episodes in the 18 patients with therapeutic shunts is indicated in table 1. Prophylactic shunts were performed in patients with cirrhosis. All shunts but one were performed as elective procedures. In one case, an emergency splenorenal shunt was done together with ligation of gastric varices in an 18 month old child with massive variceal bleeding.

Pre-operative angiography (selective arteriography of the celiac axis and superior mesenteric artery and/or splenoportography) was obtained in every child to assess the patency and the size of the portal, splenic and mesenteric veins. In 7 patients the mesenteric vein was not visualized pre-operatively. In patients with intrahepatic portal hypertension, all opacified veins were patent. In patients with extrahepatic portal hypertension, the splenic vein was always patent. The mesenteric vein was not patent in two cases. The mean size of the vein used for the shunt is indicated in table 1.

There were 20 central splenorenal anastomoses, two side to side portacaval anastomoses and one mesocaval anastomosis. Central splenorenal shunts were performed according to the technique of Clatworthy and Boles (3) and mesocaval shunt was performed according to the Farge technique (5a), using the right iliac vein anastomosed end to side to the superior mesenteric vein. During the same period, four patients were denied a shunt operation and had varices ligation. All of them were less than 2 years and one had diffuse portal thrombosis.

Disappearance of varices was controlled during the first post-operative month by barium swallow or oesophagoscopy. Patency of the shunt was tested by selective arteriography of the superior mesenteric artery in 18 patients. In addition, in the last 9 patients intra-operative ileoportography was done. All patients have been examined during the last six months. Careful search was made for neuropsychic disorders. The mean follow up is 2.5±2 years with a range of 2 months to 4 years and 7 months.

RESULTS

1. Survival. Operative mortality was nil and there have been no late deaths.

2. Post-operative complication. The only post-operative complication was intra-peritoneal hemorrhage, which occurred in a 3 year 5 month old child with mesocaval shunt for portal vein thrombosis. This was due to over-dosage of anticoagulant therapy and necessitated an emergency laparotomy on the 5th post-operative day. No precise site of bleeding was detected and the rest of the post-operative course was uneventful.

3. Recurrent bleeding. A 4 5/12 year old child with cirrhosis of unknown origin had recurrent bleeding 2 months following a splenorenal shunt. Thrombosis of the shunt was proven by angiography. He then underwent a side-to-side portacaval shunt. Recurrent bleeding again occurred a month later at which time the second shunt was also shown to be thrombosed. He eventually received a mesocaval shunt which is still patent. No other patient in this group had any recurrence.

4. Thrombosis of the shunt. Thrombosis was observed in 3 splenorenal shunts (13%). Apart from the child mentioned above in whom thrombosis was responsible for recurrent bleeding, in the other two patients it was discovered by control angiography. The obstruction of the shunt could be explained in each case. In the first patient, already described, thrombosis of the splenorenal and of the portacaval shunts was due to thrombocytosis, platelet clots being found on the vein walls even before the end of each procedure. Eventual patency of a further mesocaval shunt was obtained in this child by heparin therapy. In a second patient, thrombosis of a shunt occurred in an 18 month old girl operated upon as an emergency, in whom the diameter of the splenic veins was 2 millimeters. In the third case, stricture of the anastomosis was due to the root of the mesocolon of the splenic flexure.

Among the 20 other cases, patency of the shunt was proven in 15 by angiography (fig. 1). In the 5 other children, varices had disappeared on radiologic and oesophagoscopic examinations.

5. Neuropsychic disorders. In this group of patients, no sign of encephalopathy has been detected in any child.

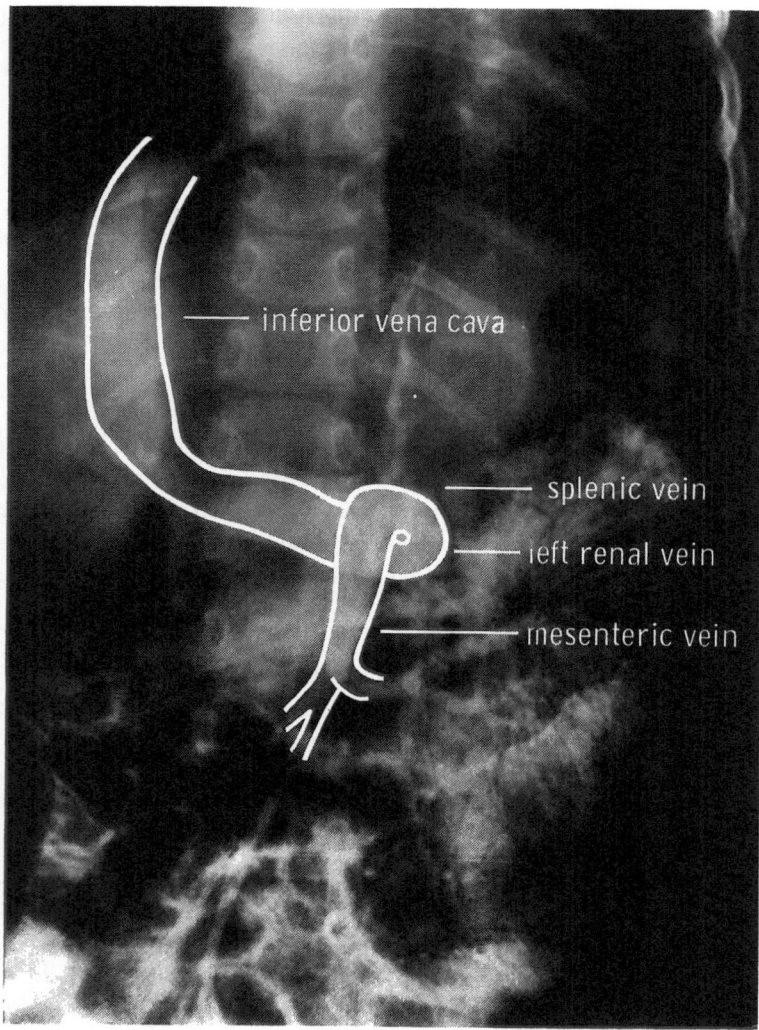

Fig. 1. Angiographic control by mesenteric arteriography of a spleno-renal shunt, six months post-operatively, on a 4 year old with hepatic cirrhosis. Dye opacifies mesenteric vein, splenic vein, left renal vein and inferior vena cava.

COMMENTS

The management of portal hypertension in childhood is still under discussion and such basic questions as the indications for surgery, the kind of operation, be done and the age at which it should be performed, remain unanswered.

Since the claim of Shaldon and Sherlock (13) that conservative treatment should always be preferred to shunt operations, the general tendency, expressed again recently by Fonkalsrud et al. (6), leans towards the non operative approach to these patients. This attitude relies on the low mortality rate in non operated patients which was 4% in the series of Voorhees et al. (14) and 3% in the series of Fonkalsrud et al. (6). However in other series, death associated with hemorrhage was more frequent, reaching 13% in the cases of Foster et al. (7), 21% of the patients of Arcari and Lynn (1) and 31% in the experience of Walker et al. (17). In the present series, two patients required emergency surgery for exsanguinating variceal bleeding. Thus the risk of death during a bleeding episode does exist in these patients. In addition, variceal hemorrhages lead to prolonged, repeated hospitalization and exposure to transfusion hepatitis (5). All these reasons favor the early active treatment of portal hypertension in children.

The choice of proper treatment must take into account the efficacy and operative risks of each surgical procedure. Direct attack on varices seems to bear a high rate of post-operative bleeding, as reported in 81% of the cases of variceal ligation in the series of Voorhees et al. (14) and 85% in the cases of Mikkelsen (10). Re-bleeding was also frequent following esogastric resection and was observed in 45% of the cases of Koop et al. (8) and 28% of the patients of Voorhees et al. (14). Also, in this last series, operative mortality was 21%. Recurrent bleeding due to thrombosis of the anastomosis is also a frequent complication of portal systemic shunts in children. Varying percentages of thromboses following spleno-renal shunts have been reported, from 18% for Clatworthy and de Lorimier (4) to 56% for Raffensperger et al. (12). The small size of the splenic vein is responsible for this high rate of thrombosis, which has led several authors as Fonkalsrud et al. (6) to abandon this type of procedure in children less than eight years of age. However, it should be possible to improve the results of peripheral portal-systemic shunts in children. Recent progress in micro-vascular surgery permits successful vascular anastomoses on small vessels. In the present series, the mean diameter of the veins used for shunts was 6.5±2.5 mn with a low rate of thrombosis (13%). In only one instance was the size of the splenic vein (2 mm) directly responsible for thrombosis of the shunt. In the two other cases, the splenic vein was 7 mm, shunt failure being due either to thrombocytosis in one case, or to mechanical obstruction in the other. Low flow through small sized anastomotic stoma may be an important cause of thrombosis. In such a case, the use of heparin as soon as the vessels are clamped should decrease the risk of clot formation. On the other hand, intra-operative angiographic control of the patency of the shunt allow the detection of any compression or stricture of the anastomosis. We now control the patency of the shunt by intra-operative portography. In an older child, not included in this series, operative angiography demonstrated a kinking of the splenic vein, so that we immediately repeated the shunt surgery with success.

Splenorenal shunt was mostly preferred in this group of patients because many children had marked splenomegaly and hypersplenism. It has been recently demonstrated (11), that the size of the spleen does not diminish following other types of shunts and that hypersplenism persists. Also, in 8 of the 14 children with extra-hepatic portal-hypertension, the splenic vein was either the largest vein or the only one available. However, if the mesenteric vein is larger than the splenic vein, mesocaval shunt may be preferred. In children, division of both iliac veins to construct a cavo-ilio-mesenteric shunt does not involve the possible risk of leg edema, as in adults (9).

It has been claimed by several authors and particularly by Fonkalsrud et al. (6) that splenorenal shunt should not be performed before 8 or 10 years. Variceal bleeding most often occurs earlier in life and, in the present series, 18 patients had experienced hemorrhage before 6 years and 5 before 3 years. The size of the splenic or mesenteric veins still appears to be the limiting factor for the decision of shunting. We have shown that spleno-renal shunt can be successfully performed on veins less than 10 mm. It would seem hazardous, at the present time, to perform spleno-renal shunts on splenic veins less than 3 mm, which usually correspond to 3 years of age although this was occasionally done in younger children.

Neuro-psychiatric abnormalities were described in 50% of shunted patients by Voorhees et al. (15). If this were really so, it would darken the prognosis of shunted children and cast doubt on the benefits of shunt operations in young patients. The significance of neurologic disorders described by these authors is not unequivocal. There is no similarity between these troubles and what is generally described, at least in adults, as post-shunt encephalopathy. Besides, the same percentage of neurologic disorders was encountered in patients with esogastric resection, without shunt (16). Fonkalsrud et al. (6) have drawn attention to the fact that neuropsychic disorders may be due, in these children, to prolonged hospitalization and multiple operations. In this case, permanent cure of portal hypertension by an early portal-systemic shunt could represent the best preventive measure against the occurrence of such troubles. Mental disorders were not observed in our series, but the follow-up may be too short to appreciate the true incidence of this serious complication.

SUMMARY

Portal systemic shunts were performed in 23 children under 6 years of age with portal hypertension. There were 20 central splenorenal, 2 portacaval and 1 mesocaval shunts, the mean size of the veins used being 7 ± 2.5 mm. There was no operative or late death. Shunts were proven to be patent in 20 patients either by angiograms (15) or by the disappearance of esophageal varices (5). Thromboses occurred in 3 patients (13%) for various causes and was responsible for recurrent bleeding in one. No other patient experienced re-bleeding. Intraoperative angiographic control of the patency of the shunt and intravenous heparin infusion have been introduced in the 9 last patients in order to lower the incidence of thrombosis of the anastomosis. These results would suggest that peripheral portal systemic shunts can be successfully performed in young children with portal hypertension. In view of the lethal risk of variceal hemorrhage in these patients, early portal diversion may represent the treatment of choice.

REFERENCES

1. Arcari, F. A. and H. B. Lynn, Bleeding esophageal varices in children. *Surg. Gynec. Obstet. 112*: 101-105 (1963).
2. Child, C. G., 3rd., *Portal hypertension*. (Saunders, Philadelphia, 1974).
3. Clatworthy, H. W., jr. and T. E. Boles jr., Extrahepatic portal bed block in children: pathogenesis and treatment. *Ann. Surg. 150*: 371-383 (1959).
4. Clatworthy, H. W. jr. and A. A. deLorimier, Portal decompression procedures in children. *Amer. J. Surg. 107*: 447-451 (1964).
5. Clatworthy, H. W., jr., Extrahepatic portal hypertension. In: *Portal hypertension*. C. G. Child (ed.), pp. 243-266 (W. B. Saunders, Philadelphia 1974).
5a. Farge, C. et J. Auvert, L'anastomose ilio-mésentérique. Procédé améliorant l'anastomose veineuse cavo-mésentérique pour l'hypertension portale. *Presse méd. 70*: 2217-2218 (1962).
6. Fonkalsrud, E. W., N. A. Myers and M. J. Robinson, Management of extrahepatic portal hypertension in children. *Ann. Surg. 180*: 487-491 (1974).
7. Foster, J. H., G. W. Holcomb and J. A. Kirtley, Results of surgical treatment of portal hypertension in children. *Ann. Surg. 157*: 868-880 (1963).
8. Koop, C. E. and A. Kavianian, Reappraisal of colonic replacement of distal eso-

phagus and proximal stomach in the management of bleeding varices in children. *Surgery 57*: 454-456 (1965).

9. Marion, P., Les obstructions portales. *Sem. Hôp. Paris 29*: 2781-2790 (1953).
10. Mikkelsen, W. P., Extrahepatic portal hypertension in children. *Amer. J. Surg. 111*: 333-340 (1966).
11. Mutchnik, M. G., E. Lerner and H. O. Conn, Effect of portacaval anastomosis on hypersplenism in cirrhosis: a prospective controlled evaluation. *Gastroenterology 68*: 1070 (1975).
12. Raffensperger, J. G., A. A. Shkolnik, J. O. Boggs and O. Swenson, Portal hypertension in children. *Arch. Surg. 105*: 249-254 (1972).
13. Shaldon, S. and S. Sherlock, Obstruction to the extrahepatic portal system in childhood. *Lancet 1*: 63-68 (1962).
14. Voorhees, A. B., jr., R. C. Harris, R. C. Britton, J. B. Price and T. V. Santulli, Portal hypertension in children: 98 cases. *Surgery 58*: 540-549 (1965).
15. Voorhees, A. B., jr., E. Chaitman, S. Schneider, J. F. Nicholson, D. S. Kornfeld and J. B. Price jr., Portal-systemic encephalopathy in the non cirrhotic patient. Effect of portal-systemic shunting. *Arch. Surg. 107*: 659-662 (1973).
16. Voorhees, A. B., jr. and J. B. Price jr., Extrahepatic portal hypertension. A retrospective analysis of 127 cases and associated clinical implications. *Arch. Surg. 108*: 338-341 (1974).
17. Walker, R. M., Treatment of portal hypertension in children. *Proc. Roy. Soc. Med. 55*: 770-772 (1962).

LIVER TUMORS

H. WILLIAM CLATWORTHY JR., M.D.

Primary tumors of the liver occur with sufficient frequency in infants and children to justify the continuing reappraisal of their management. Although nearly a quarter of a century of experience with aggressive extirpative surgery has resulted in the cure of many patients with benign lesions, most young patients with malignant tumors still die of their disease or from the surgeon's efforts to eradicate it. Therefore, clinicians must look, as we have done in the past with Wilms' tumor and more recently rhabdomyosarcoma, to non-surgical modalities of therapy which can be combined with safer and perhaps more reasonable surgical resolve in the management of future patients.

Since 1952 when the earliest successes were reported with hepatic lobectomy in adults (20, 24) many authors have recorded their results in a wide variety of childhood liver tumors as well. The first hepatic lobectomy for hepatoblastoma was performed at the Columbus Children's Hospital in 1952 and reported in 1956 (3). Since then 42 additional patients with neoplastic hepatic lesions, 29 of which were malignant, have been cared for, and many significant changes in management have taken place which have been periodically reviewed (4, 5, 6).

Diagnostic acumen has been sharpened by the radiologist's development of scanning, ultrasound, and angiography techniques suitable for small patients. Pathologists have provided a standard classification for tumors originating from hepatic cells, and more recently have developed tumor-specific laboratory tests to aid in definitive diagnosis and to follow the progress of therapy. Anatomically oriented surgeons have described many standardized operative techniques to control most diffuse angiomas or to permit the reasonably safe resection of up to 85 percent of the liver for localized disease. Simultaneously, the chemotherapists have developed a number of promising agents which can be utilized separately or in combination with radiotherapy; systematically or by intra-arterial perfusion; and for varying periods of time which are being evaluated by well controlled cancer study groups. Finally, the physiologic and immunologic factors involved in the stimulation and inhibition of liver regeneration and immunologic rejection are under continuous study in several centers.

In summarizing the 'state of the art' in 1975 I have drawn heavily from my personal experience with our own series of cases, supplemented with significant literature and occasional personal communications.

CLASSIFICATION OF TUMORS

Primary tumors of the liver in childhood are most commonly of hepatic cell origin. Thirty-two of the 43 patients in our series had mass lesions that appeared to originate from hepatic or biliary epithelium; 27 were primary malignant lesions of hepatic cell origin. As suggested by (16, 17) on the basis of histologic classification, two distinct types of hepatoma were observed: the hepatocarcinoma (similar to that seen in adults and associated with a very poor prognosis) in two older children, and the hepatoblastoma (a much more favorable lesion found in infants) in 25 patients. There was one patient with a benign cholangiohepatoma, two infants with large hepatic cysts, and two patients with nodular hyperplasia in the liver which simulated tumors and were resected, as has also been described by Hertzer et al. (14).

Nine of the patients had tumors of the supporting structures, presumably of mesodermal origin. These included five hemangiomas, two giant cystic lymphangiomas, and one each of fibroangioma and malignant mesenchymoma. There was one child with malignant teratoma and one with multiple areas of eosinophilic granuloma.

The distribution of the tumors related well to the location of liver tissue. Twenty-four lesions appeared to originate in the right lobe; 12 were central diffuse or multicentric, and seven were localized in the left lobe. The two patients with hepatocarcinoma but only one of 25 children with hepatoblastoma had extrahepatic lymph node involvement at the time of diagnosis. Four additional patients were admitted with distant (pulmonary) disease.

INCIDENCE AND SYMPTOMS

In our series and that reported by Fraumeni (11) the peak incidence of both benign and malignant primary hepatic neoplasms in children is in the first year of life and two-thirds of the patients are less than two years of age when diagnosed. This early clinical appearance and the occasional association of the infantile hepatoblastoma with other congenital defects including von Gierke's and Toni-Faconi syndromes and congenital hemihypertrophy suggests that many liver tumors are developmental aberrations. Sex distribution is nearly equal in children with hepatoma in contrast to the 2 to 1 predominance of males recorded in adult series (22).

Abdominal enlargement due to a visible or palpable mass is the only complaint in most patients. Rarely are pain, fever, weight loss, or gastrointestinal symptoms encountered. Jaundice was not observed unless hilar obstruction of the bile ducts developed. Intra-peritoneal hemorrhage due to rupture of a solid tumor, or cyanosis and congestive heart failure associated with localized angioma or diffuse hemangiomatosis are occasional but uncommon presentations.

DIAGNOSTIC STUDY

Laboratory studies of liver function are rarely altered in the absence of jaundice. Hasegawa et al. (12) have observed that serum alpha-1-feto-globulin levels are commonly elevated in all types of hepatoma. Others (15, 1, 21) have independently identified cases with increased levels of circulating gonadotropin associated with precocious puberty.

Radiographic evaluation with radiocolloid liver scans usually gives good definition of large lesions. The sonogram has a very definite ability to identify fluid filled cysts. Inferior venacavography, portovenography, and particularly arteriography, not only define the anatomical variations the surgeon may be confronted with but may also aid in lesion identification on the basis of vascular patterns depicted during the serial studies as described by Suzuki et al. (27). In patients whose disease appears to be localized to the liver, the surgeon's contribution to diagnosis usually is best deferred until a formal laparotomy when preparations for a major resection are completed. Either 'needle' or 'incisional' biopsy theoretically diminish the opportunity for cure and are generally best avoided in any patients with a resectable tumor.

TECHNIQUE OF RESECTION

The major complications associated with the resection of liver tumors are the same as those outlined by Wangensteen in 1951 (29). Liver insufficiency has not been a serious problem since adequate protein and carbohydrate replacement have been practised.

Two general types of liver resection are commonly performed for isolated primary neoplasms. The simplest and least used is the 'wedge' or 'segmental' resection of the peripheral liver substance, suitable for the left lobe lesions and pedunculated ones. Hemostasis and bile leakage can be controlled with mattress sutures. The second is the anatomically defined right or left lobectomy, or the extended right or left lobectomy, at which time the central segment of the liver is excised with the lobe. The success of each of these procedures depends primarily upon the preservation of the integrity of at least one of the major hepatic veins and the appropriate branches of the portal triad structures (portal vein - hepatic artery - bile duct) to the remaining liver segment.

The complications which lead to a reported overall mortality rate of 10 to 23 percent from such procedures are hemorrhage, air embolism, bile peritonitis, and liver failure due to injury to the remaining structures of the portal triad. A variety of procedures has been devised to circumvent these major technical difficulties. The operation popularized by Lortat-Jacobs includes individual hilar ligation of the vessels and bile ducts entering the segment to be resected and the separate ligation of all segmental hepatic veins as well. Such procedures are best performed through a thoraco-abdominal incision with caval tourniquets and temporary cross-clamping of the portal vein and hepatic artery which provides a near bloodless field in a normothermic patient for 20 minutes or, if moderate hypothermia is used, a somewhat longer period (25). Following blunt instrument or finger fracture dissection through the normal liver substance, the vessels on the transected surface are ligated or clipped before the liver wound is closed and resurfaced with flaps of peritoneum.

To obviate the tedious task of individually ligating all effluent and affluent structures entering the segment to be excised, a variety of techniques for clamping the liver mass during the transection has been recommended by Lin (19) and Doty, Kugler and Mosely (8). These vary from manual compression by the encircling hands of a cotton-gloved assistant to a variety of ingenious clamps.

For certain cases with hepatic vein involvement the intra-caval shunt has been advocated (28) and has been used to achieve a bloodless field without interfering with return flow to the heart. Recently, Fortner (9) has described his experience with a method of temporary isolation and cold perfusion of the liver developed as a by-product of the liver transplantation program

which permits a leisurely (1-2 hours) resection in a bloodless field and has
led to a very significant reduction in mortality to less than 10 percent in a
series of adult liver tumor patients treated at the Memorial Hospital in New
York City.

Obviously, individual tumor resection techniques are now sufficiently
numerous to afford the responsible surgical technician with effective methods
of removing massive primary or secondary tumors when the lesion is localized to an anatomically resectable segment or lobe of the human liver.

If the tumor is unresectable because of a central location or a diffuse involvement, such as an infant in congestive failure, ligation of the common
hepatic artery and steroid administration has been successful according to
de Lorimier (7). Indeed, Larmi (18) has reported that reasonable palliation
may be achieved by hepatic artery ligation in unresectable hepatocarcinoma
or metastatic disease, since both receive the bulk of the nourishment from
the arterial vessels. Park and Phillips (23) have reported the control of 4 of 5
hepatic hemangiomas treated with 1300-2000 rads in 14 days, and suggested
its use again for certain hemangiomatous lesions which cannot be safely
resected.

RESULTS

For nearly 25 years, surgery has been the mainstay of the treatment programs
for the major liver tumors and the results in treatment have been much better
than the results reported in adult cases. In our series of 43 patients, 10 of the
12 children with benign tumors and 13 of the 28 malignant lesions were
treated for cure by resection including 15 right lobectomies; three left lobectomies; four segmentectomies, and one wedge resection. There were three
intraoperative or postoperative deaths, all in 13 cancer cases (23%). This
compares similarly with Foster's excellent collected review of 91 cases and
21 deaths (23%) in cancer patients (10).

Similarly, and of particular significance, is the fact that all patients with
benign disease and three of the 10 with cancer who survived operation are
living and tumor free for 6, 12, 13 years. Again our data are closely supported by Foster's collected review of 74 cases who survived operation in
that 14 of the 42 (33.3%) patients followed five years are free of disease
and, in addition, there are 22 alive and well, all less than five years after
treatment.

COMMENTS ABOUT THE FUTURE

Cancer study group protocols (2) have been prepared categorizing a number of chemotherapeutic agents to establish the response in patients with malignant disease. Most studies have not been in effect sufficiently long to have produced significant data. However, a number of encouraging isolated case reports suggest that the infant hepatoblastoma may be sensitive to several standard drug programs conventionally in use for other childhood malignancies. When combined with irradiation, Herman and Lonsdale (13) have reported the conversion of an 'inoperable' case into an operable one as has Hasegawa and, still more recently, Schwartz (26) has followed a biopsy proven hepatoblastoma two years following actinomycin-vincristine and irradiation therapy for a large inoperable central tumor that has allegedly disappeared on liver scan two years ago and has not recurred. What the eventual role to be played by the operative and nonoperative modalities in the treatment of hepatoblastoma is not yet clear but it is obvious that a 'team approach' has renewed support. The surgeon needs to continue to concentrate on reducing operative mortality and serious postoperative complications as he cures benign lesions and participates in the care of the malignant ones. The chemotherapist and radiologist need to explore the role of multiple drug therapy with and without irradiation to the local lesion so that limitations of these adjunctive measures that are safe for the patient and his liver can be more precisely defined.

Finally, newer transplant techniques may permit the transplantation of segments of normal liver which will then grow to functionally replace the destroyed major structure.

SUMMARY

Primary and secondary liver tumors are sufficiently common in infants and children to warrant a continuing reappraisal of their management. Most of the primary and all metastatic lesions are malignant. In addition, there is a significant number of histologically benign congenital neoplasms or cysts which are life-threatening.

During the past quarter century, many significant contributions have been made to the care of patients harboring these lesions. Diagnostic acumen has been sharpened by scanning techniques, angiography, improved pathologic classification, tumor specific laboratory tests, and a better understanding of hepatic regeneration and transplantation. Operative procedures remain the mainstay of modern therapy and have been developed to control the blood supply of angiomas, the internal drainage of cyts, and to permit the relatively safe resection of up to 85 percent of normal liver substance. Chemotherapy and radiotherapy have proven to be of increasing value in selected cases of both metastatic and unresectable primary lesions.

The successful treatment of metastatic tumor was limited to three infants with diffuse neuroblastoma who received irradiation. The 43 children with primary liver tumors, 29 of which were malignant, fared better. These lesions included tumors derived from hepatic cells such as hepatoblastoma, cholangioma, and hepatic cysts; instances of tumor of the supporting structures such as fibromas, hemangiomas, lymphangiomas, fibroangiomas, teratoma, and hamartoma, and, finally, cases with localized giant nodular cirrhosis.

In 38 patients a laparotomy was performed, and 23 liver resections were carried out including 15 right lobectomies, 3 left lobectomies, 4 segmentectomies, and 1 wedge resection. There were 3 operative deaths due to hemorrhage, air embolism, and staphylococcal septicemia. All patients with benign tumors and 3 with hepatoblastoma are alive and well (13, 12, and 6 years). All surviving children have evidenced normal growth and developmental patterns. In the future, additional successes may be achieved, as suggested by the experience of others, by combining secondary surgery with irradiation and chemotherapy.

REFERENCES

1. Behrle, F. C., et al., Virilization accompanying hepatoblastoma. *Pediatrics 32*: 265-271 (1963).
2. Children's Cancer Study Group A, CCA-831 (Univ. of Southern California School of Medicine, Los Angeles).
3. Clatworthy, H. W., jr. and E. T. Boles jr., Right lobectomy of the liver in children. *Surgery 39*: 850-859 (1956).
4. Clatworthy, H. W., jr., E. T. Boles jr. and W. A. Newton jr., Primary tumours of the liver in infants and children. *Arch. Dis. Childh. 35*: 22-28 (1960).
5. Clatworthy, H. W., jr., E. T. Boles jr. and P. K. Kottmeier, Liver tumors in infancy and childhood. *Ann. Surg. 154*: 475-484 (1961).
6. Clatworthy, H. W., jr., M. Schiller and J. L. Grosfeld, Primary liver tumors in infancy and childhood: 41 cases variously treated. *Arch. Surg. 109*: 143-147 (1974).
7. deLorimier, A. A., et al., Hepatic-artery ligation for hepatic hemangiomatosis. *New Engl. J. Med. 277*: 333-336 (1967).
8. Doty, D. B., H. W. Kugler and R. V. Moseley, Control of hepatic parenchyma by direct compression: A new instrument. *Surgery 67*: 720-724 (1970).
9. Fortner, J. G. et al., Major hepatic resection using vascular isolation and hypothermic perfusion. *Ann. Surg. 180*: 644-652 (1974).
10. Foster, J. H., Survival after liver resection for cancer. *Cancer 26*: 493-502 (1970).

11. Fraumeni, J. F., jr., R. W. Miller and J. A. Hill, Primary carcinoma of the liver in childhood: An epidemiologic study. *J. nat. Cancer Inst. 40*: 1087-1099 (1968).
12. Hasegawa, H. et al., Embryonal carcinoma and alpha-fetoprotein with special reference to hepatoblastoma. *Gann. 14*: 129-139 (1973).
13. Herman, R. E. and D. Lonsdale, Chemotherapy, radiotherapy, and hepatic lobectomy for hepatoblastoma in infants: Report of a survival. *Surgery 68*: 383-388 (1970).
14. Hertzer, N. R., W. A. Hawk and R. E. Hermann, Inflammatory lesions of the liver which simulate tumor: Report of two cases in children. *Surgery 69*: 839-846 (1971).
15. Hung, W. et al., Precocious puberty in a boy with hepatoma and circulating gonadotropin. *J. Pediat. 63*: 895-903 (1963).
16. Ishak, K. G. and P. R. Glunz, Hepatoblastoma and hepatocarcinoma in infancy and childhood: Report of 47 cases. *Cancer 20*: 396-422 (1967).
17. Kasai, M. and I. Watanabe, Histologic classification of liver-cell carcinoma in infancy and childhood and its clinical evaluation. *Cancer 25*: 551-563 (1970).
18. Larmi, T. K. et al., Treatment of patients with hepatic tumors and jaundice by ligation of the hepatic artery. *Arch. Surg. 108*: 178-183 (1974).
19. Lin, T., Results in 107 hepatic lobectomies with preliminary report on the use of a clamp to reduce blood loss. *Ann. Surg. 177*: 413-421 (1973).
20. Lortat-Jacob, J. L. et H. G. Robert, Hepatectomie droite reglée. *Presse méd. 60*: 549 (1952).
21. Martin, L. W., Discussion of paper. Primary liver tumors in infancy and childhood. *Arch. Surg. 109*: 147 (1974).
22. Pablo Curutchet, M. et al., Primary liver cancer. *Surgery 70*: 467-479 (1971).
23. Park, W. C. and R. Philips, The role of radiation therapy in the management of hemangiomas of the liver. *J. Amer. med. Ass. 212*: 1496-1498 (1970).
24. Quattlebaum, J. K., Massive resection of the liver. *Ann. Surg. 137*: 787 (1953).
25. Raffucci, F. L., Effects of temporary occlusion of afferent hepatic circulation in dogs. *Surgery 33*: 342-351 (1953).
26. Schwartz, D. B., Personal communication.
27. Suzuki, T. et al., Study of vascularity of tumors of the liver. *Surg. Gynec. Obstet. 134*: 27-34 (1972).
28. Timmis, H. H., A. R. Rosanova jr. and W. B. Larkins, Bloodless hepatic resection with an internal caval shunt. *Surgery 65*: 109-117 (1969).
29. Wangensteen, O. H., Cancer of the esophagus and the stomach. *Amer. Cancer Soc. Inc.* p. 92 (1951).

CLOSING REMARKS

ROBERT DEBRÉ, M.D.

Je voudrais vous dire un mot avant la séparation, qui est proche.

C'est un grand problème, toujours, pour le Centre International de l'Enfance, de décider les sujets de travail, et en particulier des séminaires et colloques.

En effet, nous avons pour mission de combattre les grands fléaux de l'enfance, et ces grands fléaux sont encore très importants dans les pays heureux, mais ils sont terribles dans les pays malheureux, et nous devons prendre bien garde de ne pas détourner de son travail principal notre personnel qui est, comme vous l'avez vu, particulièrement compétent et actif. Cependant, nous pensons qu'un travail comme celui que vous avez fait, une réunion faite en collaboration entre le Centre et la Fondation Macy, comme celui qui vient de se passer, sont utiles de temps en temps.

Naturellement, les problèmes que vous envisagez sont des problèmes de biologie assez compliqués, raffinés, et qui, chez chacun de nous, excitent l'intelligence et nous passionnent, dans notre curiosité et notre désir de connaître.

Les maladies plus ou moins rares, souvent assez rares, que nous étudions maintenant dans nos hôpitaux des pays heureux, où les maladies fréquentes, banales, de l'infection des enfants ont disparu, posent des problèmes tout à fait importants, et il est bon de se réunir de temps en temps pour les étudier. Nous avons eu une très intéressante et importante réunion à propos des maladies du rein, il était just d'avoir une réunion intéressante à propos des maladies du foie de l'enfant, où la seule maladie qui constitue vraiment un grand fléau social et universel, l'hépatite virale, ne pouvait avoir qu'une place limitée, mais comme vous le savez, nous avons consacré un séminaire entier sous la présidence de Dr. John Enders à l'hépatite virale, et ce que vous avez apporté cette fois-ci s'ajoute à ce qui a été dit.

L'intérêt considérable de réunions comme celle-ci est de sortir la spécialiste trop étroit de sa spécialité, de n'envisager sa spécialité que comme une encyclopédie. En quelques heures ici même, vous avez envisagé toutes les techniques les plus récentes, de la biologie, la chimie, la culture des tissus, et les techniques chirurgicales, ceci en présence de collègues qui ne sont pas de techniciens, et cette réunion de spécialistes vivant ensemble et travaillant ensemble quelques heures, pour s'intéresser aux problèmes les uns des autres, est capital pour le développement intellectuel des médecins. La spécialité est nécessité, elle se développe de plus en plus et devient de plus en plus étroite. Cela est bien à condition qu'elle reste à caractère encyclopédique, avec le souci de toutes les disciplines et toutes les techniques qui touchent aux problèmes de la spécialité. C'est une grande leçon, et j'ai été très heureux d'apprendre que les spécialistes ici se sont intéressés chacun au travail des autres.

Bien entendu, il y a aussi les résultats pratiques importants, et nous ne pouvons pas les énumérer. Je voudrais tout de même revenir sur un lieu commun qui est la fréquence grandissante des inconvénients des accidents, des complications, dûs aux thérapeutiques que nous employons. Il suffit d'être présent quelques heures parmi vous pour entrendre parler des inconvénients des stéroïdes, ou des inconvénients des contraceptifs, ou, comme l'a indiqué M. Alagille, le fait que les hypertensions portales ont changé d'âge, si l'on peut dire. Pourquoi? Parce qu'une partie d'entre elles sont maintenant les complications des techniques de la réanimation périnatale. Il est donc très important de revenir toujours sur ce sujet; même si ces complications liées à la thérapeutique ne sont pas très fréquentes, elles sont très graves parce qu'elles sont déterminées par le médecin, et que nous en sommes moralement responsables.

Je ne veux pas continuer ces considérations, mais vous dire combien nous avons été heureux de vous recevoir tous, combien nous avons été joyeux de ces rencontres sympathiques entre médecins de différents pays passionnés pour les mêmes problèmes, et nous vous remercions pour les satisfactions que nous avons eues de cette rencontre.

Je voudrais m'associer au président pour remercier ceux qui ont préparé ce séminaire, ceux qui l'ont préparé, parmi les conseillers de la Fondation Macy. J'adresse en passant mon souvenir au Dr. John Bowers, qui regrette de ne pas être ici, comme on vous l'a dit, et vers qui vont nos pensées amicales. Les conseillers de cette fondation se sont associés aux conseillers du Centre pour la préparation de cette réunion, et ils doivent être félicités et remerciés. Remerciés aussi ceux qui ont travaillé pour son succès, c'est à dire vous tous. Rermercié aussi le personnel de cette maison qui a beaucoup travaillé pour réaliser aux mieux le succès de cette réunion, les interprètes dont la tâche est très difficile quand on discute de problèmes de biologie, de médecine, et qui ont parfaitement fait comprendre à chacun la pensée des autres.

Je voudrais terminer enfin en remerciant spécialement le Docteur Nathalie Masse qui, comme toujours, est la fée qui, non pas avec une simple baguette, mais avec un très grand effort, organise l'ensemble de ces réunions et en permet le succès.

Et maintenant, en espérant que je n'ai oublié personne dans mes remercie-ments, je vous adresse tous mes voeux de bon retour, avec l'espoir que vous reviendrez parmi nous.

INDEX